W9-CEX-683

199

Adult
Nurse Practitioner

Certification
Review Guide

EDITOR

Virginia Layng Millonig, Ph.D, R.N., C.P.N.P.
Health Leadership Associates, Inc.
Potomac, Maryland

SECOND EDITION

Health Leadership Associates, Inc.
Potomac, Maryland

Family Nurse Practitioner Set
by
Health Leadership Associates, Inc.

Adult Nurse Practitioner Certification Review Guide

Pediatric Nurse Practitioner Certification Review Guide

Women's Health Care Nurse Practitioner Certification Review Guide

Health Leadership Associates, Inc.

Production Manager: Martha M. Pounsberry
Manuscript Editors: John O'Donnell, Denise Colbert
Composition: Frances Weber, The Type House
Production: Port City Press, Inc.

Second Edition

Copyright © 1994 by Health Leadership Associates, Inc.

All rights reserved. No part of this book may be reproduced in any form or by any means, electronic, mechanical, photocopying, recording, or otherwise without prior permission in writing from the publisher.

Printed in the United States of America

Health Leadership Associates, Inc. ∎ P.O. Box 59153 ∎ Potomac, Maryland 20859

Library of Congress Cataloging-in-Publication Data

Adult nurse practitioner certification review guide / editor, Virginia Layng
   Millonig : contributing authors, Elissa Davis ... [et al.].—2nd ed.
     p.   cm.
   Includes bibliographical references and index.
   ISBN 1-878028-09-X : $43.95
     1. Nursing—Handbooks, manuals, etc.   2. Nurse
practitioners—Handbooks, manuals, etc.   3. Clinical medicine—
Handbooks, manuals, etc.   4. Nursing—Examinations, questions,
etc.   5. Nurse practitioners—Examinations, questions, etc.   6.
Clinical medicine—Examinations, questions, etc.   I. Millonig,
Virginia Layng.
   [DNLM: 1. Nurse Practitioners—examination questions.   WY 18 A244 1994]
   RT82.8.A38   1994
   610.73'076—dc20
   DNLM/DLC
   for Library of Congress   94-18462
                                CIP

10 9 8 7 6

Sixth printing July 1996

NOTICE The editors, authors and publisher of this book have taken care that the information and recommendations contained herein are accurate and compatible with standards generally accepted at the time of publication. However, the editors, authors and publisher cannot accept responsibility for errors or omissions or for the consequences from application of the information in this book and make no warranty, express or implied with respect to the contents of the book.

Contributing Authors

TEST TAKING STRATEGIES AND TECHNIQUES
Nancy Dickenson Hazard, M.S.N., C.P.N.P., F.A.A.N.
Executive Officer
Sigma Theta Tau International
Indianapolis, Indiana

HEALTH PROMOTION AND EVALUATION
Rosanne H. Pruitt, Ph.D., RN,CS
Associate Professor
College of Nursing, Clemson University
Family Nurse Practitioner
Clemson University Nursing Center
Clemson, South Carolina

DERMATOLOGICAL DISORDERS
Elissa Davis, M.S.N., RN,CS
Adult Nurse Practitioner
Clinical Associate
Family Medicine
Montefiore Medical Center
New York, New York

EYES, EARS, NOSE, THROAT DISORDERS
Madeline Turkeltaub, Ph.D., RN,CS
Adult Nurse Practitioner
Director
Clinical Nursing Research and Development
Suburban Hospital of Bethesda
Bethesda, Maryland

RESPIRATORY DISORDERS
Madeline Turkeltaub, Ph.D., RN,CS
Adult Nurse Practitioner
Director
Clinical Nursing Research and Development
Suburban Hospital of Bethesda
Bethesda, Maryland

CARDIOVASCULAR DISORDERS
Marilyn Winterton Edmunds, Ph.D., C.R.N.P.
Gerontological Nurse Practitioner
Adult Nurse Practitioner
Associate Professor
Director, Gerontological Nurse Practitioner Program
School of Nursing
University of Maryland
Baltimore, Maryland

HEMATOLOGIC/ONCOLOGIC DISORDERS
Sister Maria Salerno, O.S.F., D.N.Sc., RN,CS
Associate Professor
Director Primary Care/Adult Nurse Practitioner Program
School of Nursing
The Catholic University of America
Washington, D. C.

GASTROINTESTINAL DISORDERS
Sister Maria Salerno, O.S.F., D.N.Sc., RN,CS
Associate Professor
Director Primary Care/Adult Nurse Practitioner Program
School of Nursing
The Catholic University of America
Washington, D. C.

ENDOCRINE DISORDERS
Sister Maria Salerno, O.S.F., D.N.Sc., RN,CS
Associate Professor
Director Primary Care/Adult Nurse Practitioner Program
School of Nursing
The Catholic University of America
Washington, D. C.

GENITOURINARY and GYNECOLOGIC DISORDERS
Pamela A. Shuler, D.N.Sc., RN, CS
Assistant Professor
College of Nursing
University of Kentucky
Family Nurse Practitioner
University of Kentucky Center for Rural Health
Hazard, Kentucky

PREGNANCY, CONTRACEPTION, MENOPAUSE
Pamela A. Shuler, D.N.Sc., RN, CS
Assistant Professor
College of Nursing
University of Kentucky
Family Nurse Practitioner
University of Kentucky Center for Rural Health
Hazard, Kentucky

MUSCULOSKELETAL DISORDERS
Madeline Turkeltaub, Ph.D., RN,CS
Adult Nurse Practitioner
Director
Clinical Nursing Research and Development
Suburban Hospital of Bethesda
Bethesda, Maryland

NEUROLOGICAL DISORDERS
Marilyn Winterton Edmunds, Ph.D., C.R.N.P.
Gerontological Nurse Practitioner
Adult Nurse Practitioner
Associate Professor
Director, Gerontological Nurse Practitioner Program
School of Nursing
University of Maryland
Baltimore, Maryland

PSYCHOSOCIAL DISORDERS
Sister Maria Salerno, O.S.F., D.N.Sc., RN,CS
Associate Professor
Director Primary Care/Adult Nurse Practitioner Program
School of Nursing
The Catholic University of America
Washington, D. C.

CARE OF THE AGING ADULT
Catharine A. Kopac, Ph.D., RN,CS
Gerontological Nurse Practitioner
Assistant Professor
The Catholic University of America
Washington, D. C.

TRENDS, PROFESSIONAL ISSUES, HEALTH POLICY
Marilyn Winterton Edmunds, Ph.D., C.R.N.P.
Gerontological Nurse Practitioner
Adult Nurse Practitioner
Associate Professor
Director, Gerontological Nurse Practitioner Program
School of Nursing
University of Maryland
Baltimore, Maryland

Debra Hardy Havens, B.S.N., R.N., F.N.P.
Vice President, Chief Executive Officer
Capitol Associates, Inc.
Washington, D. C.

HEALTH LEADERSHIP ASSOCIATES, INC.
POTOMAC, MARYLAND

Reviewers

Kathryn Blair, PhD., RN,CS
Family Nurse Practitioner
Instructor of Clinical Nursing
University of Missouri-Columbia
Columbia, Missouri

Margaret A. Fitzgerald, MS, RN,CS
Assistant Professor
Graduate School for Health Studies
Coordinator Adult Primary Health Care Nursing
Simmons College
Boston, Massachusetts
Family Nurse Practitioner
The Family Health Center
Lawrence, Massachusetts

L. Colette Jones, Ph.D., RN,CS., F.A.A.N.
Professor and Associate Dean
Philip Y. Hahn School of Nursing
University of San Diego
San Diego, California

Carolyn M. Sutton, MS, RNC
Director
Women's Health Care Advanced Nurse Practitioner Program
The University of Texas
Southwest Medical Center at Dallas
Dallas, Texas

Joan Swiatek, MS., RN,CS
Adult Nurse Practitioner
Day Surgicenter
Chicago, Illinois

Preface

The second edition of this book has been developed especially for adult and family nurse practitioners preparing to take Certification Examinations. The second edition differs substantially from the first edition in several respects. All sections have been expanded and updated. The number of questions have been increased and the bibliographies enhanced. The new addition to this edition is the chapter on health promotion and evaluation. It brings together much of what is the essence of nurse practitioner practice by a well known expert in the field of health promotion.

The purpose of the book is twofold. This book will assist individuals engaged in self study preparation for Certification Examinations, and may be used as a brief reference guide in the practice setting. It is also one of three books that comprises the "Family Nurse Practitioner Series," the others being the Pediatric Nurse Practitioner Certification Review Guide and the Ob-Gyn Nurse Practitioner Certification Review Guide.

The book has been organized to provide the reader with test taking strategies first. This is followed by the chapter on health promotion. The next 13 chapters address common disorders and provide succinct summaries of definitions, etiology, signs and symptoms, physical findings, differential diagnoses, diagnostic tests/findings and management/treatment. The final chapter addresses health policy, role, trends and professional issues for the nurse practitioner in the health care industry at large.

Following each chapter are test questions, which are intended to serve as an introduction to the testing arena. In addition a bibliography is included for those who need a more in depth discussion of the subject matter in each chapter. These references can serve as additional instructional material for the reader.

Many nurses preparing for certification examinations find that reviewing an extensive body of scientific knowledge requires a very difficult search of many sources that must be synthesized to provide a review base for the examination. This publication provides a succinct, yet comprehensive review of the core material.

The editor and contributing authors are certified nurse practitioners. They have designed this book to assist potential examinees to prepare for success in the certification examination process.

It is assumed that the reader of this review guide has completed a course of study in either an adult or family nurse practitioner program. The Adult Nurse Practitioner Certification Review Guide is not intended to be a basic learning tool.

Certification is a process that is gaining recognition both within and outside the profession. For the professional it is a means of gaining special recognition as a certified nurse practitioner which not only demonstrates a level of competency, but may also enhance professional opportunities and advancement. For the consumer, it means that a certified nurse has met certain predetermined standards set by the profession.

Acknowledgements

The editor and authors wish to express their appreciation to the Centers for Disease Control for permission to use the sexually transmitted disease treatment regimens in the Genitourinary and Gynecolologic Disorders chapter which are based on the *1993 Sexually Transmitted Disease Treatment Guidelines published by the Centers for Disease Control.*

Appreciation is also extended to the authors, reviewers and the many nurse practitioners throughout the country who have provided suggestions and direction in the development of the second edition of this Review Guide. And finally, to the nurse practitioners who have found this review guide not only responsible for success in the certification process, but also as a useful tool in the clinical setting.

CONTENTS

TEST TAKING STRATEGIES AND TECHNIQUES

Nancy A. Dickenson Hazard

We all respond to testing situations in different ways. What separates the successful test taker from the unsuccessful one is knowing how to prepare for and take a test. Preparing yourself as a successful test taker is as important as studying for the test. Each person needs to assess and develop their own test taking strategies and skills. The primary goal of this chapter is to assist potential examinees in knowing how to study for and take a test.

STRATEGY #1 Know Yourself

When faced with an examination, do you feel threatened, experience butterflies or sweaty palms, have trouble keeping your mind focused on studying or on the test question? These common symptoms of test anxiety plague many of us, but can be used advantageously if understood and handled correctly (Divine & Kylen, 1979). Over the years of test taking, each of us have developed certain testing behaviors, some of which are beneficial, while others present obstacles to successful test taking. You can take control of the test taking situation by identifying the undesirable behaviors, maintaining the desirable ones and developing skills to improve test performance.

Technique #1: From the following descriptions of test taking personalities, find yourself (Table 1). Write down those characteristics which describe you even if they are from different personality types. Carefully review the problem list associated with your test taking personality characteristics. Write down the problems which are most troublesome. Then make a list of how you can remedy these problems from the improvement strategies list. Be sure to use these strategies as you prepare for and take examinations.

STRATEGY #2 Develop Your Thinking Skills

Understanding Thought Processes: In order to improve your thinking skills and subsequent test performance, it is best to understand the types of thinking as well as the techniques to enhance the thought process.

Everyone has their own learning style, but we all must proceed through the same process to think.

Thinking occurs on two levels—the lower level of memory and comprehension and the higher level of application and analysis (ABP, 1989). Memory is the ability to recall facts. Without adequate retrieval of facts, progression through the higher levels of thinking can not occur easily. Comprehension is the ability to understand memorized facts. To be effective, comprehension skills must allow the person to translate recalled information from one context to another. Application, or the process of using information to know why it occurs, is a higher form of learning. Effective application relies on the use of understood memorized facts to verify intended action. Analysis is the ability to use abstract or logical forms of thought to show relationships and to distinguish the cause and effect between the variables in a situation.

Table 1

Test Taker Profile

Type	Characteristics	Pitfalls	Improvement Strategies
The Rusher	• Rushes to complete the test before the studied facts are forgotten • Arrives at test site early and waits anxiously • Mumbles studied facts • Tense body posture • Accelerated pulse, respiration and neuromuscular excitement • Answers questions rapidly and is generally one of the first to complete • Experiences exhaustion once test is over	• Unable to read question and situation completely • At high risk for misreading, misinterpreting and mistakes • Difficult items heighten anxiety • Likely to make quick, not well-thought-out guesses	• Practice progressive relaxation techniques • Develop a study plan with sufficient time to review important content • Avoid cramming and last minute studying • Take practice tests focusing on slowing down and reading and answering each option carefully • Read instructions and questions slowly
The Turtle	• Moves slowly, methodically, deliberately through each question • Repeated re-reading, underlining and checking • Takes 60 to 90 seconds per question versus an average of 45 to 60 seconds	• Last to finish; often does not complete the exam • Has to quickly complete questions in last part of exam, increasing errors • Has difficulty completing timed examinations	• Take practice tests focusing on time spent per item • Place watch in front of examination paper to keep track of time • Mark answer sheet for where one should be halfway through exam based on total number of questions and total amount of time for exam • Study concepts, not details • Attempt to answer each question as you progress through the exam

Adult Nurse Practitioner

Type	Characteristics	Pitfalls	Improvement Strategies
The Personalizer	• Mature person who has personal knowledge and insight from life experiences	• Runs risk in relying on what has been learned through observation and experience since one may develop false understandings and stereotypes	• Focus on principles and standards that support nursing practice
		• Personal beliefs and experiences are frequently not the norm or standard tested	• Avoid making connections between patients in exam clinical situations and personal clinical experience
		• Has difficulty identifying expected standards measured by standardized examination	• Focus on generalities not experiences
The Squisher	• View exams as threat, rather than an expected event in education	• Procrastinates studying for exams	• Establish a plan of progressive, disciplined study
	• Preoccupied with grades and personal accomplishment	• Unable to study effectively since waits until last minute	• Use defined time frames for studying content and taking practice exams
	• Attempts to avoid responsibility and accountability associated with testing in order to reduce anxiety	• Increased anxiety over test since procrastinating in the study effort impairs ability to learn and perform	• Use relaxation techniques • Return to difficult items • Read carefully
The Philosopher	• Academically successful person who is well disciplined and structured in study habits	• Over analysis causes loss of sight of actual intent of question	• Focus on questions as they are written
	• Displays great intensity and concentration during exam	• Reads information into questions answering with their own added information rather than answering the actual intent of question	• Work on self confidence and not on question. Initial response is usually correct
	• Searches for questions hidden or unintended meaning		• Avoid multiple re-readings of questions
	• Experiences anxiety over not knowing everything		• Avoid adding own information and unintended meanings
			• Practice, practice, practice with sample tests
The Second Guesser	• Answers questions twice, first as an examinee, second as an examiner	• Altering an initial response frequently results in an incorrect answer	Re-read only the few items of which one is unsure. Avoid changing initial responses

Type	Characteristics	Pitfalls	Improvement Strategies
	• Believes second look will allow one to find and correct errors	• Frequently changes answers because the pattern of response appears incorrect (i.e. too many "true" or too many correct responses)	• Take exam carefully and progressively first time, allowing little or no time for re-reading
			• Study facts
			• Avoid reading into the question
The Lawyer	• Frequently changes initial responses (i.e. grades own test)		
	• Attempts to place words or ideas into the question (leads the witness)	• Veers from the obvious answer and provides response from own point of view	• Focus on distinguishing what patient is saying in question and not on what is read into question
	• Occurs most frequently with psychosocial or communication questions which ask for the most appropriate response	• Reads a question, jumps to a conclusion then finds a response that leads to predetermined conclusion	• Avoid formulating responses aimed at obtaining certain information
			• Choose responses that allow patient to express feelings which encourage hope, not catastrophe, those which are intended to clarify, which identify feeling tone of patient or which avoid negating or confronting patient feelings
			• Carefully read entire question before selecting a response

From: "Making the grades as a test-taker," by N. Dickenson-Hazard, (1989) *Pediatric Nursing* 15, p.303. Adapted from: *Nurse's guide to successful test-taking*, by M. B. Sides and N. B. Cailles, 1989. Philadelphia: J. B. Lippincott, Co., pp 59-70, 199-203. Copyright 1989 by A. J. Jannetti, Inc. Reprinted by permission.

As related to testing situations, the thought process from memory to analysis occurs quite quickly. Some examination items are designed to test memory and comprehension while others test application and analysis. An example of a memory question is as follows:

Non insulin dependent diabetes results from dysfunction of the:

   a)   liver
   b)   *pancreas*
   c)   adrenal glands
   d)   kidneys
   e)   pituitary gland

To answer this question correctly, the individual has to retrieve a memorized fact. Understanding the fact, knowing why it is important or analyzing what should be done in this situation is not needed. An example of a question which tests comprehension is as follows:

> You are taking a history on a 47 year old white female during a routine health assessment visit. She reports that in the past month she has experienced increased thirst and needs to urinate frequently. She reports recurrent episodes of vaginitis and is concerned about an abrasion on her leg which will not heal. You note that her blood pressure is recorded at 150/90 and that she is overweight. You would most likely suspect which of the following?
>
> a) Urinary tract infection
> b) Hyperthyroidism
> c) Type I diabetes mellitus
> d) Essential hypertension
> e) *Type II diabetes mellitus*

In order to answer this question correctly, an individual must retrieve the facts about the physiology of diabetes mellitus in order to understand and differentiate the presenting symptoms.

In a higher level of thinking examination question, individuals must be able to recall a fact, understand that fact in the context of the question, apply this understanding to explaining why one answer is correct, after analyzing the answer choices as they relate to the situation (Sides & Cailles, 1989). An example of an application analysis question is as follows:

> A 48 year old diabetic woman wants to enroll in a low-impact aerobics class. Her diabetes is being well managed with twice daily insulin injections. Your best advice is to:
>
> a) Increase daily doses of insulin
> b) *Have an extra snack before exercise class*
> c) Administer a dose of regular insulin after exercise is completed
> d) Tell her participating in the class is not advisable

To answer this question correctly, the individual must recall physiologic facts of insulin dependent diabetes, understand what is happening in this situation, consider each option and how it applies to the patient's condition and analyze why each advice option works or doesn't work for this patient. Application/analysis questions require the examinee to use logical rationale, which demonstrates the ability to analyze a relationship, based on a well defined principle or fact. Problem solving ability becomes important as the examinee must think through each question option, deciding its relevance and importance to the situation of the question.

Building your thinking skills: Effective memorization is the cornerstone to learning and building thinking skills (Olney, 1989). We have all experienced "memory power outages" at some time, due in part to trying to memorize too much, too fast, too ineffectively. Developing skills to improve memorization is important to increasing the effectiveness of your thinking and subsequent test performance.

Technique #1: Quantity is NOT quality, so concentrate on learning important content. For example, it is important to know the various pharmacologic agents appropriate for the management of chronic obstructive pulmonary disease (COPD), not the specific dosages for each medication.

Technique #2: Memory from repetition, or saying something over and over again to remember it, usually fades. Developing memory skills which trigger retrieval of needed facts is more useful. Such skills are as follows:

Acronyms: These are mental crutches which facilitate recall. Some are already established such as PERRL (pupils equal, round, reactive to light), CHF for (congestive heart failure), or TIA for (transient ischemic attack). Developing your own acronyms can be particularly useful since they are your own word association arrangements in a singular word. Nonsense words or funny, unusual ones are often more useful since they attract your attention.

Acrostics: This mental tool arranges words into catchy phrases. The first letter of each word stands for something which is recalled as the phrase is said. Your own acrostics are most valuable in triggering recall of learned information since they are your individual situation associations. An example of an acrostic is as follows:

Sam **E**xercises **B**y **W**eight-lifting and **R**unning stands for the aspects of non-drug therapy/management for hypertension: **S**alt restriction, **E**xercise, **B**iofeedback, **W**eight reduction, and **R**elaxation techniques.

ABCs: This technique facilitates information retrieval by using the alphabet as a crutch. Each letter stands for a symptom, which when put together creates a picture of the clinical presentation of the disease. For example the characteristics of peptic ulcer disease using the ABC technique is as follows:

a) Antacids relieve pain
b) Burning epigastric pain
c) Cycle of pain two hours after eating
d) Discomfort awakens at night
e) Experiences weight loss
f) Food sometimes aggravates pain

Imaging: This technique can be used in two ways. The first is to develop a nickname for a clinical problem which when said produces a mental picture. For example, "thin, barrel-chested pink puffer" might be used to visualize a patient with emphysema who has a muscle wasted body appearance, absent central cyanosis, hypertrophy of respiratory accessory muscles and an AP chest diameter greater than the transverse chest. A second form of imaging is to visualize a specific patient while you are trying to understand or solve a clinical problem when studying or answering a question. For example, imagine a young man who is experiencing an acute asthma attack. You are trying to analyze the situation and place him in a position which maximizes respiratory effort. In your mind you visualize him in various positions of sidelying, angular and forward, imaging what will happen to the man and his respiratory effort in each position.

Rhymes,   The absurd is easier to remember than the most common. Rhymes,
music   music or links can add absurdity and humor to learning and remembering
& links: (Olney, 1989). These retrieval tools are developed by the individual for specific content. For example, making up a rhyme about diabetes may be helpful in remembering the predominant female incidence, origin of disease, primary symptoms and management as illustrated by:

> There once was a woman
>   whose beta cells failed
> She grew quite thirsty
>   and her glucose levels sailed
> Her lack of insulin caused her to
>   increase her intake
> And her increased urinary output
>   was certainly not fake
> So she learned to watch her diet
>   and administer injections
> That kept her healthy, happy
>   and free of complications.

Setting content to music is sometimes useful to remembering. Melodies which are repetitious jog the memory by the ups and downs of the notes and the rhythm of the music.

Links connect key words from the content by using them in a story. An example given by Olney (1989) for remembering the parts of an eye is: IRIS watched a PUPIL through the LENS of a RED TIN telescope while eating CORN-EA on the cob.

Additional memory aids may also include the use of color or drawing for improving recall. Use different colored pens or paper to accentuate the material being learned. For example, highlight or make notes in blue for content about respiratory problems and in red for cardiovascular content. Drawing assists with visualizing content as well. This is particularly helpful for remembering the pathophysiology of the specific health problem.

The important thing to remember about remembering is to use good recall techniques.

Technique #3: Improving higher level thinking skills involves exercising the application and analysis of memorized fact. Small group review is particularly useful for enhancing these high level skills. It allows verbalization of thought processes and receipt of input about content and thought process from others (Sides and Cailles, 1989). Individuals not only hear how they think, but how others think as well. This interaction allows individuals to identify flaws in their thought process as well as to strengthen their positive points.

Taking practice tests are also helpful in developing application/analysis thinking skills. They permit the individual to analyze thinking patterns as well as the cause and effect relationships between the question and its options. The problem solving skills needed to answer application/analysis questions are tested, giving the individual more experience through practice (Dickenson-Hazard, 1990).

STRATEGY #3 Know The Content

Your ability to study is directly influenced by organization and concentration (Dickenson-Hazard, 1990). If effort is spent on both of these aspects of exam preparation, examination success can be increased.

Preparation for studying: Getting organized. Study habits are developed early in our education experiences. Some of our habits enhance learning while others do not. To increase study effectiveness, organization of study materials and time is essential. Organization decreases frustration, allows for easy resumption of study and increases concentrated study time.

Technique #1: Create your own study space. Select a study area that is yours alone, free from distractions, comfortable and well lighted. The ventilation and room temperature should be comfortable since a cold room makes it difficult to concentrate and a warm room makes you sleepy (Burkle & Marshak, 1989). All your study materials should be left in your study space. The basic premise of a study space is that it facilitates a mind set that you are there to study. When you interrupt study, it is best to leave your materials just as they are. Don't close books or put away notes as you will just have to relocate them, wasting your study time, when you do resume study.

Technique #2: Define and organize the content. From the test giver, secure an outline or the content parameters which are to be examined. If the test giver's outline is sketchy, develop a more detailed one for yourself using the recommended text as a guideline. Next, identify your available study resources: class notes, old exams, handouts, textbooks, review courses, or study groups. For national standardized exams, such as initial licensing or certification, it is best to identify one or two study resources which cover the content being tested and stick to them. Attempting to review all available resources is not only mind boggling, but increases anxiety and frustration as well. Make your selections and stay with them.

Technique #3: Conduct a content assessment. Using a simple rating scale of

> 1 = requires no review
> 2 = requires minimal review
> 3 = requires intensive review
> 4 = start from the beginning

Read through the content outline and rate each content area (Dickenson-Hazard, 1990). Table 2 provides a sample exam content assessment. Be honest with your assessment. It is far better to recognize your content weaknesses when you can study and remedy them, rather than wishing during the exam that you had studied more. Likewise with content strengths: if you know the material, don't waste time studying it.

Table 2

Sample Content Assessment

Exam Content: Gastrointestinal Health Problems of the Adult	
Category: Provided by Test Giver	*Rating: Provided by Examinee*

I. Peptic Ulcer Disease
    A. Etiology 4
    B. Pathophysiology 3
    C. Symptomatology 3
    D. Management 4
    E. Nursing Interventions 3

II. Esophagitis
    A. Etiology 3
    B. Pathophysiology 3
    C. Symptomatology 3
    D. Management 3
    E. Nursing Interventions 2

III. Cholecystitis
    A. Etiology 4
    B. Pathophysiology 3
    C. Symptomatology 3
    D. Management 3
    E. Nursing Interventions 2

IV. Appendicitis
    A. Etiology 2
    B. Pathophysiology 2
    C. Symptomatology 1
    D. Management 1
    E. Nursing interventions 1

V. Diverticulitis
    A. Etiology 4
    B. Pathophysiology 3
    C. Symptomatology 3
    D. Management 4
    E. Nursing Interventions 4

VI. Hepatitis
    A. Etiology 3
    B. Pathophysiology 2
    C. Symptomatology 1
    D. Management 2
    E. Nursing Interventions 1

VII. Acute Gastroenteritis
    A. Etiology 1
    B. Pathophysiology 2
    C. Symptomatology 1
    D. Management 1
    E. Nursing Interventions 1

VIII. Irritable Bowel Syndrome
    A. Etiology 4
    B. Pathophysiology 3
    C. Symptomatology 2
    D. Management 2
    E. Nursing Interventions 2

Technique #4: Develop a study plan. Coordinate the content which needs to be studied with the time available (Sides and Cailles, 1989). Prioritize your study needs, starting with weak areas first. Allow for a general review at the end of the study plan. Lastly establish an overall goal for yourself; something that will motivate you when brought to mind.

Table 3 illustrates a study plan developed on the basis of the exam content assessment in Table 2. Conducting an assessment and developing a study plan should require no more than 50 minutes. It is a wise investment of time with potential payoffs of reduced study stress and exam success.

Technique #5: Begin now and use your time wisely. The smart test taker begins the study process early (Olney, 1989). Sit down, conduct the content assessment and develop a study plan as soon as you know about the exam. DON'T PROCRASTINATE!

Getting Down To Business—The Actual Studying: There is no better way to prepare for an examination than individual study (Dickenson-Hazard, 1989). The responsibility to achieve the goal you set for this exam lies with you alone. The means you employ to achieve this goal do vary and should begin with identifying your peak study times and using techniques to maximize them.

Technique #1: Study in short bursts. Each of us have our own biologic clock which dictates when we are at our peak during the day. If you are a morning person, you are generally active and alert early in the day, slowing down and becoming drowsy by evening. If you are an evening person, you don't completely wake up until late morning and hit your peak in the afternoon and evening. Each person generally has several peaks during the day. It is best to study during those times when your alertness is at its peak (Dickenson-Hazard, 1990).

During our concentration peaks, there are mini peaks, or bursts of alertness (Olney, 1989). These alertness peaks of a concentration peak occur because levels of concentration are at their highest during the first part and last part of a study period. These bursts can vary from ten minutes to one hour depending on the extent of concentration. If studying is sustained for one hour there are only two mini peaks; one at the beginning and one at the end. There are eight mini peaks if that same hour is divided into four, 10-minute intervals. Hence it is more helpful to study in short bursts (Olney, 1989). More can be learned in less time.

Table 3

Sample Study Plan

Goal: Achieve a "B" on the Gastrointestinal Problems of the Adult Patient. Test Time Available: 2 Weeks

Objective	Activity	Date Accomplished
Master Content on diverticulitis	Read Chapter 26. Take notes on chapter content according to outline	Feb. 5 & 6, 1 hour
	Review class notes combined with chapter notes	Feb. 6, 1 hour
	Review sample test questions	Feb. 6, 1 hour
Understand content on peptic ulcer disease	Read Chapter 25. Take notes on chapter content according to content outline	Feb. 7, 2 hours
	Review class notes combined with chapter notes	Feb. 8, 1½ hours
Master content on cholecystitis	Read Chapter 24. Take notes on chapter content according to content outline	Feb. 10, 2 hours
	Review class notes combined with chapter notes	Feb. 11, ½ hours
	Review sample test questions	Feb. 12, 1½ hours
Know material on irritable bowel syndrome	Scan Chapter 27. Review class notes supplementing with text notes	Feb. 14, 2 hours
Know material on esophagitis	Scan Chapter 23. Review class notes supplementing with text notes	Feb. 15, 2 hours
Know material on hepatitis	Scan Chapter 28. Review highlights and important concepts	Feb. 16, 2 hours
Know material on appendicitis and acute gastroenteritis	Scan Chapter 29. Review highlights and important concepts	Feb. 17, 2 hours
Demonstrate understanding of all material	Review with another person	Feb. 18, 2 hours
	Review all notes	Feb. 19, 1½ hours
	Take sample test questions	Feb. 19, 1½ hours
Think positively	SMILE	ON GOING
	Take frequent breaks	
	Reward myself after each study session	
	Keep my goal in mind	

Technique #2: Cramming can be useful. Since concentration ability is highly variable, some individuals can sustain their mini-peaks for 15, 20 or even 30 minutes at a time. Pushing your concentration beyond its peak is fruitless and verges on cramming, which in general is a poor study technique. There are, however, times when cramming, a short term memory tool, is useful. Short term memory generally is at its best in the morning. A quick review or cram of content in the morning can be useful the day of the exam (Olney, 1989). Most studying, however, is best accomplished in the afternoon or evening when long term memory functions at its peak.

Technique #3: Give your brain breaks. Regular times during study to rest and absorb the content is needed by the brain. The best approach to breaks is to plan them and give yourself a conscious break (Dickenson-Hazard, 1990). This approach eliminates the "day dreaming" or "wandering thought" approach to breaks that many of us use. It is better to get up, leave the study area and do something non-study related for longer breaks. For shorter breaks of five minutes or so, leave your desk, gaze out the window or do some stretching exercises. When your brain says to give it a rest, accommodate it! You'll learn more in less stress free time.

Technique #4: Study the correct content. It is easy for all of us to become bogged down in the detail of the content we are studying. However, it is best to focus on the major concepts or the "state of the art" content. Leave the details, the suppositions and the experience at the door of your study area. Concentrate on the major textbook facts and concepts which revolve around the subject matter being tested.

Technique #5: Fit your studying to the test type. The best way to prepare for an objective test is to study facts, particularly anything printed in italics. Memory enhancing techniques are particularly useful when preparing for an objective test. If preparing for an essay test, study generalities, examples and concepts. Application techniques are helpful when studying for this type of an exam (Burkle and Marshak, 1989).

Technique #6: Use your study plan wisely. Your study plan is meant to be a guide, not a rigid schedule. You should take your time with studying. Don't rush through the content just to remain on schedule. Occasionally study plans need revision. If you take more or less time than planned, readjust the plan for the time gained or lost. The plan can guide you, but you must go at your own pace.

Technique #7: Actively study. Being an active participant in study rather than trying to absorb the printed word is also helpful. Ways to be active include: taking notes on the content as you study; constructing questions then answering them; taking practice tests or; discussing the content with yourself. Also using your individual study quirks are encouraged. Some people stand, others walk around and some play background music. Whatever helps you to concentrate and study better, you should use.

Technique #8: Use study aids. While there is no substitute for individual studying, several resources, if available, are useful in facilitating learning. Review courses are an excellent means for organizing or summarizing your individual study. They generally provide the content parameters and the major concepts of the content which you need to know. Review courses also provide an opportunity to clarify not-well-understood content, as well as to review known material (Dickenson-Hazard, 1990). Study guides are useful for organizing study. They provide detail on the content which is important to the exam. Study groups are an excellent resource for summarizing and refining content. They provide an opportunity for thinking through your knowledge base, with the advantage of hearing another person's point of view. Each of these study aids increases understanding of content and when used correctly increase effectiveness of knowledge application.

Technique #9: Know when to quit. It is best to stop studying when your concentration ebbs. It is unproductive and frustrating to force yourself to study. It is far better to rest or unwind, then resume at a later point in the day. Avoid studying outside your A.M. or P.M. concentration peaks and focus your study energy on your right time of day or evening.

STRATEGY #4 Become Test-wise

Most nursing examinations are composed of multiple choice questions (MCQs). This type of question requires the examinee to select the best response(s) for a specific circumstance or condition. Successful test taking is dependent not only on content knowledge but on test taking skill as well. If you are unable to impart your knowledge through the vehicle used for its conveyance, i.e. the MCQ, your test taking success is in jeopardy.

Technique #1: Recognize the purpose of a test question. Most test questions are developed to examine knowledge at two separate levels: memory (or recall) and comprehension (or application). A memory question requires the examinee to recall facts from their knowledge base while an application question requires the examinee to use and apply the knowledge (ABP, 1989). Memory questions test recall while application questions test synthesis and problem solving skills. When taking a test you need to be aware of whether you are being asked a fact or to use that fact.

Table 4

Anatomy Of A Test Question

Background Statement:	A 32 year old black female is being seen for a complaint of sores in the vaginal area. She has been experiencing a low grade fever, headache and malaise over the past five days. Physical examination reveals inguinal lymphadehopathy, vaginal erythema and multiple labial and vaginal vesicular lesions.
	Stem: Which of the following causative organisms woulld you most likely suspect?
	Options: (A) *Herpes simplex virus 2*
	(B) Condylomata lata
	(C) Herpes simplex virus 1
	(D) Treponema pallidum

Table 5

Test Question Key Words And Phrases

First	Significant	Counseling
Best	Immediate	Facilitative
Most	Helpful	Indicative
Initial	Closely	Suggestive
Important	Priority	Appropriate
Major	Advice	Accurately
Common	Approach	Likely
Least	Consideration	Characteristics
Except	Management	True Statements
Not	Expectation	Correct Statements
Greatest	Intervention	Contributing to
Earliest	Assessment	Of the following
Useful	Contraindication	Which of the following
Leading	Evaluation	Each of the following

From "Anatomy of a test question" by N. Dickenson-Hazard, 1989, *Pediatric Nursing 15*, p. 395. Copyright 1989 by A. J. Jannetti, Inc. Reprinted by permission.

Technique #2: Recognize the components of a test question. Multiple choice questions may include the basic components of a background statement, a stem and a list of options. The background statement presents information which facilitates the examinee in answering the question. The stem asks or states the intent of the question. The options are 4 or 5 possible responses to the question. The correct option is called the keyed response and all other options are called distractors (ABP, 1989). Knowing the components of a test question helps you sift through the information presented and focus on the questions intent (see Table 4).

Technique #3: Identify the key word(s) in a test question. Key words are generally included in the stem of a test question, whereas key concepts or conditions appear in the background statement. You should pay particular attention to the key words in the stem and their impact on the intent of the question (See Table 5).

Technique #4: Recognize the item types. Basically two styles of MCQs are used for examinations. One requires the examinee to select the one best answer; the other requires selection of multiple correct answers. Among the one best answer styles there are three types. The A type requires the selection of the best response among those offered. The B type requires the examinee to match the options with the appropriate statement. C type items require the examinee to compare or contrast two related conditions. The X type asks the examinee to respond either true or false to each option (ABP, 1989). Table 6 illustrates these item types. **Most standardized tests, such as those used for nursing licensure and certification, are composed of four or five option-A type questions.**

Technique #5: Read the directions to the questions carefully. Since an examination may have several types of questions, it is imperative to read the directions carefully. If different item types are used on an exam, they are generally grouped together by type and marked clearly with directions. Be on the lookout for changing item types and be sure you understand how you are to answer before you begin reading the question.

Technique #6: Apply the basic rules of test taking. Examination candidates can avert many problems associated with test taking if they give thought to the mechanics of sitting down, reading the question and noting their answers. Timing yourself to avoid spending too much time on a question, returning to difficult questions, and not changing your answers are all techniques that can improve performance. Table 7 provides helpful hints for the basic rules of test-taking. Review these and apply them to the testing situation.

Technique #7: Practice, practice, practice. Taking practice tests can improve performance. While they can assist in evaluation of your knowledge, their primary benefit is to assist you with test taking skills. You should use them to evaluate your thinking process, your ability to read, understand and interpret questions, and your skills in completing the mechanics of the test.

Technique #8: Be prepared for exam day. It is important to familiarize yourself with the test site, the building, the parking and travel route prior to the exam day. If you must travel, arrive early to allow time for this familiarization. It is helpful to make a list of things you need on the exam day: pencils, admission card, watch and a few pieces of hard candy as a quick energy source. On exam day allow yourself plenty of time to arrive at the site. Wear comfortable clothes and have a good breakfast that morning. The night before the exam, go to bed at a reasonable hour; avoid last minute cramming; and avoid excessive drinking or eating (Sides & Cailles, 1989). The idea is to arrive on time at the test site, prepared and as rested as possible.

Table 6
Item Type Examples

A TYPE

Directions for One Best Choice Items: This item-type requires that you indicate the one best answer from the lettered alternatives offered for each item. After you have decided on the one BEST answer, completely blacken the corresponding lettered circle on the answer sheet.

   #1 A 46 year old white female is being seen in follow-up for the treatment of migrane headaches. Your management plan would most appropriately include counseling on which of the following preventive techniques?

   a. Limiting intake of high calcium foods
   b. Encouraging additional sleep hours
   c. *Learning biofeedback techniques*
   d. Massaging posterior head and neck areas regularly
   e. Developing a rigorous exercise routine

B TYPE

Directions: Each group of questions below consists of five lettered headings followed by a list of numbered words or statements. For each numbered word or statement, select the one lettered heading that is most closely associated with it and fill in the circle beneath the corresponding letter on the answer sheet. Each lettered heading may be selected once, more than once, or not at all.

   #2-4
   Medication types:
   a. Beta-adrenergic blockers
   b. Diuretics
   c. Digoxin
   d. Angiotension-converting enzyme inhibitors
   e. Calcium antagonists

   Most useful for treatment of:
   2. Supraventricular tachyarrhythmias (E)
   3. Congestive heart failure (B)
   4. Myocardial infarction (A)

C TYPE

Directions: Each set of lettered headings below is followed by a list of numbered words or phrases. For each numbered word or phrase fill in the circle on the answer sheet under A if the item is associated with (A) only, B if the item is associated with (B) only, C if the item is associated with both (A) and (B), D if the item is associated with neither (A) nor (B).

   (A) Diabetic acidosis
   (B) Insulin shock
   (C) Both
   (D) Neither

   #5 - Elevated bicarbonate level in serum (D)
   #6 - The duration of the condition before proper treatment is begun may influence the prognosis (C)
   #7 - Deep breathing (A)
   #8 - Coma (C)
   #9 - Moist skin (B)

X TYPE

Directions: Each of the questions or incomplete statements below is followed by five suggested answers or completions. For EACH let .ed alternative completely blacken one lettered circle in either column T or F on the answer sheet.

   Which of the following tests are useful for differentiating anemia associated with a chronic disease from iron deficiency anemia?
   a. Serum iron levels (F)
   b. Bone marrow examination (T)
   c. Reticulocyte count (F)
   d. Serum transferrin level (F)
   e. Serum ferritin level (T)

Adapted from "Anatomy of a test question." by N. Dickenson-Hazard, 1989, *Pediatric Nursing 15*, p. 396. Copyright 1989 by A. J. Jannetti, Inc. Adapted by permission.

Table 7

Basic Rules For Test Taking

Basic Rule	Helpful Hints
Use time wisely and effectively	Allow no more than 1 minute per question—If you can't answer question, make an intelligent guess

Know the parts of a question
    Background statement: Informational scenario
    Stem: Specific question or intent statement
	Select the option that best completes question or solves the problem
	Relate options to question and balance against each other
	Consider all options

Read question carefully	Understand stem first, then look for answer Underline key words in background information and stem (i.e. first, best, initial, early, most, appropriate, except, least, not).
Identify intent of item based on information given	Don't assume any information not given Don't read in or add any information not given Actively reason through question
Answer difficult questions by eliminating obviously incorrect options first	Select the best of the viable, options available using logical thought Re-read stem; select stongest option Skip difficult questions and return to them later or make an educated guess
Select responses guided by principles of communication	Choose therapeutic, respectful, communication enhancing options Avoid inappropriate, punitive responses
Know the principles of nursing practice	Select options that relate to common need or the population in general Select options that are correct without exception Select options which reflect nursing judgement
Know and use test-taking principles	Avoid changing answers without good reason Attempt every question Don't rely on flaws in test construction Be systematic and use problem-solving technique in answering questions

From "Making the grade as a test-taker" by N. Dickenson-Hazard, 1989. *Pediatric Nursing 15*, p. 304. Adapted from *How to Take Tests*. (pp 15-57) by J. Millman and W. Paul, 1969, New York: McGraw-Hill Co. and from *Nurses's guide to successful test taking*. (pp 43-53) by M. B. Sides and N. B. Cailles, 1989, Philadelphia: J. B. Lippincott Co. Copyright 1989 A. J. Jannetti, Inc. Reprinted and Adapted by permission.

Strategy #5 Psych Yourself Up: Taking tests is stressful

While a little stress can be productive, too much can incapacitate you in your studying and test taking (Divine & Kylen, 1979). Your attitude and approach to test-taking and studying can influence your outcomes. Psyching yourself up can have a positive affect and make examinations a non-anxiety laden experience (Dickenson-Hazard, 1990). The following techniques are based on the principles of successful test taking as presented by Sides & Cailles (1989). Incorporation of these techniques can improve response and performance in examination situations.

Technique #1: Adopt an "I can" attitude. Believing you can succeed is the key to success. Self belief inspires and gives you the power to achieve your goals. Without a success attitude, the road to your goal is much harder. We all stand an equal chance of success in this world. It is those who believe they can who achieve it. This "I can" attitude must permeate all your efforts in test taking from studying to improving your skills to actually writing the test.

Technique #2: Take control. By identifying your goal, deciding how to accomplish it and developing a plan for achieving it, you take control. Do not leave your success or failure to chance; control it through action and attitude.

Technique #3: Think positively. Examinations are generally based on a standard which is the same for all individuals. Everyone can potentially pass. Performance is influenced not only by knowledge and skill but attitude as well. Those individuals who regard an exam as an opportunity or challenge will be more successful.

Technique #4: Project a positive self-fulfilling prophecy. While preparing for an examination, project thoughts of the positive outcomes you will experience when you succeed. Self-talk is self-fulfilling. Expect success, not failure, of yourself.

Technique #5: Feel good about yourself. Without feeling a sense of positive self worth, passing an examination is difficult. Recognize your professional contributions and give yourself credit for your accomplishments. Think "I will pass," not "I suppose I can."

Technique #6: Know yourself. Focus exam preparation and test taking on your strengths. Try to alter your weaknesses instead of becoming hung up on them. If you tend to overanalyze, study and read test questions at face value. If you're a speed demon when taking a test, slow down and read more carefully.

Technique #7: Failure is a possibility. We all have failed at something at some point in our lives. Rather than dwelling on the failure, making excuses and believing you'll fail again, recognize your mistakes and remedy them. Failure is a time to begin again; use it as a motivator to do better. It is not the end of the world unless you allow it to be. It is best to deal with the failure and move on, otherwise it interferes with your success.

Technique #8: Persevere, persevere, persevere! Endurance must underlie all your efforts. Call forth those reserve energies when you've had all you think you can take. Rely upon yourself and your support systems to help you maintain a sense of direction and keep your goal in the forefront.

Technique #9: Motivation is muscle. Most individuals are motivated by fear or desire. The fear in an exam situation may be one of failure, the unknown or discovery of imperfection. Put your fear into perspective; realize you are not the only one with fear and that all have an equal opportunity for success. Develop strategies to reduce fear and use fear to your advantage by improving the imperfections. Desire is a powerful motivator and you should keep the rewards of your desire foremost in your mind. Whatever motivates you, use it to make you successful. Reward yourself during your exam preparation and once the exam has been completed. You alone hold the key to success; use what you have wisely.

This chapter has provided concepts, strategies and techniques for improving study and test taking skills. Your first task in improvement is to know yourself: how you study and how you take a test. You should use your strengths and remedy the weaknesses. Next you need to develop your thinking skills. Work on techniques to improve memory and reasoning. Now you need to organize your study and concentrate on using these new and used skills to be successful. Create a study space, develop a plan of action, then implement that plan during your periods of peak concentration. Before taking the exam be sure you understand the components of a test question, can identify key words and phrases and have practiced. Apply the test taking rules during the exam process. Finally, believe in yourself, your knowledge and your talent. Believing you can accomplish your goal facilitates the fact that you will.

Bibliography

American Board of Pediatrics, (1989). *Developing questions and critiques*. Unpublished material.

Burke, M. M., & Walsh, M.B. (1992). *Gerontologic Nursing*, St. Louis: Mosby Year Book.

Burkle, C. A., & Marshak, D. (1989). *Study Program: Level 1*. Reston, Va: National Association of Secondary School Principals.

Dickenson-Hazard, N. (1989). Making the grade as a test taker. *Pediatric Nursing*, 15, 302-304.

Dickenson-Hazard, N. (1989). Anatomy of a test question. *Pediatric Nursing*, 15, 395-399.

Dickenson-Hazard, N. (1990). The psychology of successful test taking. *Pediatric Nursing*, 16, 66-67.

Dickenson-Hazard, N. (1990). Study smart. *Pediatric Nursing*, 16, 314-316.

Dickenson-Hazard, N. (1990). Study effectiveness: are you 10 a.m. or p.m. scholar? *Pediatric Nursing*, 16, 419-420.

Dickenson-Hazard, N. (1990). Develop your thinking skills for improved test taking. *Pediatric Nursing*, 16, 480-481.

Divine, J. H., & Kylen, D. W. (1979). *How to beat test anxiety*. New York: Barrons Educational Series.

Goroll, A., May, L., & Mulley, A (Eds.) (1988). *Primary care medicine* (2nd ed.). Philadelphia: J. B. Lippincott.

Millman, J., & Paul, W. (1969). *How to take tests*. New York: McGraw-Hill Book Co.

Millonig, V. L. (Ed). (1991). *The adult nurse practitioner certification review guide*. Potomac, MD: Health Leadership Associates.

Olney, C. W. (1989). *Where there's a will, there's an A*. New Jersey: Chesterbrook Educational Publishers.

Sides, M., & Cailles, N. B. (1989). *Nurse's guide to successful test taking*. Philadelphia: J. B. Lippincott.

Health Promotion and Evaluation

Rosanne H. Pruitt

Theoretical Aspects

- Health Promotion Theories

    1. High Level Wellness—a continuum that demonstrates dynamic interaction of health and environment as one moves toward high level wellness. Health is dynamic with a continuous need for health promoting activity to maintain and improve one's health (Dunn 1971)

    2. Maslow's Hierarchy of Need

        a. Self actualization-achievement of personal potential

        b. Self esteem-sense of self worth, recognition

        c. Love and belonging-affection, companionship

        d. Safety and security-protection from physical hazards

        e. Survival needs-food, water, sleep (Health promotion activities usually address self actualization and self esteem needs)

    3. Health Belief Model—health is influenced by age, sex, race, ethnicity, and income

        a. Threats to health

            (1) Perceived susceptibility

            (2) Perceived seriousness of condition

        b. Outcome expectation of health action

            (1) Perceived benefits of action

            (2) Perceived barriers to taking action

            (3) Efficacy expectations—conviction about one's ability to carry out recommended action (self-efficacy) (Glanz, Lewis & Rimer, 1990)

    4. Social Learning Theory—explains human behavior in terms of a dynamic reciprocal interaction between behavior, personal factors, and environmental influences. Key concepts

        a. Personal factors which include the ability to symbolize behavior meaning, to foresee outcomes of given behavior, to learn by observing others, to self-determine and self regulate, and to reflect and analyze experience

        b. Reciprocal determinism refers to behavior as dynamic and dependent on environmental and personal constructs that influence each other simultaneously (Bandura, 1977)

5. Health Promotion Model—developed as an explanation for health promoting behaviors using multiple cognitive-perceptual factors such as the importance of health and perceived benefits, perceived control of health and self efficacy modified by factors such as demographics and interpersonal influences (Pender, 1994)

■ System Theories

1. General Systems Theory—views world in terms of sets of integrated reactions in an effort to see parts in relation to the whole. Key concepts

    a. System is a goal directed unit with interdependent, interacting parts

    b. Boundaries regulate exchange of energy, information, and matter between systems and may be open or closed depending on interaction with surrounding environment

    c. Input, output, and the feedback loop which provide for an exchange of energy, information, and matter (Bertalanffy, 1969)

2. Neuman's Systems Model—uses a systems format and includes the levels of prevention as well as the multiple dimensions of health promotion (physical, psychological, spiritual, and social). Health promotion efforts are used to strengthen the line barriers of defense (Neuman, 1989)

■ Life Span Developmental Theories

1. Erikson's Stages of Psychosocial Development—the degree of success experienced in accomplishing developmental tasks influences accomplishments of tasks of older adults

    a. Trust versus mistrust-trust of self and others

    b. Autonomy versus shame and doubt-self expression and cooperation with others

    c. Initiative versus guilt-focus on purposeful behavior

    d. Industry versus inferiority-belief in one's ability

    e. Identity versus role confusion-clear sense of self

    f. Intimacy versus role confusion-capacity for reciprocal love relationships

    g. Generativity versus stagnation— creativity and productivity

    h. Ego identity versus despair—acceptance of one's life as worthwhile and unique (Erikson, 1963)

- Family Theory
  1. Systems Theory—the family is viewed as an open social system
  2. Structural-Functional Theory— families are viewed as having an internal and external environment, recognizing the importance of interaction between members, and focusing on outcomes
  3. Family Developmental Theory—family life is described over time in a series of discrete stages based on age of oldest child. Theory is a blend of developmental theory, such as Erikson, with concepts of role and interpersonal interaction.
  4. Institutional-Historical Approach—families are analyzed as institutions with certain functions in society at some point in time. The theory includes cross-cultural considerations. A central focus is how the family unit influences and is affected by social change in society (Friedman, 1992)

Related Concepts

- Levels of Prevention from public health science are used by most authorities when differentiating health promotion activities from other interventions. *Healthy People 2000* and other federal documents use a broader interpretation which include health protection, such as specific screenings and safety factors
  1. Primary prevention includes measures to promote optimum health prior to the onset of any problems (health promotion), e.g., promoting a healthy diet, immunization, exercise, or the identification of occupational or environmental hazards
  2. Secondary prevention focuses on early identification and treatment of existing health problems, e.g., routine Pap smear or mammogram
  3. Tertiary Prevention is the rehabilitation and restoration to health, e.g., cardiac rehabilitation
- Cultural influence must be considered with any health encounter. Cultural beliefs of disease causation influence health practices, (e.g., magic or evil spirits (Latino); violation of a natural law (American Indian); imbalance between 'hot' or "cold" forces (Asian, Latino); varied beliefs affect the acceptance of practices such as handwashing and immunizations (Leininger, 1985, Creasia & Parker, 1992)

Lifestyle/Health Behaviors

■ Stress Management— stress is an imbalance between environmental demands and one's individual and social resources required to cope with those demands

1. Types of stressors

    a. Major life events-discrete events that disrupt normal functioning

    b. Daily hassles-minor daily events perceived as frustrating

    c. Chronic strains-challenges, hardships, and problems

    d. Cataclysmic events-sudden disasters that require major adaptive responses

    e. Ambient stressors-continuous and often unchanging conditions in physical environment, such as chronic pollution or noise

2. Theoretical basis of stress

    a. General Adaptation Syndrome—Selye's stress continuum demonstrates how small amounts of stress are motivating and improve the quality of life (eustress or good stress), however beyond a certain point the stress becomes psychologically and physically debilitating (distress). (Goldberger & Breznitz, 1993)

3. Physical indicators of stress

    a. GI symptoms—upset stomach, change of appetite

    b. Headache, muscle tension, elevated blood pressure (BP)

    c. Restlessness—cold and sweaty palms

4. Emotional indicators of stress

    a. Irritability, emotional outbursts, crying

    b. Depression, withdrawal

    c. Hostility, tendency to blame others

    d. Anxiety, suspiciousness

5. Behavioral indicators of stress

    a. Lethargy, loss of interest

    b. Poor concentration, forgetfulness

    c. Decreased productivity, absenteeism

        d. Sleep disturbance

6.   Related indicators—Karoshi (Japanese) death by overwork; associated with long hours and stressful working conditions

7.   Stress Management Intervention Techniques

    a. Stress reduction techniques

        (1)   Time management—determine goals and priorities, set time priorities, and learn to say no to non-goal related activities

        (2)   Time blocking—set aside time to adapt to change and incorporate it into daily routine

        (3)   Change avoidance—during periods of high life change, avoid unnecessary change to prevent need to make multiple adjustments simultaneously

        (4)   Habituation—make aspects of day routine, during a stressful situation, (e.g., park in the usual place to avoid having to look for car upon return)

        (5)   Environmental modification—identify experiences and/or personalities that are abrasive or stress producing and minimize contact as much as possible

        (6)   Involvement with activities of interest-doing something for others and helping with activities that interest one to decrease focus on self

    b. Behavioral aspects to build stress resistance

        (1)   Increase self esteem—focus on own strengths and attributes

        (2)   Increase assertiveness—substitute positive assertive behavior for negative passive actions

        (3)   Meditation/prayer—includes Zen and yoga

    c. Counter conditioning to lower stress response

        (1)   Autogenic training—repetition of autogenic suggestions such as "my arms and legs are heavy"

        (2)   Imagery—image visualization used to relax or assist with past frightening experiences

        (3)   Tension/relaxation exercises—tense muscles for 8-10 seconds, then relax; longer training sessions are usually required initially to enhance benefits

(4) Biofeedback—awareness and control to influence response that is not ordinarily under voluntary control

(5) Exercise—produces physiological changes that counteract the effects of stress

8. Contraindications for stress management

   a. Severe depression—may stimulate further withdrawal

   b. Hallucinations or delusions

   c. Temporary hypotensive or hypoglycemic states

   d. Severe pain—may increase awareness

   e. Tensing of large muscle groups with severe heart disease

■ Social Support

1. Four types of supporting behaviors

   a. Emotional support—provision of empathy, love, trust and caring (strongest, most consistent relationship to positive health status)

   b. Instrumental support—direct assistance or services

   c. Informational support—advice, suggestions and information for problem solving

   d. Appraisal support or provision of information—useful for self-evaluation purposes (feedback, affirmation)

2. Related research

   a. Research evidence suggests that the quality of supportive relationships is a better predictor of health than quantity. Relationships are thought to provide buffering effects to protect people from negative consequences of stressful situations

   b. The importance of social support has been demonstrated in multiple studies related to recovery from illness, disaster, success with weight loss and other positive life changes

   c. Support groups provide encouragement for those without a strong positive social network (Glanz, Lewis, & Rimer, 1990)

■ Nutrition

1. Healthy diet guidelines

   a. The Food Guide Pyramid is the official graphic of federal dietary guidance for daily food group selection

       (1)   Milk, yogurt, and cheese—2 to 4 servings

       (2)   Meat, poultry, fish, dry beans, eggs, and nuts—2 to 3 servings

       (3)   Vegetables—3 to 5 servings

       (4)   Fruits—2·to 4 servings

       (5)   Bread, cereal, rice—6 to 11 servings

       (6)   Oils, sweets, and fats are to be used sparingly

  b. Eat a variety of foods

       (1)   Eat foods from all five food groups every day

       (2)   Select *different* foods from each group every day

  c. Limit total fat to less than 30% of total calories and saturated fat to less than 10% of total calories

  d. Limit cholesterol intake to less than 300 mg/day

  e. Limit consumption of salt-cured, smoked, or nitrite preserved food (limit sodium to no more than 3 grams); limit use of salt in cooking and avoid adding it to food at the table

  f. Calorie breakdown 55 to 60% carbohydrates 30% fat with remainder protein

2. Assessment for weight loss

  a. Initially identify any symptoms which are associated with and/or aggravated by excessive weight and indicative of underlying pathology requiring different action

       (1)   Polyuria/polyphagia/polydipsia—diabetes

       (2)   Joint pain or marked swelling—osteoarthritis or gout

       (3)   Angina/palpitations/dyspnea— cardiovascular disease

       (4)   Edema/cold intolerance— hypothyroidism

       (5)   Recent weight gain with edema, pruritus—renal disease

  b. Recommended laboratory tests

       (1)   EKG

       (2)   Blood chemistry profile— blood lipids, glucose, uric acid, thyroid (T_3, T_4)

  c. Contraindications for weight loss

(1) Pregnancy

(2) Chemotherapy—due to already compromised nutritional status and potential impact on therapy

3. Body weight determinations

a. Determine ideal body weight (IBW) using an anthropometric chart or the following formula

Determination of IBW		
Build	**Women**	**Men**
Medium	Allow 100 lbs for first 5 ft plus 5 lb for each add. inch e.g., 5 ft 5 in = 125 (100+25)	Allow 106 lbs for first 5 ft plus 6 lb for each add. inch e.g., 5 ft 9in = 160 (105+54)
Small	Subtract 10%	Subtract 10%
Large	Add 10%	Add 10%

b. Estimate percentage of ideal body weight (IBW) by dividing present weight (PW) by IBW   PW/IBW = % IBW

$$\text{e.g., } 160(PW)/120(IBW) = 1.33\ (\%IBW) \text{ or } 33\% \text{ over Ideal Body Weight}$$

c. Use growth chart for height and weight comparisons for adolescents

4. Guidelines for healthy weight loss

a. Diet deficient in calories, not nutrients

b. Balanced—a variety of foods

c. Should not depend on vitamins, weight loss pills, or prepared liquids

d. Should supply all essential vitamins and minerals

e. Should provide adequate fiber for proper GI functioning

f. Should provide adequate fluid for renal functioning

g. Should provide enough fat to supply essential fatty acid, linoleic acid

h. Should contain a variety of highly nutritious foods

    i. Should set a goal of 1 to 2 lb/week (gradual)

    j. Should focus on regular meals, avoiding snacks and modifying bad eating habits

5. Weight Control Strategies

    a. Regular physical activity for calorie use and assistance in regulating appetite

    b. Social support by family, friends, colleagues, and support groups

    c. Focus on internal motivation for loss, e.g., control, personal goals, and positive health benefits

    d. Smaller, more frequent meals to maintain blood sugar levels and avoid feelings of hunger

    e. Control home environment, e.g., limit eating to one room, sit down at table; don't eat while watching television

    f. Control snacking, e.g., keep low calorie snacks available/ready to eat

    g. Control eating environment, e.g., avoid serving bowls at the table, use smaller plates and glasses, and eat slowly

    h. Control work environment, e.g., eat away from your desk, don't store food near your work area, and take exercise breaks

    i. Use a shopping list, do not shop when hungry

6. Yo-Yo syndrome associated with severe dieting efforts (metabolic response to starvation)

    a. Lowers metabolic rate making permanent weight loss more difficult to achieve

    b. Lower metabolic rate also results in a tendency to gain weight easier once individual returns to usual diet

7. Weight loss prognostic factors

    a. Stability of present weight (# years)

    b. Motivation to change, conditions making weight loss a high priority

    c. Realistic expectations

8. Diet prescription components

    a. Determine ideal body weight using the formula or anthropometric chart

b. Estimate caloric needs by adding basal calories (IBW $\times$ 10) and activity calories, sedentary IBW $\times$ 3, moderate IBW $\times$ 5, strenuous $\times$ 10

c. IBW = 125 lb
125 $\times$ 10 = 1250 (basal calories)
125 $\times$ 3 = 375 (activity calories)
1250 + 375 = 1625 (total calories needed per day)

■ Physical Fitness

1. Psychological benefits

   a. Increased alertness

   b. Improved self esteem

   c. Decreased depression

   d. Reduced stress and tension

2. Physical benefits

   a. Heart—increases efficiency, lowers heart rate, lowers BP, increases oxygen capacity

   b. Decreases LDL, increases HDL

   c. Improves muscles tone (strength and endurance)

   d. Improves flexibility

   e. Increases BMR during and after exercise

   f. Promotes loss of body fat while retaining muscle tissue

   g. Anti-aging effect

   h. Minimizes bone mineral loss to some degree in postmenopausal women

3. Physical fitness evaluation

   a. Cardiorespiratory endurance or aerobic fitness—usually measured by performance on 1.5 mile run, step test (5 minute pulse recovery step test), bicycle ergometer test or swimming test

   b. Skinfold test or other determination of body fat composition, (e.g., body mass index)

   c. Flexibility of back—hyperextension, sit and reach tests

   d. Muscle strength—tested by determining the maximum amount of weight that can be lifted comfortably a single time by four different muscle groups. This test is usually delayed until after approximately six weeks in a training program

e. Muscle endurance—determined by push-ups (shoulder, arm and chest muscle endurance) and bent knee sit-ups (abdominals)

f. Leg power—tested by height of vertical jump from squat position

4. Exercise—the following guidelines should be met for full psychological and physical benefits, including cardiovascular and respiratory conditioning*

a. Components of effective exercise

(1) Performed at least 3 to 5 times/week

(2) Enjoyable for the participant

(3) Rhythmic movement, alternating relaxation and contraction of large muscle groups

(4) Energy expenditure of approximately 300 calories over usual activities (see Table 1)

(5) Sustained heart rate in the target heart zone 20 to 30 minutes; Heart rate (HR) is used as the external indicator of oxygen consumption of muscles necessary for aerobic fitness

(6) Maximum heart rate (MHR) is estimated by subtracting one's age from 220. A target heart zone of 70 to 85% is then estimated, e.g., 220—age=maximum heart rate; multiply maximum MHR by .7 and .85, (e.g., 220-20=200, 200 x .7= 140; 200 x .85 = 170 for range 140-170)

*"Those who engage in limited exercise on a regular basis are better off than those who do almost nothing (Haskell, 1992, p. 42)." Therefore, it is not necessary to meet all of the above criteria consistently.

Table 1
Calorie Expenditure for Various Activities (Sharkey, 1990)

Work Intensity	Pulse rate	Calories/min	Examples
Light	Below 120	< 5	Golf, walk (1-2 mph)
Moderate	120 to 150	5 to 10	Brisk walk, jog, biking, tennis
Heavy	Above 150	Above 10	Running, fast swim

   b. Components of an exercise plan

     (1) Warm up—increases blood flow, loosens and strengthens muscles, e.g., brisk walk and deep breathing

     (2) Stretch—maintains and increases flexibility, e.g., stretch slowly and hold position several seconds to point of tightness, not pain, do not bounce

     (3) Endurance—select a variety of activities to work different muscle groups; start slow and build up gradually

     (4) Cool down—allows body temperature and heart rate to decrease slowly, prevents pooling of blood in the extremities and decreases muscle soreness, e.g., walk, deep breathe and loosely shake extremities

   d. Exercise counseling

     (1) Exercises to avoid

       (a) Bouncing while stretching strains involved joints

       (b) Sit-ups with legs straight or double leg lifts strain the lower back

       (c) Duck walk—(walk with bent knees) stresses knee joint

       (d) Toe touching—stresses hamstrings

       (e) Leg splits and leg thrusts in kneeling position—stresses legs and groin area and also creates potential hip strain

     (2) Exercise self care

       (a) Appropriate clothing with layers in winter

       (b) Caps for cold weather and summer heat

       (c) Appropriate footwear, snug socks

(d) Avoid weather extremes

(e) Plenty of fluids before, during and after exercise

(f) Monitor pulse rate every 5 minutes, as soon as labored breathing begins. Take a six second pulse and multiply number by ten at any site except carotids to minimize disruption of exercise. Slow exercise rate if heart's target zone is exceeded

(3) Tolerance barometer refers to potentially dangerous physical symptoms or early signs of injury

(a) Breathlessness—inability to talk while exercising

(b) Excessive fatigue—fatigue for more that one hour after exercise

(c) Other symptoms, such as chest discomfort, dizziness, faintness, exertional dyspnea, nausea or vomiting, muscle or joint problems

(d) Stiffness in joint with slight loss of motion

(e) Swelling and localized pain

5. Exercise prescription components

a. Specify type, duration, intensity, and frequency

b. Progression of exercise

c. Individualized to client capabilities

d. Client motivation, goals, and interest

e. Based on available time, equipment, and facilities

f. Categories for exercise prescription

(1) Under 35 asymptomatic—gradual onset increasing in intensity and duration; if jogging is preferred, one should initially begin with brisk walk and gradually replace with jog

(2) Over 35 or symptomatic—start with complete history, physical examination and exercise stress test (bicycle ergometer or treadmill); with normal results, proceed with category (1) prescription, otherwise refer

(3) Contraindications—congestive heart failure, third degree heart block, recent pulmonary embolism, aortic embolism, active or recent myocarditis, congenital heart disease with

cyanosis, artificial pacemaker

(4) Precautions—positive personal or family history of heart disease, hyperlipidemia, hypertension, severe anemia, first degree heart block, diabetes, obesity, heart valve or large vessel disease, phlebothrombosis, current use of beta blockers, digitalis, or cigarettes. (American College of Sports Medicine, 1988)

- Safety and Environment
  1. General
     a. Fire safety—smoke alarms, fire extinguishers
     b. Home safety—secure locks on doors and windows
     c. Automobile—use of safety belts, harnesses, safe driving strategies
     d. Helmets—for bikes, motorcycles, roller blades
     e. Personal safety
     f. Violence—precautions appropriate for client and community
  2. Safety for aging adult
     a. Home safety
        (1) Adequate lighting especially around stairs
        (2) Assessment for objects that might create walking hazards (furniture placement, cords, loose rugs)
        (3) Nightlight or flashlight by bed to avoid falls or disorientation in the dark
     b. Personal safety
        (1) Avoid dangers of hypothermia with adequate heat; and adequate caloric intake
        (2) Set up daily communication system with others
     c. Physical deficits and related environmental hazards
        (1) Gait and balance problems
           (a) Slippery or irregular surfaces
           (b) Clutter or obstructions
           (c) Stairs, steep or without rails
           (d) Lack of space to maneuver assistive device, (e.g.,

walker)

        (e) Bathtub without rail or slip guards

    (2) Decreased vision

        (a) Inadequate lighting

        (b) Poorly marked stairs

    (3) Decreased sensitivity to pain/heat

        (a) Hot water bottle/heating pad

        (b) Hot bath water

    (4) Potential driving/traffic hazards

        (a) Decreased visual acuity and hearing

        (b) Decreased reaction time

        (c) Decreased mobility

3. Four categories of environmental hazards

    a. Biological—e.g., viruses, microorganisms

    b. Chemical—e.g., lead, asbestos

    c. Physical—e.g., natural disasters

    d. Sociological and psychological hazards, e.g., overcrowding, lack of resources

4. Components of an environmental assessment

    a. Home hazards—fire safety, pest control, inadequate heat or toileting facilities

    b. Work site hazards and protection—noise, inhalants, and lifting

    c. Neighborhood hazards—noise, air/water pollution, inadequate police protection, overcrowding or isolation from neighbors

    d. Community hazards—lack of availability of food stores, pharmacies, public transportation

5. Additional Research Findings (Pender, 1994)—Research over the past 20 years has identified factors associated with physical health and longer healthier life

    a. Exercise (regular)

    b. Non-smoker

    c. Seven to eight hours of sleep

   d. Moderate or no alcohol

   e. Regular and moderate eating (including breakfast)

   f. Weight control—life expectancy is reduced by one year for every 10 lb overweight

   g. Ample exercise, good nutrition and healthy lifestyle will slow aging process

Health Evaluation Across the Lifespan

- Health History—the health history is important in identifying risk behaviors and need for health education

  1. Demographics and biographical data

  2. History of present illness

    a. Symptom analysis (if appropriate)

      (1) Location and radiation

      (2) Quality or character description

      (3) Quantity, frequency, intensity, duration, effect on daily activities

      (4) Onset, course, length of time, pattern, gradual or abrupt onset

      (5) Aggravating and alleviating factors

      (6) Associated symptom/manifestations

    b. Reason for seeking health care

  3. Past medical history

    a. Childhood illnesses, child abuse

    b. Immunizations

    c. Adult illnesses

    d. Emotional health—past problems including support system, history of domestic violence

    e. Sexual health—obstetric and contraceptive history, number of partners, sexual problems

    f. Food or drug allergies—specify reaction and treatment, if any

    g. Current medication use—prescription and over the counter

    h. Past injuries, surgery—dates, treatment, and follow-up

      i.   Time period since last examinations/tests—physical, dental, vision, hearing, radiography, electrocardiogram (EKG) and cancer screenings

   4.   Personal habits

      a.   Tobacco use—cigarettes, pipe, cigars and smokeless; pack years (number of packs per day multiplied by number of years); if stopped, how long ago

      b.   Alcohol and drug use

      c.   Use of caffeine, coffee, colas, etc.

      d.   Exercise—type of exercise, frequency

      e.   Leisure/social activities

   5.   Dietary intake—including nutritional supplements and health food

   6.   Occupational history with possible exposure to environmental toxins

   7.   Family history—include age, health status or cause of death of parents, siblings, and children in a genogram; diabetes, heart disease, cancer, hypertension, lung disease, alcoholism, and any other illnesses that are hereditary

   8.   Review of systems—with symptom analysis as needed

■ Age Related Health Monitoring (if asymptomatic)

   1.   Adolescence—12 to 19 years of age

      a.   Complete physical examination every two years (American Academy of Pediatrics, 1994) including

        (1)   Height and weight

        (2)   Complete skin examination

        (3)   Assessment for gingivitis, caries, and malalignment

        (4)   Assessment for signs of abuse or neglect

        (5)   Hearing and vision—hearing may be assessed subjectively unless acuity problems are suspected

      b.   Blood pressure (BP)

      c.   Tuberculin skin test (PPD)—tested once during adolescence with annual tests for high-risk groups

      d.   Urinalysis, hemoglobin, hematocrit—tested once during

adolescence unless indicated otherwise

   e. Female

      (1) Breast examination

      (2) Teach self breast examination (SBE)

   f. Sexually active female

      (1) Papanicolaou (Pap) smear

      (2) Gonorrhea (GC) and chlamydia culture

      (3) RPR or VDRL (male and female)

   g. Male

      (1) Testicular examination

      (2) Teach self testicular examination (STE)

   h. If high risk, counseling and test for human immunodeficiency virus (HIV)

   i. Immunization—see immunization guidelines

      (1) Tetanus-diptheria booster (Td)

      (2) Measles-mumps-rubella (MMR)—if needed second MMR recommended at age 11 to 12

      (3) Hepatitis B—series of 3 recommended if resources permit if not previously immunized

   j. Dental/oral hygiene every 6 to 12 months

   k. Remain alert for depressive symptoms and any suicide risk factors

2. Young adult—20 to 39 years of age

   a. Complete physical examination—age 20, then every 5 to 6 years

   b. BP

   c. Total cholesterol with additional tests if cholesterol exceeds 200 mg/dl

   d. Female

      (1) SBE monthly

      (2) Pap and pelvic examination, GC and chlamydia

   e. Male—STE monthly

   f. PPD if exposed to tuberculosis

     g. Immunizations—Td every ten years

     h. Self skin examination

     i. Dental/oral hygiene every 6 to 12 months

3. Middle-aged adult—40 to 59 years of age

     a. Complete physical examination every 5 to 6 years

     b. BP, cholesterol, EKG

     c. Female—SBE monthly

     d. Mammogram every 2 years, 40 to 50, then yearly

     e. Male—STE monthly

     f. Sigmoidoscopy age 50, then every 3 to 5 years

     g. Stool guaiac age 50, then yearly

     h. Tonometry (glaucoma screen) annually

     i. Immunizations—tetanus every 10 years

     j. Dental/oral hygiene every 6 to 12 months

4. Elderly adult—60 + years of age

     a. Complete physical examination every 2 years

     b. BP, cholesterol

     c. Female—SBE monthly, annual mammogram

     d. Male—STE monthly

     e. Female—annual Pap and pelvic examination

     f. Sigmoidoscopy every 3 to 5 years

     g. Stool guaiac yearly

     h. Tonometry (glaucoma screen) annually

     i. Immunizations

         (1) Tetanus every 10 years

         (2) Pneumococcal and Influenza

     j. Dental/oral hygiene every 6 to 12 months

■ Wellness/risk factor identification

Adults 18 years and older
(National Heart, Lung and Blood Institute, 1993)

Blood Pressure	Systolic (mm Hg)	Diastolic (mm Hg)
Normal	under 130	under 85
High Normal	130 to 139	85 to 89
Hypertension		
Stage 1 (mild)	140 to 159	90 to 99
Stage 2 (moderate)	160 to 179	100 to 109
Stage 3 (severe)	180 to 209	110 to 119
Stage 4 (very severe)	210 and above	120 and above

Adolescents

Blood Pressure	Systolic (mm Hg)	Diastolic (mm Hg)
High Normal (90-94th percentile)		
13 to 15 years	130 to 135	80 to 85
16 to 18 years	136 to 141	84 to 91
Significant Hypertension (95-99th percentile)		
13 to 15 years	136 to 143	86 to 91
16 to 18 years	142 to 149	92 to 97
Severe Hypertension (> 99th percentile)		
13 to 15 years	144 or greater	92 or greater
16 to 18 years	150 or greater	98 or greater

Other Risk Factors

	High Risk	Moderate Risk	Low Risk
Body Fat Composition			
Men	over 27%	22-26%	below 22%
Women	over 33%	27-32%	below 26%
Weight	21+ lb overweight	5-21 lb over	within 5 lb
Exercise	sedentary		
Cholesterol	> 240 mg/dl	200-239 mg/dl	<200 mg/dl
LDL	> 160 mg/dl	130-159 mg/dl	< 130 mg/dl
HDL	< 35 mg/dl		≥ 60 mg/dl
(National Cholesterol Education Program, 1993)			
Tobacco Use	> 9 cigs/day	1-9 cigs/day	non-smoker

■ American Cancer Society Guidelines for Periodic Screening if individual is asymptomatic (Jan 1994)

Test or procedure	Gender	Age	Frequency
Sigmoidoscopy	M, F	over 50	Every 3-5 years
Stool guaiac	M, F	over 50	Every year
Digital rectal exam	M, F	over 40	Every year
Pap test/pelvic exam	F	age 18	Annually x 3, if normal decrease frequency*
	F	18-40	Every 1-3 years
	F	over 40	Every year
Endometrial tissue sample	F	at menopause	with hx of infertility, abnormal bleeding or estrogen therapy
Breast self exam	F	20 +	Every month
Breast physical exam	F	20-40	Every 3 years
	F	over 40	Every year
Mammography	F	40-49	Every 1-2 years
	F	50 +	Every year
Chest Xray	— — —	— — —	Not recommended
Sputum cytology	— — —	— — —	Not recommended
Health counseling and cancer check-up	M, F	over 20	Every 3 years
	M, F	over 40	Every year

*The American College of Obstetrics and Gynecology continues to recommend a yearly Pap test. (Hale, 1991)

■ Age related anticipatory guidance (U.S. Preventative Services Task Force, 1989)

1. Adolescence (12 to 19 years of age)—leading causes of death are motor vehicle accidents, homicide, suicide, injuries, heart disease

   a. Nutrition and healthy diet

   b. Physical activity-selection of exercise program

   c. Skin care/skin protection

   d. Dental care (brushing and flossing)

      (1) Fluoride supplementation

      (2) Dental visits

   e. Injury prevention

      (1)   Athletics

      (2)   Safety belts/safety helmets

      (3)   Firearm safety

      (4)   Safe driving strategies

      (5)   Violent behavior, awareness of violence in environment

  f. Substance use/abuse

      (1)   Tobacco cessation/primary prevention

      (2)   Alcohol and other drugs

  g. Sexual practices

      (1)   Sexual development and behavior

      (2)   Family planning, contraception

      (3)   Risk factors, sexually transmitted diseases

  h. Challenges for discussion

      (1)   Dating, marriage, sexual practices

      (2)   Education, career choice

      (3)   Confrontation with drugs, violent behavior

2.   Young adult (20 to 39 years of age)—leading causes of death are motor vehicle accidents, homicide, suicide, injuries, heart disease

  a. Nutrition and exercise

      (1)   Weight management with changing basal metabolic rate

      (2)   selection of exercise program

  b. Dental care

  c. Sex education

      (1)   Family planning, contraception

      (2)   Sexually transmitted diseases

  d. Cancer warning signs/skin protection

  e. Substance use/abuse

      (1)   Tobacco cessation/primary prevention

      (2)   Alcohol and other drugs

  f. Injury prevention

      (1)   Athletics

      (2)   Safety belts/safety helmets

      (3)   Firearm safety

      (4)   Defensive driving

      (5)   Violent behavior, awareness of violence in environment

  g. Lifestyle choices

      (1)   Family and parenting skills

      (2)   Stress management

      (3)   Safety and environmental health

3.   Middle aged adult (40 to 59 years of age)—leading causes of death are heart disease, lung cancer, cerebrovascular disease, breast cancer, colorectal cancer, obstructive lung disease

  a. Health education (same as age 20 to 39 plus)

      (1)   Menopause

      (2)   Sexual changes due to aging

  b. Midlife changes

      (1)   "Empty nest" syndrome

      (2)   Grandparenting

      (3)   Planning for retirement

4.   Elderly adult (age 60+ years of age)—leading causes of death are heart disease, cerebrovascular disease, obstructive lung disease, pneumonia and/or influenza, lung cancer, colorectal cancer

  a. Health education (same as 40-59 plus)

      (1)   Home safety

      (2)   Personal safety

  b. Life changes

      (1)   Retirement

      (2)   Loss of spouse, friends

      (3)   Changes in vision, hearing reaction time

      (4)   Alterations of bowel and bladder habits

- Immunization Guidelines

  1. Td—primary series is recommended if not complete during childhood with two doses at lease four weeks a part and a third dose six to twelve months after the second dose. The Td booster is recommended every ten years (CDC, 1991)

  2. MMR administered initially after the first birthday and a second dose for persons born after 1956 (CDC, 1993)

  3. Recommended schedule for individual with unknown or uncertain immunization history

     a. First visit—Td, MMR, PPD

     b. One month later—Td

     c. Six to 12 months later—Td

     d. Every 10 years—Td

  4. Influenza vaccine—recommended annually for any person over six months of age with underlying medical conditions which pose increased risk for complications; persons 65 years of age or older and persons with any chronic health condition are considered at increased risk

     a. Groups that can transmit influenza to high risk persons should be immunized, e.g., health care workers and household members

     b. Optimal time for immunization—mid October to mid November

     c. Contraindication—history of anaphylactic hypersensitivity to eggs or other components; refer to physician for appropriate therapy and possible allergy evaluation (CDC, 1992)

  5. Pneumococcal vaccine—recommended for any person over two years of age who is at increased risk of complications due to chronic illness; revaccination after six or more years is recommended for those at highest risk of antibody decline, e.g., renal disease, organ transplant (CDC, 1993)

  6. Hepatitis B vaccine consists of a three dose regimen recommended for all individuals who are or will be at increased risk of infection. A second dose is given one month after the first with a third dose six months later. Categories include health care workers, individuals at high risk of exposure to blood and blood products, and individuals at increased risk of exposure due to sexual practices. The timing and need for periodic boosters is determined by serologic testing. The

American Academy of Pediatrics (1994) recommends that the series be given to previously unimmunized adolescents when resources are available

7. Individuals with altered immunocompetence (such as HIV, leukemia, or chemotherapy) refer to immunization guidelines (CDC, 1993: MMWR April 1993)

■ Resources

American Association for Retired Persons
1909 K Street N.W. Fifth Floor
Washington, D. C. 20049
(202) 872-4700
Services for age 50 and older, includes lobby for senior citizens, mail-order pharmacy and bimonthly magazine

National Council on Aging 1-800-424-9046
Information/publications related to seniors (9am-5pm EST)

National Institute on Aging
Information Officer
Building 31, Room 5C-35, 900 Rockville Pike
Bethesda, MD 20205
Self-care and self-help groups for the elderly (Directory)

U.S. Consumer Product Safety Commission
Washington DC 20207 Hotline 1-800-2772
Provides information on consumer product safety. Pamphlet "Safety for older consumers: Home safety check list"

National Safety Council 1-800-621-7619 (Central)
Provides posters, brochures, videocassettes, and booklets on safety and accident prevention

American Dietetic Hotline 1-800-366-1655
Provides dietetic and nutrition information (9am-4pm)

National Clearinghouse for alcohol and drug information
Provides prevention and education publications, also provides literature searches
1-800-729-668

Aerobics and Fitness Foundation 1-800-233-4886
Answers questions on safe and effective exercise and certification of instructors

Check the telephone directory for local chapters of:

American Cancer Society
4 West 35th Street
New York, NY 10001 (212) 736-0303
Response Line 1-800-227-2345 Publications and information

American Heart Association
7320 Greenville Avenue
Dallas TX 75231 (214) 373-6300

American Lung Association
1740 Broadway, P.O. Box 596
New York, NY 10019 (212) 315-8700

Questions

Select the best answer

1. Health promotion activities are most consistent with which level of Maslow's hierarchy?

   a. Self actualization
   b. Love and belonging
   c. Communication needs
   d. Survival needs

2. Using the Health Belief Model (1990), determine which of the following individuals would be the most motivated for behavior change

   a. Forty two year old married female, excess weight for over 20 years
   b. Sixteen year old female with poorly controlled sugar levels and poor dietary habits consistent with her friends
   c. Fifty year old male with recent myocardial infarction, prognosis good with weight loss and exercise
   d. Forty year old who reports spouse wants him to lose weight

3. Which of the following activities would be most appropriate for the individual planning retirement to successfully complete the final 2 stages of Erikson's psychosocial development

   a. Plan to simultaneously complete any community obligations
   b. Get involved with enjoyable activities in the community
   c. Plan several extended trips early in retirement while still active and mobile
   d. Do not make any commitments initially, wait for opportunities to come along

4. Which of the family theories will most likely be congruent with the assessment of a family from another culture?

   a. Family development theory
   b. Institutional-historical
   c. Systems theory
   d. Structural-functional

5. Screening for breast cancer is which level of prevention

   a. Primary
   b. Secondary
   c. Tertiary
   d. Preliminary

6. Jim, age 32, is ready to start exercising and wants to jog. Guidelines should include which one of the following?

   a. A complete sports physical examination
   b. Jog at least once a week for 30 minutes to condition heart and lungs
   c. Begin with brisk walking and gradually replace with jogging
   d. Exercise stress test

7. Gloria, age 70, comes into your clinic the first week of November for health screening. Her last dT was ten years age. Which immunization will you recommend?

   a. dT, influenza, and pneumococcal
   b. dT and pneumococcal
   c. dT and influenza
   d. dT only

8. According to research, which type of social support has the strongest relationship with health status

   a. Emotional
   b. Instrumental
   c. Informational
   d. Appraisal

9. Which of the following conditions may be associated with rapid weight gain?

   a. Renal disease
   b. Diabetes mellitus
   c. Cerebrovascular disease
   d. Arthritis

10. According to research, how much sleep is associated with a longer healthier life?

    a. 5-6 hours
    b. 6-7 hours
    c. 7-8 hours
    d. 8-9 hours

11. Which test for physical fitness is delayed until the individual has been in training approximately six weeks to reduce injury risk?

    a. Trunk flexibility
    b. Muscle endurance
    c. Body composition
    d. Muscle strength

12. Body fat composition above what percentage puts a woman in the high risk

category?

    a. Over 20%
    b. Over 33%
    c. Over 38%
    d. Over 40%

13. What cholesterol level poses a moderate risk?

    a. 180-199 mg/dl
    b. 200-239 mg/dl
    c. over 300 mg/dl
    d. over 240 mg/dl

14 Meg, age 42, has just had a normal mammogram. She asks when she should get her next mammogram

    a. Every 1 to 2 years until 50, then annually
    b. Every other year from age 40 to 49, then every two years
    c. Every three years until age 50, then annually
    d. Every 5 years for the remainder of her life

15. Joe, age 15, has just moved to your community and is staying in a temporary foster home. He has no record of any immunizations. Which of the following does Joe need today?

    a. Tuberculin skin test
    b. Measles-Mumps-Rubella
    c. Td
    d. All of the above

16. Joe is given a temporary certificate for school attendance. When will he need to return for more immunizations?

    a. six months
    b. four to six weeks
    c. one year
    d. four months

17. Cardiac rehabilitation is which level of prevention?

    a. Primary
    b. Seconday
    c. Tertiary
    d. Restorative

18. What is the approximate target heart zone for an individual 40 years old?

    a. 100-150

b. 110-160
c. 120-170
d. 125-155

19. Jim asks why cooling down is necessary for an exercise plan?

 a. Allows body temperature and heart rate to decrease slowly
 b. Prevents pooling of blood in extremities
 c. Decreases muscle soreness
 d. All of the above

20. Jim asks about "no pain, no gain" in advancing his training program. Your best response(s) would be?

 a. Some pain is necessary for you to physically improve
 b. Pain is often an indicator of injury
 c. Young people are less likely to have pain with exercise
 d. Strenuous daily workouts will lead to improvement

21. Which stress management technique would be most appropriate for a newly diagnosed diabetic?

 a. Change avoidance
 b. Habituation
 c. Time blocking
 d. Imagery

22. Stress management is contraindicated for clients with which of the following conditions?

 a. Anxiety related to job placement change
 b. Depression
 c. Boredom
 d. Hyperventilation

Answer Key

1. a.	12. b.
2. c.	13. b.
3. b.	14. a.
4. b.	15. d.
5. b.	16. b.
6. c.	17. c.
7. c.	18. d.
8. a.	19. d.
9. a.	20. b.
10. c.	21. c.
11. d.	22. b.

Bibliography

American Academy of Pediatrics. (1994). *Report of the committee on infectious disease* (23rd ed.). Elk Grove Village, IL: American Academy of Pediatrics.

American Cancer Society (1994). *Summary of the American Cancer Society recommendations for the early detection of cancer in asymptomatic people.*

American College of Sports Medicine (1988). *Resource manual for guidelines for exercise testing and prescription.* Philadelphia: Lea and Febiger.

Bandura, A. (1977). *Social learning theory.* Englewood Cliffs, NJ: Prentice-Hall.

Bertalanffy, L. (1969). *General system theory.* NY: G. Braziller.

Bowers, A., & Thompson, J. (1992). *Clinical manual of health assessment.* St. Louis: Mosby Year Book.

Centers for Disease Control and Prevention (1993). *Standards for pediatric immunization practices. Morbidity and mortality weekly report.* 42 (RR-5)

Centers for Disease Control and Prevention (1993). *Emerging infectious diseases. Morbidity and Mortality Weekly Report.* 42(14)

Centers for Disease Control and Prevention (1992). *Prevention and control of influenza. Morbidity and Mortality Weekly Report.* 42, (RR-12)

Centers for Disease Control and Prevention (1991). Update on adult immunization. *Morbidity and Mortality Weekly Report.* 40 (RR-12)

Clark, M. (1992). *Nursing in the community.* Norwalk, CT: Appleton & Lange.

Creasia, J., & Parker, B. (1991). *Conceptual foundations of professional nursing practice.* St. Louis, MO: Mosby Year Book.

Dunn, H. (1971). *High level wellness.* Arlington, VA: Beatty.

Edlin, G., & Golanty, E. (1992). *Health and wellness* (4th ed.). Boston: Jones & Bartlett.

Erikson, E. (1963). *Childhood and society.* NY: Norton.

Friedman, M. (1992). *Family nursing: Theory and practice.* Norwalk, CT: Appleton & Lange.

Gilchrist, V. (1991). Preventive health care for the adolescent. *American Family Physician.* 43(3), 869-878.

Glanz, K., Lewis, F., & Rimer, B. (1990). *Health behavior and health education:*

Theory, research, and practice. San Francisco: Jossey-Bass.

Goldberger, L., & Breznitz, S. (1993). *Handbook of stress: Theoretical and clinical aspects*. NY: The Free Press.

Grubbs, L. (1993). The critical role of exercise in weight control. *Nurse Practitioner*. 18(4), 20-29.

Hales, D. (1991). *Your health*. NY: Benjamin/Cummings.

Haskell, W. L. (1992). Exercise and health. In J. W. Wyngaarder, L. H. Smith, & J. C. Bennett (eds). *Cecil textbook of medicine* (pp. 42-44). (19th ed.) Philadelphia: W. B. Saunders.

Lawson, D. (1992). *Safety & accident prevention*. Guilford, CT: Duchkin

Leininger, M. (1985). *Handbook of crosscultural counseling and therapy*. Westport, CT: Greenwood.

McGlynn, G. (1990). *Dynamics of fitness* (2nd ed.). Dubuque, IA: Brown.

National Cholesterol Education Program. (in press, 1994). *Second report of the expert panel on detection, evaluation, and treatment of high blood cholesterol in adults*. NIH 94, Washington, DC: U.S. Department of Health and Human Services.

National Heart, Lung, and Blood Institute. (1993). *The fifth report of the joint national committee on detection, evaluation, and treatment of high blood pressure*. U.S. Department of Health and Human Services, (NIH Publication No. 93-1088). January 1993. Bethesda, MD: National Institutes of Health.

Neuman, B. (1989). *The Neuman systems model* (2nd ed.). Norwalk, CT: Appleton & Lange.

Pender, N. (1994). *Health promotion in nursing practice (3rd ed.)*. Norwalk, CT: Appleton & Lange.

Public Health Service. (1990). *Healthy People 2000*. (DHHS Publication No. PHS 91-50212), Washington, DC: U.S. Government Printing Office.

Sharkey, B. (1990). *Physiology of fitness* (3rd ed.). Champaign, IL: Human Kinetics

U.S. Preventative Services Task Force (1989). Assessment of the effectiveness of 169 interventions: Report of the U.S. Preventative Services Task Force. Baltimore: Williams & Wilkins.

Dermatological Disorders

Elissa Davis

Acne

- Definition: A disorder of the sebaceous glands, characterized by comedones, papules, and pustules
- Etiology/Incidence
  1. Increased sebum retained in duct, obstructing it
  2. Contributing factors include
     a. Increased androgen production
     b. *Propionibacterium acnes*, a normal skin inhabitant, breaks down sebum, leading to an inflammatory reaction
     c. External sources of oils
        (1) Topical applications of oily products
        (2) Increased oil particles in the environment
     d. Medications, especially
        (1) Androgenic oral contraceptives
        (2) Steroids
        (3). Anticonvulsants
     e. Stress
     f. Food has not been shown to be a contributing factor
  3. Very common among teenagers
     a. Affects sexes equally
     b. Earlier onset in females
  4. Rarely persists into third or fourth decade
- Signs and Symptoms
  1. Usually only complaint is concern about appearance
     a. Rarely may report mild discomfort related to an isolated swollen lesion
     b. Non-pruritic
  2. May report increased symptoms before menses
- Differential Diagnosis
  1. Rosacea
  2. Pyogenic folliculitis

3. Hidradenitis suppurativa

- Physical Findings

    1. Distribution

        a. Face

        b. Shoulders

        c. Upper back

        d. Chest

    2. Lesions, mild acne

        a. Open comedones (blackheads)

        b. Closed comedones (whiteheads)

    3. Lesions, moderate to severe acne

        a. Inflammatory papules, red solid elevated areas

        b. Pustules, raised lesions containing purulent material

        c. Cysts, fluid-filled sacs

        d. Depressed or hypertrophic scars

- Diagnostic Tests/Findings: None indicated except rarely, culture to rule out causative organism

- Management/Treatment

    1. Mild acne needs only topical treatment

        a. Benzoyl peroxide, 2.5% or 5% to involved area

            (1) Apply at bedtime

            (2) If well tolerated, increase to 10%

        b. If not effective, prescribe retinoic acid, .025% or .05% cream to entire affected area

            (1) Apply to dry skin at bedtime

            (2) If too irritating, use every other night

            (3) May use stronger, but more irritating, gel

        c. In addition, may prescribe topical antibiotic

            (1) Cleocin-T lotion every morning

            (2) Tetracycline 2.2% solution

2. Lesions on chest or back, or severe acne requires systemic antibiotic therapy, such as one of the following

    a. Tetracycline 250 mg. q.i.d. before meals

    b. Erythromycin 250 mg. q.i.d. after meals

3. Severe acne requires systemic isotretinoin

    a. Prescribe in consultation with a dermatologist

    b. Do not use if pregnancy is a possibility

4. Patient education

    a. Dietary modification is unnecessary

    b. Avoid squeezing or picking lesions

    c. Wash gently twice a day with a mild non-oily soap

    d. Response to therapy takes at least a month and must be continued for effective treatment

5. Follow-up monthly

Bacterial Skin Infections

- Definition: Infection of skin, usually due to streptococcus or staphylococcus

1. Furuncle (boil)

    a. Deep abscess

    b. Very tender

2. Cellulitis-diffuse spreading infection

3. Folliculitis

    a. Pustules or inflamed nodules

    b. Within hair follicles

4. Carbuncle

    a. Large coalescence of deep boils

    b. Usually has several drainage points

5. Hidradenitis suppurativa

    a. Painful abscess of sweat glands

    b. Occurs in young adults

        (1) Axillae in women

      (2)   Anogenital glands in men

  6. Impetigo

     a. Honey colored crusts

     b. Highly contagious

  7. Paronychia—Infection at margin of nail

- Etiology/Incidence

  1. Caused by skin bacteria, especially

     a. *Staphylococcus aureus*

     b. Group A ßeta hemolytic streptococcus

  2. Incidence increased by

     a. Break in skin integrity

     b. Close contact with infected persons

        (1)   Contact may be asymptomatic carrier

        (2)   Impetigo is especially contagious

     c. Sharing of personal items, especially razors

     d. Recent upper respiratory infection

     e. Poor hygiene

     f. Immunocompromised individuals, especially diabetics

- Signs and Symptoms

  1. Mild infections and most cases of impetigo have only local symptoms

     a. Pain

     b. Swelling

     c. Warmth

     d. Redness

  2. Occasional regional lymphadenopathy

  3. Severe infection may have systemic symptoms

     a. Fever

     b. Chills

     c. Malaise

- Differential Diagnosis
  1. Contact dermatitis
  2. Allergic dermatitis
  3. Foreign body with inflammation
  4. Fungal dermatitis
  5. Herpes simplex
  6. Herpes zoster
  7. Varicella
- Physical Findings
  1. If severe, infection may present with
     a. Fever
     b. Regional lymphadenopathy
  2. Findings which typify specific infections
     a. Carbuncle
        (1) Swollen painful area due to inflammation of deeper layers of skin
        (2) Several openings in taut reddened skin
        (3) Purulent drainage
     b. Cellulitis
        (1) Edema with taut shiny skin
        (2) Erythema which may be spreading
        (3) Warmth
        (4) May have no discrete lesion or opening
     c. Folliculitis
        (1) One or more small superficial lesions
            (a) Pustules
            (b) Nodules
            (c) May be crusted
        (2) Erythema
     d. Furuncle

      (1)   One or two tender nodules

      (2)   Very tender

      (3)   May be punctate, i.e., have pinpoint punctures

      (4)   Located in hair follicles

  e. Hidradenitis suppurativa

      (1)   May be single large lesion

          (a) Cyst

          (b) Nodule

      (2)   May have multiple lesions

          (a) Papules

          (b) Pustules

      (3)   Located in sweat glands

          (a) Axillae, especially in women

          (b) Groin

  f. Impetigo

      (1)   Starts as thin-walled vesicle

          (a) Vesicle ruptures

          (b) Extending denuded area

      (2)   Exudate forms yellow crusts

      (3)   Crusted lesions may heal centrally, leaving crusted ring

  g. Paronychia

      (1)   Swollen red infected area

      (2)   May have purulent discharge

      (3)   Involves tissue surrounding the fingernail

■ Diagnostic Tests/Findings

  1. Usually not necessary

  2. Culture and sensitivity of discharge will identify causative organism and most appropriate antibiotic

  3. Microscopic examination of scraping with KOH would be negative

  4. No fluorescence with Wood's light

- Management/Treatment
    1. Minor superficial lesions
        a. Warm soaks 20 minutes q.i.d. to increase circulation
        b. Topical antimicrobial
            (1) Mucopirocin (Bactroban) t.i.d.
            (2) Bacitracin
    2. More severe infections
        a. Systemic antibiotics
            (1) Dicloxacillin 125-500 mg q.i.d. for 7-10 days
            (2) Cephalexin (Keflex) 500 mg b.i.d. for 10 days
        b. For impetigo, soak crusts t.i.d. with Burow's solution to soften, in addition to antibiotic therapy
        c. Deep abscesses require incision and drainage as well as antibiotic therapy
        d. Severe cellulitis requires IV antibiotic therapy
    3. Wash area well with soap and water
    4. If frequent recurrences
        a. Wash with phisohex or hibiclens to decrease skin flora
        b. Consider treatment of close contact who may be carrier
        c. Bacitracin to nares to eradicate streptococcus
        d. Systemic antibiotics
        e. Order appropriate laboratory tests to rule out causes of immunocompromise
            (1) Diabetes
            (2) AIDS
    5. Folliculitis may be due to shaving too closely, causing an ingrown hair—instruct patient regarding prevention
    6. Advise patient to avoid sharing personal items such as razors
    7. Follow-up in three days unless minor superficial lesion

Cancer of the Skin

- Definition: Malignancy of the epidermis or dermis
- Etiology/Incidence
  1. Most common malignancy
  2. Increased incidence
     a. Fair-skinned people
     b. Sun damaged skin, especially with history of severe sunburn during childhood or adolescence
     c. Exposure to carcinogens
        (1) Photosensitizing pitch, tar, and oils
        (2) Ultraviolet radiation
        (3) Arsenic, formerly used in "tonics"
     d. Scars due to radiation, vaccination, or trauma
  3. Some families have predisposition to skin cancer
- Signs and Symptoms
  1. A painless sore that does not heal
  2. A change in a wart or mole
     a. Enlarging
     b. Darkening
  3. Non-pruritic
- Differential Diagnosis
  1. Melanocytic nevus
  2. Giant molluscum contagiosum
  3. Seborrheic keratosis
- Physical Findings
  1. Basal cell carcinoma
     a. Location
        (1) Most common on face or ear
        (2) Also found on head, neck, or trunk

  b. Pearly dome shaped

  c. Irregular shape

  d. Telangiectatic vessels

  e. Center may ulcerate and crust

2. Squamous cell carcinoma

  a. Location

   (1) Common lower lip and mouth

   (2) Also found

    (a) Scalp and face

    (b) Pinna of ear

  b. Soft and freely moveable tumor on a red base

3. Kaposi's sarcoma

  a. Macular, gradually becomes raised

  b. Purple

4. Malignant melanoma, characterized by A,B,C,D,E

  a. Asymmetry

  b. Border irregular

  c. Color variability

  d. Diameter generally greater than 5 mm

  e. Elevation irregular

  f. Most common locations

   (1) Back of male

   (2) Leg of female

  g. Also found on palms, soles, face, and arms

■ Diagnostic Tests/Findings: Biopsy is imperative

■ Management/Treatment: Refer to dermatologist

1. Teach all patients to avoid sun exposure especially during the hours of 10 a.m. to 3 p.m.

  a. Use sunscreen with a sun protective factor (SPF) of at least 15

  b. Wear protective clothing

    c. Educate about risks of tanning salons

  2. Monitor nevi for changes

    a. Examine entire skin surface, using mirror or helper

    b. Measure and photograph nevi for future comparison

    c. Any change in nevus or sore that doesn't heal needs evaluation

Contact Dermatitis

- Definition: An acute pruritic rash confined to areas where an irritating or allergenic substance has come in contact with the skin

- Etiology/Incidence

  1. Contact with an irritating substance

    a. Plants, e.g., poison ivy or oak

    b. Household chemical, soap, or detergent

    c. Occupational chemicals

    d. Excreta or urine in incontinent patients

  2. Contact with allergenic substance such as

    a. Cosmetics, perfumes, and hair sprays

    b. Chemicals in certain leather

    c. Pets

    d. Nickel in jewelry or belt buckle

- Signs and Symptoms

  1. Symptoms occur after exposure to substance and often subside within hours or days after initial contact

  2. Rash is pruritic and occasionally causes burning sensation

- Differential Diagnosis

  1. Eczema

  2. Psoriasis

  3. Fungal infections

  4. Scabies

  5. Pediculosis

  6. Pityriasis rosea

7. Secondary syphilis

8. Drug reactions

9. Viral infections

■ Physical Findings

1. Maculopapular rash in a distribution which may suggest the precipitating substance

2. No lymphadenopathy

3. Normal oropharynx

4. Normal vital signs

■ Diagnostic Tests/Findings

1. Usually not necessary, unless to rule out other diagnosis

2. KOH preparation of skin scraping is negative

3. Culture of lesion is negative

4. VDRL to rule out syphilis if history and distribution of rash suggestive of syphilis

■ Management/Treatment

1. Soak affected area in saline or Burow's solution or use cool compresses for 20 minutes q.i.d.

2. Colloidal oatmeal baths are soothing

3. Topical steroids sparingly to affected area b.i.d.

   a. Non-fluorinated (mild) steroid, such as 1% hydrocortisone to face

   b. More potent steroid, such as valisone .5% cream to other areas

4. If pruritus is severe or disturbs sleep, may prescribe an antihistamine, such as hydroxyzine 25 mg t.i.d., advising patient regarding drowsiness

5. For very severe cases, consult with physician concerning tapering course of prednisone

6. Patient education

   a. Avoid precipitating substance

   b. Keep nails short and try to avoid scratching

7. Follow-up

a. Severe cases one week

b. Failure to improve in one week would require a consultation or referral

c. Signs of infection

Eczema

- Definition: Chronic pruritic dermatitis, characterized by hyperkeratosis and lichenification.

- Etiology/Incidence

  1. Most common in infancy, but milder adult form occurs, especially at times of stress

  2. Contributing factors include

     a. Familial tendency toward allergic diseases

     b. Hypersensitivity to certain proteins

     c. Skin sensitivity to heat, cold, or emotional stress

- Signs and Symptoms

  1. Pruritus

  2. Leathery dryness, especially on limb flexures

- Differential Diagnosis

  1. Contact dermatitis

  2. Drug reaction

  3. Fungal dermatitis

  4. Scabies

  5. Impetigo

- Physical Findings

  1. Patches with varying degrees of erythema and indistinct borders. May also include

     a. Papules

     b. Vesicles

     c. Fine scaling

     d. Lichenification

2. Distribution of lesions

    a. Flexures of limbs

    b. Dorsum of feet

    c. Forearms

    d. Anus

    e. Scalp

3. No lymphadenopathy

4. Normal vital signs

■ Diagnostic Tests/Findings: Usually not necessary unless to rule out other etiology

1. Culture to rule out infection is negative

2. Microscopic examination of skin scraping with KOH is negative for hyphae

3. Skin testing for specific allergens

4. Skin scraping negative for burrows of scabies is indicated only if sudden onset, close contacts are affected, or itching increases at night

■ Management/Treatment

1. Bland emollients to the skin or in bath water

2. Occlusive dressing with 1% icthammol paste

3. Topical steroids applied sparingly b.i.d.

    a. Mild non-fluorinated cream, e.g., 1% hydrocortisone for facial lesions

    b. Moderate potency steroid such as valisone to inner thighs or to wrists

    c. Potent steroid such as lidex or aclovate if no response to milder steroid

    d. Oral antihistamine such as hydroxyzine

4. Patient education

    a. Stress management exercises

    b. Avoidance of allergens, especially wool

    c. Use of light clothing

      d. Keep skin lubricated

  5. Follow-up long term to assess response to treatment and signs of infection

Herpes Zoster ("Shingles")

- Definition: Vesicular dermatomal eruption due to a reactivation of latent varicella virus in the dorsal sensory ganglia of a partially immune host.

- Etiology/Incidence

  1. Cause is varicella zoster virus

  2. Increases in immunocompromised individuals

  3. Increases with advanced age

  4. Affects 10-20% of U.S. adult population at some time

- Signs and Symptoms

  1. Prodrome lasts 1 to 4 days

      a. Burning pain and paresthesia along 1 or 2 dermatomes which do not cross the midline

      b. Fever

      c. Malaise

      d. Headache

  2. Vesicular stage lasts 2 to 3 weeks

      a. Very painful vesicles grouped along 1 or 2 dermatomes

         (1) Initially clear or blood filled

         (2) Become purulent

      b. Area along dermatome is erythematous

      c. Vesicles crust, then scab

      d. Scabs separate, may leave hypopigmented scars

  3. Post herpetic pain may persist months after lesions resolve

- Differential Diagnosis

  1. Prodromal period resembles visceral pain

      a. Migraine

      b. Pleurisy

      c. Ulcer

      d. Kidney stone

  2. Vesicular period-herpes simplex

- Physical Findings

  1. None during prodromal period

  2. Unilateral distribution along 1 to 2 dermatomes

      a. Red swollen plaques of various sizes

      b. Clusters of cloudy vesicles of various sizes

      c. Vesicles appear in successive crops

      d. Vesicles may umbilicate or rupture before crusting

  3. May have 20 or more vesicles scattered outside the affected dermatome

  4. Lymphadenopathy

- Diagnostic Tests/Findings

  1. Not generally needed to make diagnosis

  2. Tzanck smear is positive, but not specific for herpes zoster, also positive in herpes simplex

- Management/Treatment

  1. Condition is self-limited and will resolve without treatment

  2. Symptomatic treatment

      a. Analgesics

         (1) Acetaminophen with codeine

         (2) Percodan or percocet

      b. Burow's solution 1:40 to area q.i.d. for 15 minutes

  3. Antimicrobials to prevent secondary infection

         (1) Polysporin q.i.d.

         (2) Silvadene q.i.d.

  4. Antiviral therapy with Acyclovir 800 mg 5 times per day for seven days may speed healing if started within 2 to 3 days of onset, especially in immunocompromised individuals.

  5. Corticosteroid therapy decreases incidence of post-herpetic neuralgia,

especially in the elderly

    a. May increase incidence of disseminated infection

    b. Prednisone 60 mg daily, taper dose over 2 to 3 weeks

6. Patient education

    a. Varicella is contagious—isolate from contact with susceptible persons, especially if immunocompromised

    b. Herpes zoster may recur

7. Refer to ophthalmologist if lesions involve eye or tip of nose

8. Follow-up weekly, more frequently if

    a. Immunocompromised

    b. Eye or sacral involvement

Tinea

- Definition: A fungal infection of the dead keratin layers of the epidermis characterized by itching
- Etiology/Incidence

1. Common infection caused by dermatophyte

2. Species varies with location

    a. Tinea capitis on scalp

    b. Tinea corporis on trunk, limbs, or face

    c. Tinea cruris on groin

    d. Tinea pedis on feet

3. Increased incidence related to contact with warm moist surfaces

    a. Locker room floors

    b. Athletic equipment

    c. Towels

    d. Swimming pools

4. Occlusive footwear increases tinea pedis

5. Contagious if contaminated articles are shared

- Signs and Symptoms

1. Pruritis

2. Inflammation and tenderness

3. Lesions may have been present for an extended period of time

■ Differential Diagnosis

1. Intertrigo

2. Candida

3. Pityriasis rosea

4. Eczema

■ Physical Findings

1. Erythematous plaques

2. Active border

a. Scaly

b. Raised

c. May be scalloped or irregular

3. Scalp

a. Patchy hair loss

b. Scaly inflammation

4. Body and face

a. Annular lesions

b. Raised border

5. Groin

a. Bilateral half moon lesions on medial aspects of thighs

b. May involve scrotum in males

6. Feet

a. Toe webs either

(1) Dry, scaly, and fissured or

(2) White and macerated

b. Soles

(1) Vesicular

(2) Inflamed

- Diagnostic Tests/Findings

  1. Tinea capitis may show pale green fluorescence if examined with Wood's light

  2. Microscopic exam of skin scraping with KOH shows hyphae ("spaghetti and meatballs")

- Management/Treatment

  1. Topical antifungal cream sparingly b.i.d. until resolved

     a. Clotrimazole (Lotrimin)

     b. Ketoconazole (Nizoral)

     c. Miconazole (Micatin, Monistat-Derm)

  2. If inflamed

     a. Use Lotrisone b.i.d.

     b. Do not use with signs of bacterial coinfection

  3. If scalp or nails are involved, consult regarding use of oral griseofulvin for at least six weeks

  4. Patient education

     a. Keep area clean and dry

     b. Avoid sharing personal care items

     c. Carefully launder all clothing and linen

     d. Continue treatment for several weeks until resolved

     e. For tinea pedis, socks should be put on before underwear to avoid possibility of transferring organism to groin

  5. Follow-up if erythema, swelling, discharge

Tinea Versicolor

- Definition: Common superficial benign fungus infection characterized by changes in skin pigmentation

- Etiology/Incidence

  1. Caused by *Pityrosporon orbiculare*

  2. Increased incidence related to

     a. Warm humid environment

     b. Steroid therapy

    c. Poor hygiene

- Signs and Symptoms
    1. Rarely, mild pruritus
    2. Scaling oval patches
    3. Color of lesions may be red, brown, or white
    4. Rash may involve neck, trunk, upper arms
- Differential Diagnosis
    1. Seborrheic dermatitis
    2. Vitiligo
    3. Pityriasis
- Physical Findings
    1. Hypo- or hyperpigmented discrete macules
    2. Color varies from white to tan or brown
    3. Light scratching produces fine scales
- Diagnostic Tests/Findings
    1. Microscopic exam of skin scraping with KOH reveals black clusters of spores and hyphae ("spaghetti and meatballs")
    2. Wood's light may show yellow orange fluorescence
- Management/Treatment
    1. Selenium sulfide shampoo (Selsun) to skin after shower, avoiding broken skin
        a. Allow to dry
        b. Leave on overnight
        c. Vigorously scrub off in a.m.
        d. Repeat in one week, then every three months
    2. Topical antifungals, e.g., clotrimazole, may be used but are more expensive and no more effective than selenium sulfide shampoo
    3. Skin should be kept clean and dry
    4. Advise patients that resolution takes 3 to 6 months, but may be hastened by careful sun exposure, avoiding sun burn

Lyme disease

- Definition: Acute or chronic infection carried by ticks

    1. Characterized by

        a. Erythema migrans skin lesion (80% of cases)

        b. Flu-like illness

    2. May progress to late stage, which may feature

        a. Arthritis

        b. Neurological symptoms

        c. Cardiac symptoms

- Etiology/Incidence

    1. Caused by spirochete, *Borrelia burgdorferi*

    2. Transmitted by deer tick, *Ixodes dammini*

    3. Increased incidence in coastal states and northern Midwestern states

    4. Incidence increased by

        a. Outdoor activities such as hiking, golf, gardening

        b. Exposure to pets which may harbor deer ticks

- Signs and Symptoms

    1. Erythema migrans lesion at site of tick bite

        a. 50% of patients recall tick bite 4 to 20 days earlier

        b. Large annular macule with central pallor

        c. Non-pruritic

    2. Flu-like symptoms

        a. Fever and chills

        b. Malaise

        c. Headache, stiff neck, and backache

    3. Symptoms resolve in 3 to 4 weeks

    4. If untreated, secondary symptoms may appear

        a. Arthritis of one or more large joints

        b. Cardiac palpitations

        c. Neurological

            (1)   Bell's palsy

       (2)   Headache

       (3)   Photophobia

- Differential Diagnosis
  1. Tinea corporis
  2. Insect bite
  3. Cellulitis
  4. Arthritis
  5. Cardiac disease
  6. Neurologic disease

- Physical Findings
  1. One to three weeks after tick bite
     a. Target-like lesion at site of bite
        (1) Macule with central pallor
        (2) May be up to 10 centimeters
     b. May have multiple annular lesions at other sites
     c. Occasional regional or general lymphadenopathy
  2. Three to twenty-four weeks after tick bite
     a. Joint pain and swelling
        (1) Affects 60% of untreated cases
        (2) One or more large joints, especially knees
     b. Cardiac arrhythmia and tachycardia
     c. Neurological signs
        (1) Bell's palsy
        (2) Nuchal rigidity

- Diagnostic Tests/Findings
  1. Lyme titer
     a. Becomes positive twenty days after onset of symptoms
     b. High incidence of false negatives, especially if treatment is started early
  2. Elevated erythrocyte sedimentation rate

■ Management/Treatment

1. Amoxicillin 500 mg t.i.d. plus probenecid 500 mg t.i.d. for 21 days

2. Tetracycline 500 mg q.i.d. for 21 days

3. Doxycycline 100 mg b.i.d. for 21 days

4. Secondary disease requires IV ceftriaxone for 14 days

5. Prevention of tick bites

  a. Avoid contact with foliage

  b. Dress for outdoor activities

   (1) Wear light colors to make ticks visible

   (2) Wear long sleeves and long pants tucked into socks

  c. Use tick repellent containing DEET

  d. Check skin and clothing carefully for ticks after being outdoors

6. Remove ticks from skin promptly

  a. Grasp firmly with tweezers close to skin

  b. Pull tick straight out

  c. Avoid crushing embedded tick, which releases spirochetes

7. Brush ticks off pets promptly

8. Asymptomatic tick bites do not require treatment

  a. Not all deer ticks are infected with Lyme disease

  b. Ticks must remain on skin for hours to transmit Lyme disease

9. Follow-up

  a. Repeat Lyme titer 1 to 2 months after treatment to determine possible need for continued therapy

  b. Report any arthritic, cardiac, or neurological symptoms

Pityriasis Rosea

■ Definition: A common acute or subacute, self-limited, exanthematous disease

■ Etiology/Incidence

1. Unknown etiology

2. Common in young adults

3. Greatest incidence during winter months

- Signs and Symptoms

    1. Herald patch

        a. Single large bright red macule can occur anywhere but often appears on the neck or lower trunk

        b. Precedes the general rash by several days to a week

        c. Commonly misdiagnosed as "ringworm"

    2. May be mildly pruritic

- Differential Diagnosis

    1. Drug reaction

    2. Secondary syphilis

    3. Psoriasis

    4. Erythema chronicum

- Physical Findings

    1. Lesions

        a. Oval or round tannish pink or salmon colored scaling papules and plaques

        b. Discrete oval patches have an unusual fine white scale located near the border, forming a "collarette"

    2. Distribution

        a. Follows skin cleavage lines in Christmas tree pattern

        b. Neck, trunk, and upper arms and legs

- Diagnostic Tests/Findings

    1. VDRL to rule out syphilis

    2. Lyme titer if rash looks like erythema migrans

    3. Biopsy only if symptoms persist more than six weeks

- Management/Treatment

    1. Treatment is usually not necessary

    2. Ultraviolet (UVB) light therapy given as three to five treatments eliciting a mild erythematous reaction which often clears the rash

    3. Assure patient that condition is benign

4. Inform patient that rash will subside in 6 to 12 weeks without treatment

Psoriasis

- **Definition**
    1. Genetically determined, chronic, epidermal, proliferative disease of unpredictable course
    2. Characterized by
        a. Raised erythematous plaques
        b. Dull silvery scales
    3. Chronic condition with
        a. Exacerbations
        b. Remissions
- **Etiology/Incidence**
    1. Etiology not fully understood
        a. Genetic predisposition in some families
            (1) Polygenic or autosomal dominant
            (2) Incomplete penetrance, i.e., condition does not always appear even if the gene has been transmitted
        b. Altered epidermal metabolism
            (1) Increased epidermal proliferation
                (a) Increased number of cells in cell cycle
                (b) Rapid cell turnover
            (2) Altered cell membrane metabolism
        c. Epidermal inflammation
            (1) Increased neutrophils
            (2) Erythema
            (3) Edema
        d. Abnormal dermis with tortuous capillary loops
    2. Precipitating factors
        a. Trauma, especially scratches and surgical wounds
        b. Infection, especially streptococcal tonsillitis

     c. Sunlight in 10% of patients

     d. Medications

        (1)   Antimalarials

        (2)   Beta blockers

        (3)   Lithium

        (4)   May rebound following completion of steroid therapy

     e. Emotional stress

3. Increased prevalence

     a. Northern climates, especially during winter

     b. Caucasians

4. Incidence

     a. Affects 1 to 3% of population

     b. Affects males and females equally

     c. Age range

        (1)   Onset at any age, but rare before 10

        (2)   Peak incidence ages 15 to 40 years

■ Signs and Symptoms

1. Major complaint is cosmetic appearance

2. May have no complaint

3. May be slightly pruritic

4. Gradual onset

5. Lesions

     a. Most patients have plaques on skin

     b. A few patients have no dermal lesions but have

        (1)   Pitted fingernails with onycholysis

        (2)   Polyarthritis (5% incidence)

■ Differential Diagnosis

1. Cutaneous T cell lymphoma

2. Discoid eczema

3. Lyme disease

4. Pityriasis rosea

5. Seborrheic eczema

6. Secondary syphilis

7. Tinea corporis

■ Physical Findings

1. Sharply demarcated erythematous papules or plaques with overlapping silvery scales.

2. Lesions sometimes extend and coalesce and produce large plaques

3. Lesions are usually distributed over areas of bony prominence such as elbows and knees; also commonly occur on trunk, scalp and intergluteal cleft; palms and soles may be involved

4. Scalp may be affected

   a. Areas of scaling interspersed with normal skin

   b. Scalp feels lumpy and firm

5. Nails may be affected

   a. Pitted surface, like a thimble

   b. Onycholysis (separation of nail from nail bed)

6. Flexures may be affected

   a. Distribution

      (1) Submammary

      (2) Axillary

      (3) Anogenital folds

   b. Glistening red plaques

      (1) Not scaly

      (2) Fissures in depths of folds

■ Diagnostic Tests/Findings

1. Biopsy rarely indicated

2. Microscopic exam of skin to rule out tinea; would show hyphae in tinea, but not in psoriasis

3. Throat culture for streptococcus only if lesions are small round red macules, which gradually become scaly

4. VDRL to rule out secondary syphilis

5. If patient has arthropathies, rule out other causes of arthritis

    a. Rheumatoid factor

    b. Antinuclear antibody

    c. Lyme titer

    d. X-rays

■ Management/Treatment

1. Coal tar to inhibit DNA synthesis

    a. Estar gel to plaques

    b. Bath additives

        (1) Polytar

        (2) Balnatar

2. Dithranol, an irritant which also inhibits DNA synthesis, possibly by forming oxygen free radicals

    a. Start with a weak (0.1%) cream

        (1) Increase strength at weekly intervals

        (2) Greater than 1% is rarely indicated

    b. Protect surrounding skin with zinc oxide

    c. If left on longer than 30 minutes, cover with gauze

    d. Apply five days per week

    e. Avoid use on face, inner thighs, genitalia

    f. Will cause purple-brown stain

        (1) Stain on skin will peel off in a few days

        (2) Stains on clothing and bathtub are permanent

3. Topical steroids

    a. Use only where coal tar or dithranol are contraindicated or if no response to treatment

    b. For face, use mild preparation such as hydrocortisone 0.5% or 1%

    c. For other areas use a moderate potency cream

        (1) Kenalog

          (2)   Valisone

      d. May cause rebound exacerbation when discontinued

  4. Ultraviolet light therapy

      a. Natural sunlight

      b. Artificial ultraviolet in slowly increasing increments to produce mild erythema

          (1)   Use twice a week for eight weeks

          (2)   Protect eyes with goggles

  5. Refer refractory cases for systemic therapy

      a. Retinoids, such as isotretinoin

      b. Antimetabolites

      c. Psoralens, used with high-intensity ultraviolet A (PUVA)

  6. Provide emotional support

  7. Patient education

      a. Adequate rest will help to control symptoms

      b. Stress management

      c. Counselling regarding chronicity

      d. Reassurance patient that condition is not contagious

Seborrheic Dermatitis

- Definition

  1. Chronic dermatosis characterized by

      a. Redness

      b. Scaling

  2. Occurs in areas of high concentrations of sebaceous glands

      a. Face

      b. Scalp

      c. Body folds

      d. Genitalia

- Etiology/Incidence

   1. Very common
   2. Increased incidence
      a. Males
      b. Persons with genetic predisposition
      c. Immunocompromised individuals, especially HIV positive
      d. In those individuals who perspire profusely
      e. Individuals with Parkinson's disease
      f. Individuals with zinc deficiency

■ Signs and Symptoms
   1. Gradual onset
   2. Pruritus variable, increased during winter

■ Differential Diagnosis
   1. Psoriasis
   2. Tinea
   3. Candidiasis
   4. Lupus

■ Physical Findings
   1. Lesions
      a. Scattered and discrete
      b. Appearance either
         (1) Yellowish-red and greasy or
         (2) Dry white scaly macules
   2. Sharply defined borders
   3. Distribution
      a. Hairy areas of head
         (1) Scalp
         (2) Eyebrows and lashes
         (3) Beard
      b. Face
         (1) Butterfly pattern (malar flush)

(2) Behind ears

(3) Forehead

(4) Nasolabial fold

  c. Presternal areas

  d. Body folds

  e. Genitalia

- Diagnostic Tests/Findings

1. Microscopic examination of skin scraping with KOH will be negative

2. Lupus erythematosus (LE) prep will be negative (only needed with malar rash)

3. Biopsy is rarely needed when diagnosis is unclear

- Management/Treatment

1. Scalp or other hirsute areas

  a. Selenium sulfide shampoo

  b. Zinc pyrithione shampoo

2. Other areas

  a. May apply foam from selenium sulfide shampoo for mild cases

  b. Short course of low potency steroid, such as 1% hydrocortisone

  c. Ketoconazole cream

  d. 2% salicylic acid cream

3. Advise that treatment may be prolonged

4. Inform patient that recurrences are common

Seborrheic Keratosis

- Definition: Benign neoplasms of epidermal cells of face and trunk, also called
  1. Basal cell papilloma
  2. Seborrheic wart
  3. Senile wart, a term which could be offensive to patient
- Etiology/Incidence
  1. Cause is unknown but may
     a. Be inherited as an autosomal dominant trait
     b. Follow an inflammatory dermatitis
  2. Common after age 50, but small ones may be visible earlier
  3. Affects men and women equally
- Signs and Symptoms
  1. Usually multiple lesions
  2. Patient reports lesions are multiplying with age
  3. Patient may be concerned because lesions are
     a. Ugly
     b. Easily traumatized
- Differential Diagnosis
  1. Pigmented nevus
  2. Basal cell carcinoma
  3. Malignant melanoma
- Physical Findings
  1. Lesions are most common on the face or trunk
  2. Have characteristic "stuck on" appearance
  3. Shape may be
     a. Flat
     b. Raised
     c. Pedunculated

4. Color ranges from yellow to almost black

5. Surface may be greasy and scaly, described as like a "currant bun"

- Diagnostic Tests/Findings

    1. Usually diagnosed by clinical appearance

    2. Biopsy is rarely needed to confirm diagnosis

- Management/Treatment

    1. No treatment is required, unless patient is concerned about cosmetic effect or lesion is easily traumatized due to its location

    2. Curettage

    3. Liquid nitrogen cryotherapy

    4. Reassure patient that lesion is not malignant

    5. Lesion may be photographed for future comparison so that rapidly expanding lesions may be biopsied

    6. Instruct patient to return to clinic if lesion changes or grows

Warts (*Verrucae*)

- Definition: Benign, common contagious epithelial tumors

    1. Common wart

        a. Starts as a smooth flesh colored papule; can be light gray, yellow, brown, or grayish-black

        b. Enlarges to develop irregular surface with "warty" appearance

        c. More common on hands, but also found on face or genitals

    2. Plantar warts

        a. Painful papules on the soles of the feet

        b. Covered by a thick callus with black puncta within the lesion

    3. Flat warts (also called plane warts)

        a. Flat-topped painless papules

        b. Most common on face, brow, and dorsum of hands

    4. Facial warts

        a. Cauliflower or fingerlike projections

        b. Found in beard area of men and probably related to shaving

    5. Genital warts (condylomata acuminata) are discussed with sexually transmitted diseases

- Etiology/Incidence
  1. Caused by various strains of human papillomavirus (HPV)
  2. Only genital warts are considered to be contagious
  3. Other kinds of warts are common in children and young adults
  4. Increased incidence
     a. After trauma, particularly a scratch
     b. Among immunocompromised patients
        (1) AIDS
        (2) Lymphoma
        (3) Atopic dermatitis

- Signs and Symptoms
  1. Generally painless except a plantar wart which is subjected to pressure
  2. Begins as a flesh-colored papule
  3. May become a dome shaped grayish bump

- Differential Diagnosis
  1. Amelanotic melanoma, especially after age 40
  2. Calluses
  3. Condylomata
  4. Molluscum contagiosum
  5. Plantar corns
  6. Nevi

- Physical Findings
  1. Dome shaped hyperkeratotic
  2. Usually flesh-colored, but may be grayish
  3. Plantar warts have central black dot which may only be visible after paring lesion
  4. Normal skin markings are obscured
  5. No inflammation except for resolving flat warts

- Diagnostic Tests/Findings

    1. Laboratory studies are not required except a biopsy to rule out possible melanoma in a patient over age 40 or in younger patients whose physical findings are consistent with melanoma

    2. Diagnosis may be confirmed by scraping surface to expose central black dot

    3. VDRL to rule out syphilis if wart is genital

- Management/Treatment

    1. Common warts—salicylic acid and lactic acid applications; liquid nitrogen

    2. Plantar warts—abrade with pumice stone or emery board; salicylic acid tape; surgery if medical treatment is not effective

    3. Flat warts—tretinoin (retinoic acid)

    4. Facial warts—surgery

    5. Warts frequently resolve without treatment, except in immunocompromised patients

    6. Flat warts on the face should be allowed to resolve spontaneously to avoid scarring

    7. Refer for curettage, cryotherapy, or electrocautery

        a. Solitary warts

        b. Stubborn warts

        c. Painful warts

        d. Facial common warts

    8. Patients with facial common warts should avoid shaving or use a brushless foam and disposable razor to avoid spreading the warts

    9. Advise patients that home treatment is prolonged and requires consistency

    10. Patients engaging in home treatment need follow-up every 2 weeks

Questions

Select the best answer

1. Tom, age 17, has moderately severe acne on his face, chest, and back. He tells the clinician that he works at the grill in a fast food hamburger restaurant, washes twice a day with a mild soap, and enjoys outdoor exercise. Which lifestyle modification should the clinician suggest to control Tom's acne?

    a. Avoid the use of soap
    b. Avoid eating chocolate
    c. Consider a change of employment
    d. Avoid sun exposure

2. The therapeutic regimen which would be prescribed to control Tom's acne might include

    a. Retin-A and topical antibiotics
    b. Accutane
    c. Topical steroids
    d. Systemic steroids

3. Sarah, age 18, has a slightly pruritic scaling red maculpapular rash on her trunk. The oval lesions are arranged along lines of skin cleavage. She recalls a single large red macule which appeared before the rash. The probable diagnosis is

    a. Tinea versicolor
    b. Acne
    c. Pityriasis rosea
    d. Seborrheic dermatitis

4. Mrs. Ramirez has a maculopapular rash in straight linear bands across the dorsum of both feet. She states that this rash is very pruritic. It has been present all summer. A probable diagnosis for Mrs. Ramirez' rash is

    a. Eczema
    b. Contact dermatitis
    c. Herpes zoster
    d. Tinea corporis

5. Mrs. Cohen, age 35, has marked swelling, erythema, and warmth to the touch from her right ankle to her knee. The area is very tender but not pruritic. There is no discrete lesion or discharge, but the skin of the involved leg is taut and shiny. The diagnosis is probably

   a. Allergic dermatitis
   b. Contact dermatitis
   c. Furuncle
   d. Cellulitis

6. Appropriate therapy for Mrs. Cohen would include

   a. Warm soaks and IV antibiotics
   b. Systemic steroids
   c. Topical steroids
   d. Excisional biopsy

7. Mrs. Smith, age 28, has recurrent epidermal abscesses. They always respond to appropriate treatment, but recur within one to two months. Lab work which should be considered might include

   a. Two hour post-prandial blood sugar to rule out diabetes
   b. Culture the nose and throat of her close contacts to detect a possible asymptomatic carrier of the causative organism
   c. CBC with differential to look for possible leukopenia
   d. All of the above

8. Mr. Sorensen, a fair-skinned farmer, has noted an irregular pearly dome-shaped lesion on the dorsum of his hand for several months. The primary care provider should advise

   a. Duoplast nightly to the lesion
   b. Topical steroids
   c. Podophyllin to the lesion
   d. Prompt referral to a dermatologist

9. Mr. Chin has a severe case of contact dermatitis due to poison ivy. His symptoms will be relieved by

   a. Cool soaks with Burow's solution
   b. Warm compresses
   c. Bactroban ointment
   d. Sun exposure

10. Because severe pruritus disturbs Mr. Chin's sleep, the clinician may prescribe

   a. Hydroxyzine (Atarax)
   b. Retinoic acid
   c. Acyclovir
   d. Dicloxacillin

11. Mr. Becker, age 55, has a painful vesicular rash. The vesicles are arranged in a line on just one side of his trunk. He also has a fever and malaise. The most likely diagnosis is

   a. Herpes simplex
   b. Herpes zoster
   c. Impetigo
   d. Lyme disease

12. Prevention for Lyme disease includes

   a. Immunization against the causative spirochete
   b. Avoidance of persons with symptoms of the disease
   c. Wearing long pants tucked into socks for outdoor activities
   d. Avoidance of sharing personal care items

13. Treatment for mild psoriasis is likely to start with

   a. Coal tar preparations such as estar gel
   b. Topical steroids
   c. Retinoids
   d. Psoralen with UV light (PUVA)

14. William, age 19, has annular lesions with a raised border on his trunk. They are mildly pruritic. A skin scraping viewed with KOH under the microscope shows hyphae. The probable diagnosis is

   a. Tinea corporis
   b. Tinea cruris
   c. Tinea pedis
   d. Lyme disease

15. Treatment for tinea versicolor might include

   a. Selenium sulfide applied to body and left on overnight
   b. Topical steroids

c. Dithranol

d. Coal tar preparations in the bath water

16. Miss Bradshaw has a number of moles on her back. The clinician would be most concerned about a lesion which

   a. Appears to be "stuck on"
   b. Is port wine colored
   c. Is variably colored and asymmetrical
   d. Has a red scaly border

17. The patient has an irregular rough flesh-colored lesion on the sole of his foot. Gentle scraping exposes a central black dot. The clinician should

   a. Refer to a dermatologist for biopsy
   b. Order diagnostic tests for diabetes and HIV
   c. Prescribe a salicylic acid tape
   d. Prescribe a topical antifungal

18. The patient has tender lesions with honey colored crusts on her chin. Appropriate treatment might include

   a. Topical steroids
   b. An oral penicillin, such as dicloxacillin
   c. A topical antifungal
   d. Acyclovir

19. Mr. Clark has a large red macule with a pale center on his thigh. It is not painful or pruritic. He also complains of fever, myalgia, and malaise. A probable diagnosis is

   a. Tinea corporis
   b. Herpes zoster
   c. Malignant melanoma
   d. Lyme disease

20. Mrs. Thompson has pruritic dry patches on her forearms. The normal skin markings are accentuated and the skin seems leathery. Her close contacts are not affected. Appropriate therapy would be

   a. Retinoic acid
   b. Topical steroids
   c. Systemic steroids
   d. Topical antifungals

Answers.

1. c
2. a
3. c
4. b
5. d
6. a
7. d
8. d
9. a
10. a
11. b
12. c
13. a
14. a
15. a
16. c
17. c
18. b
19. d
20. b

Bibliography

Abramowitz, M. (Ed.). (1989). Treatment of Lyme disease. *Medical Letter*, 31(794), 57-60.

Burk, P. (1990). Diagnosing skin infections while they're superficial. *Emergency Medicine*. 22(5), 74-84.

Davis, E., & Rich, E. (Eds.). (1991). *Clinical protocols manual*. Pleasantville, NY: Pace University Center for Nursing Research and Clinical Practice.

Fitzpatrick, T., Johnson, R., Polano, M., Suurmond, D., & Wolff, K. (1992). *Color atlas and synopsis of clinical dermatology* (2nd ed.). New York: McGraw-Hill.

Habif, T. (1990). *Clinical dermatology, a color guide to diagnosis and therapy* (2nd ed.). St. Louis: C. V. Mosby.

Hunter, J., Savin, J., & Dahl, M. (1989). *Clinical dermatology*. London: Blackwell Scientific.

Jordan, R. (Ed.). (1991). *Immunologic diseases of the skin*. East Norwalk: Appleton and Lange.

Sams, W., Jr., & Lynch, P. (Eds.). (1990). *Principles and practice of dermatology*. New York: Churchill Livingstone.

Sauer, G. (1985). *Manual of skin diseases* (5th ed.). Philadelphia: J. B. Lippincott.

Thomas, C. (Ed.). (1993). *Taber's Cyclopedic Medical Dictionary* (17th ed.). Philadelphia: F. A. Davis.

Woodley, M. & Whelan, A. (Eds.). (1992). *Manual of medical therapeutics*. (27th ed.). St. Louis: Washington University Press.

Eyes, Ears, Nose, Throat Disorders

Madeline Turkeltaub

The Common Cold

- Definition: Acute upper respiratory infection
- Etiology/Incidence
    1. A variety of viruses that cause the same manifestations
    2. Incidence decreases with age
        a. Children—6 to 8 per year
        b. Adults—2 to 4 per year
    3. Transmitted by contact with respiratory secretions
    4. Incubation period is 48 to 72 hours
    5. Usually lasts one week
- Signs and Symptoms
    1. Nasal discharge and obstruction
    2. Sneezing
    3. Sore throat
    4. Cough
    5. Hoarseness
    6. Mild malaise
    7. Loss of taste and smell
    8. Watery eyes
- Differential Diagnosis
    1. Influenza
    2. Bacterial sinusitis
    3. Otitis media
    4. Pneumonitis
    5. Pharyngitis
- Physical Findings
    1. Occasional 1 °F temperature elevation
    2. Injected conjunctiva
    3. Erythematous and edematous nasal mucosa

4. Erythematous oropharynx

5. Lungs clear

■ Diagnostic Tests/Findings

1. Non-specific

2. Throat culture if Group A ß-hemolytic streptococci infection is suggested by history and/or physical examination

3. Chest radiograph if chest tightness or wheezes are present

■ Management/Treatment: Symptomatic treatment is the only treatment available

1. Aspirin for fever and myalgias

2. Steam or cool mist to liquify secretions

3. Topical decongestants for nasal congestion (drops or sprays)

4. Oral decongestants for congestion

5. Counsel patients that transmission can be minimized by handwashing and reduced finger-to-nose contact

6. Caution against using decongestant drops or sprays for more than five days to decrease rebound effect

7. Oral decongestants should be used with caution in hypertensive patients

8. Instruct patient to report ear pain (otitis media), chest pain (pneumonitis) or discolored nasal discharge (bacterial sinusitis)

Influenza (Flu Syndrome)

■ Definition: An acute self-limiting febrile illness that occurs in outbreaks of varying severity

■ Etiology/Incidence

1. Influenza virus A and B

2. 85% of cases are seen during an epidemic

3. Those infected with influenza virus may be coinfected with

a. Parainfluenza

b. Respiratory syncytial virus

c. Adenovirus

4. Influenza A is responsible for increased mortality

5. Transmitted by virus-containing respiratory secretions by way of

    a. Sneezing

    b. Talking

    c. Coughing

6. Incubation period—18 to 72 hours

7. Occurs primarily during winter months

■ Signs and Symptoms

1. Acute onset of

    a. Fever up to 106 °F lasting three days

    b. Chills

    c. Headache

    d. Myalgias

    e. Malaise

    f. Anorexia

    g. Athralgias

    h. Cough at onset and again as systemic signs and symptoms decrease in intensity; may persist for two or more weeks

■ Differential Diagnosis

1. Pneumonia

2. Airway hyperreactivity

3. Bronchitis

4. Infectious mononucleosis

5. Early HIV infection

■ Physical Findings

1. Flushed face

2. Hot skin

3. Watery red eyes

4. Clear nasal discharge

5. Tender cervical lymph nodes

6. Chest—occasional localized rales

■ Diagnostic Tests/Findings

1. WBC

    a. Granulocytopenia

    b. Mild neutropenia

    c. Relative lymphocytosis

2. Monospot—negative

3. Rapid plasma reagin (RPR)—negative

■ Management/Treatment

1. Antiviral agent—Amantadine (200 mg x 1, then 100 mg b.i.d. for 5 days)

    a. Most effective within 24 to 48 hours of onset of symptoms

    b. Reduces fever by 50%, shortens illness by 1 to 2 days

2. Monitor for complications

    a. Pulmonary

        (1) Spectrum from wheezing to Acute Respiratory Disease Syndrome (ARDS)

        (2) Pneumonia incidence high in those over 70 years of age

    b. Non-pulmonary

        (1) Myositis

        (2) Acute renal failure

        (3) Guillain-Barr syndrome

        (4) Encephalitis

        (5) Transverse myelitis

        (6) Reye syndrome—not associated with ASA in adults

3. General considerations

    a. Review side effects of Amantadine, including

        (1) Insomnia

        (2) Nervousness

        (3) Dizziness

          (4)   Difficulty concentrating

  4. Decrease exposure to droplets

  5. Non-pulmonary complications require hospitalization for differential diagnosis

  6. Prevention

    a. Influenza vaccine, given in fall before epidemic occurs, recommended for

      (1)   People over 60 years of age

      (2)   Pre-existing heart, lung, or debilitating disease

      (3)   People in critical jobs or high exposure—teachers, hospital personnel, policemen, firemen

    b. Amantadine prophylaxis against influenza A in high risk populations not receiving vaccine (100 to 200 mg orally every day for 2 weeks)

Pharyngitis

- Definition: Inflammation of the Pharynx. (Sore throat)
- Etiology/Incidence

  1. Fourth most common symptom seen in medical practice

  2. No pathogens are found in 1/3 of cases

  3. Common pathogens include

    a. Usually viral

    b. Group A ß-hemolytic streptococcus

    c. *Mycoplasma pneumoniae*

    d. *Chlamydia pneumoniae*

    e. *Neisseria gonorrhoea*

- Signs and Symptoms

  1. Sore throat

  2. Fever

  3. Malaise

- Differential Diagnosis

  1. Mononucleosis

2. Peritonsillar abscess

3. Pharyngeal abscess

4. Epiglottitis

5. Tonsillitis

6. U.R.I.

■ Physical Findings

1. Red inflamed posterior pharynx with or without exudate

2. Tender cervical lymph nodes

■ Diagnostic Tests/Findings

1. Throat cultures are indicated if the following is suspected

a. Group A streptococci

b. Gonococcal pharyngitis

2. No clinical distinction can be made between streptococcal and nonstreptococcal pharyngitis—throat culture or rapid detection method for streptococcal antigens are usually confirmatory

3. WBC—leukocytosis with group A ß-hemolytic infection

4. Monospot—negative

■ Management/Treatment

1. Streptococcal pharyngitis

a. Benzathine penicillin 1.2 million units IM one time only or

b. Penicillin V 250 mg orally t.i.d. for 10 days

c. Post treatment culture if history of rheumatic fever

d. Erythromycin for penicillin sensitive patients

2. Gonococcal pharyngitis

a. Ceftriaxone 250 mg IM as a single dose plus

b. Doxycycline 100 mg orally b.i.d. for 7 days

c. Culture 7 days post-treatment

d. Cotreat for chlamydia—doxycycline 100 mg orally b.i.d. for 7 days

3. General therapy

a. Force fluids to 3,000 cc/day

b. Gargle with warm saline solution

c. Throat lozenges

Infectious Mononucleosis

- Definition: An acute disease characterized by fever, pharyngitis and lymphadenopathy

- Etiology/Incidence

  1. Epstein-Barr Virus (EBV), a member of the herpes virus group is principal cause

  2. May occur during childhood, adolescence or adulthood

     a. Rare in children under two years and adults over 40 years of age

     b. Overall incidence is approximately 50:100,000 persons per year

     c. In young adults incidence is about 1:1,000 per year

  3. Transmitted in saliva

- Signs and Symptoms

  1. Patients may have all or only some of the characteristic features

  2. Often, patient experiences malaise for several days followed by fever, pharyngitis with lymphadenopathy

  3. Pharyngitis can be severe with exudate and edema

- Differential Diagnosis

  1. EBV infection without heterophil antibody response

  2. CMV infection

  3. Toxoplasmosis

  4. Acute HIV infection

  5. Infectious hepatitis (hepatitis A)

  6. Streptococcal pharyngitis

- Physical Findings

  1. Moderate to severe erythematous findings in throat with marked tonsillar enlargement with exudate

  2. Lymphadenopathy, which is striking, can be limited to the cervical

nodes, but can be so extensive that all lymph node groups are involved

3. Splenomegaly—maximal during 2nd and 3rd weeks of illness

4. Hepatomegaly may also be present

- Diagnostic Tests/Findings

1. WBC—leukocytosis with approximately two thirds lymphocytes

2. Monospot test—positive

3. Heterophil titer—titers greater than 1:28 or 1:40 considered positive; usually rise during the 2nd and 3rd week of illness (magnitude of heterophil titer does not correlate with severity of illness)

- Management/Treatment

1. Mostly supportive; no specific therapy indicated

2. Rest during acute phase of illness when fever, pharyngitis and malaise are present

3. Strenuous exercise and contact sports should be avoided if splenomegaly is present

4. Corticosteroids useful only for significant airway obstruction due to edema and tonsillar hypertrophy

5. Use of ampicillin—should be avoided due to ampicillin-related rash which develops frequently with individuals diagnosed with infectious mononucleosis

Epistaxis

- Definition: Bleeding from the nose

- Etiology/Incidence

1. Most bleeding occurs in the vascular plexus in the anteroinferior septum (Kiesselbach plexus)

2. Can occur secondary to rhinitis, sinusitis; dryness of nasal mucosa; trauma; systemic infections; arteriosclerosis; hypertension; bleeding disorders; tumors; medications

- Signs and Symptoms

1. Bleeding from nose

2. Nausea and/or coffee ground emesis, secondary to swallowing blood

- Differential Diagnosis: See etiology
- Physical Findings
  1. Usually unilateral bloody discharge from nose secondary to irritation or minor trauma
  2. Bilateral bloody discharge from nose may be due to a bleeding disorder, systemic cause or severe craniofacial trauma
- Diagnostic Tests/Findings: Based upon suspected etiologic factors
- Management/Treatment
  1. Compress the nasal alae together for 10 minutes
  2. Keep patient quiet and in a forward leaning position or in reclining position with head and shoulders elevated
  3. If bleeding fails to stop then bleeding site must be found; a pledget of cotton with a vasoconstricter such as phenylephrine 0.25% placed in the nose will stop most bleeding from Kiesselbach's area
  4. Referral if bleeding does not stop
  5. For severe bleeding or bleeding which fails to stop check vital signs
  6. For infrequent controlled epistaxis patients should be instructed not to pick nose nor blow nose for approximately 12 to 24 hours
  7. Recurrence of epistaxis requires investigative measures to determine cause and preventive measures

Allergic Rhinitis

- Definition: Noninfectious allergic manifestation, characterized by rhinorrhea, nasal congestion, pruritus
- Etiology/Incidence
  1. Allergens most often responsible—pollens, molds, animal danders, dust mites
  2. Prevalence differs in geographical regions; affects 10% of population between 16 to 64 years of age
  3. Seasonal allergy—at the same time every year, associated with pollen count
  4. Perennial allergy—year round, related to indoor inhalants, animal dander, and mold

■ Signs and Symptoms

1. Nasal congestion

2. Dry mouth—from breathing through mouth

3. Clear nasal discharge

4. Itching nose

5. Sneezing

6. Cough—from postnasal drip

7. Allergic conjunctivitis

8. Loss of smell and taste

■ Differential Diagnosis

1. Nasal polyps

2. U.R.I.

3. Deviated nasal septum

4. Flu

5. Syphilis—2nd stage

■ Physical Findings

1. Nasal mucosa pale and swollen

2. Enlarged turbinates

■ Diagnostic Tests/Findings

1. Allergic rhinitis—allergy skin testing to identify specific allergens

2. Eosinophils often seen on Wright's stain of nasal secretions

■ Management/Treatment

1. Seasonal rhinitis

    a. Avoid exposure to allergens

    b. Air conditioner in home and car

2. Perennial rhinitis

    a. Environmental controls

    b. Air filtration

3. Pharmacologic—depends on duration of symptoms, severity of condition, convenience, patient preference

a. Antihistamines

b. Sympathomimetic nasal sprays—Afrin Nasal Spray 0.05% two sprays each nostril b.i.d. only for 3 days

c. Topical corticosteroids

    (1) Decadron (Turbinaire)—1 inhalation q.i.d. or two inhalations b.i.d.

    (2) Beclomethasone dipropionate (Vancenase)—1 inhalation q.i.d. or two inhalations b.i.d.

d. Systemic corticosteroids may be indicated until nasal preparations are effective

e. Intranasal cromolyn sodium—Nasalcrom one spray each nostril, 3 to 6 times daily

f. Seldane, Hismanal

g. Immunotherapy following identification of offending allergens may be prescribed by an allergist

4. Discourage abuse of topical decongestants leading to rebound rhinitis (rhinitis medicamentosa)

5. Review environmental controls, including

    a. Air filtration

    b. Bare floors

    c. Washable curtains

    d. No books or stuffed animals in room

    e. Allergy-proof encasements for bedding

6. Advise patients taking seldane to *not take* erythromycin due to arrythmia potential

7. Patients receiving immunotherapy must be aware of signs and symptoms of anaphylactic reaction

Sinusitis

■ Definition: Bacterial infection of one or more paranasal sinuses

■ Etiology/Incidence

1. Complication associated with about 0.5% of viral U.R.I.

2. Ten percent of cases are associated with dental abscess

3. Nursing home patients with long term nasogastric tubes develop occult sinusitis

- Signs and Symptoms

   1. Pain—dull, progressing to throbbing especially when head is dependent

   2. Coughing increases pain

   3. Cold symptoms lasting more than two weeks

   4. Headache

   5. Purulent nasal discharge and post-nasal drip

   6. Malaise

- Differential Diagnosis

   1. Dental abscess

   2. Migraine and cluster headaches

   3. Trigeminal neuralgia

   4. Optic neuritis

   5. Allergic rhinitis

- Physical Findings

   1. Percussing over affected area exacerbates pain

   2. Examination of the pharynx, nose, ears, for edema and erythema

   3. Examination of the teeth for uneven surfaces associated with grinding

   4. Transillumination of the sinuses, although not definitive, does not reflect light

   5. Nontender edema of eyelids associated with maxillary sinusitis

- Management/Treatment

   1. Antimicrobials

      a. Ampicillin or Amoxicillin 250 to 500 mg q.i.d. for 10 days

      b. Trimethoprim—sulfamethoxazole 2 tablets b.i.d. for 10 days as an alternative for penicillin allergic patients

   2. Symptomatic relief

      a. Decongestant spray to improve sinus drainage

      b. Steam in inhalation to liquify secretions

    c. Analgesics for facial pain and headache

3. Advise patients who plan to fly to take an oral decongestant prior to takeoff

4. If symptoms worsen or do not improve after 48 hours of treatment, refer to M.D. Instruct patients to report symptoms of complications such as increased fever, stiff neck (meningitis) tender periorbital edema (orbital cellulitis)

Hearing Loss

- Definition: Diminished ability to detect pure tone in decibels of 30 or greater
- Etiology/Incidence

    1. Hearing loss is a common complaint in older people

    2. About 10 percent of U.S. population has a degree of hearing loss

    3. Hearing loss is conductive or sensorineural

    4. Conductive hearing loss results from dysfunction of the external or middle ear, due to

        a. Obstruction—cerumen impaction, foreign body

        b. Increased mass—middle ear effusion, chronic otitis media

        c. Stiffness effect—otosclerosis, scarring of tympanic membrane

        d. Discontinuity—ossicular disruption

    5. Sensorineural hearing loss (SNHL) results from deterioration of the cochlea and/or involvement of the eighth cranial nerve

- Signs and Symptoms

    1. Conductive hearing loss—decreased ability to detect low tones and vowels

    2. Sensorineural hearing loss—high frequency loss with loss of speech discrimination of consonants, female pitch voices, difficulty with background noises

    3. Presbycusis—the SNHL associated with tinnitus that occurs as a part of normal aging; high frequency hearing loss initially, intolerance of high pitched and loud sounds; gradually moves into lower frequency loss; some research show smokers have greater loss

- Differential Diagnosis

    1. Conductive hearing loss—cerumen impaction, foreign body, otitis

externa, serous otitis media, acute otitis media, chronic otitis media, otosclerosis

2. Mixed conductive and sensorineural loss—barotrauma; traumatic injury, otosclerosis, although typically conductive in most cases, can lead to sensorineural loss too

3. Sensorineural loss—presbycusis; acoustic trauma; drug induced, e.g., streptomycin; Meniere's Syndrome; acoustic neuroma; chronic noise exposure

- Physical Findings

  1. Rinne test—compares air-to-bone conduction

     a. Normal—AC > BC

     b. Conductive loss—BC > AC in affected ear(s)

     c. Sensorineural loss—AC > BC bilaterally

  2. Weber test—confirms results of Rinne test; determines if sound is louder on one side

     a. Normal—midline

     b. Conductive loss—lateralized to poorer ear

     c. Sensorineural loss—lateralized to better ear

  3. Whisper test—examiner stands one to two feet to the side of patient and speaks in a whisper; patient is asked to repeat examiner's words on request; ear not being tested is masked

  4. Physical examination of ear—normal

- Diagnostic Tests/Findings

  1. Pure tone audiometry conducted by an audiologist

     a. Air conduction and bone conduction are both measured with masking in opposite ear

     b. Intensity is measured in decibels, frequency is measured in Hertz

     c. Threshold of normal hearing—0 to 20 dB

        (1) Mild hearing loss threshold—20 to 40 dB (equivalent to soft voice)

        (2) Moderate loss threshold—40 to 60 dB (equivalent to normal voice)

        (3) Severe loss threshold—60 to 80 dB (equivalent to loud voice)

(4)   Profound loss—80 dB

2.   Speech discrimination testing

    a. Detects impaired clarity of hearing related to sensorineural loss

    b. Reported as percentage correct

    c. 90 to 100% is normal

3.   Cranial radiograph to detect tumors, such as acoustic neuroma

■ Management/Treatment: Treatment depends on the disease condition causing the symptoms

1.   Refer patient to an otolaryngologist for

    a. Further evaluation of sensorineural hearing loss

    b. Conductive disorders not responding to treatment

2.   Avoid activities which increase hearing loss, such as

    a. Swimming—"swimmer's ear"

    b. Exposure to loud noise—music, drills, etc.; use earplugs

3.   Discontinue medications which are ototoxic if patient complains of tinnitus or decreased hearing

4.   Monitor occupational exposure yearly with audiograms

Vertigo

■ Definition: Subjective impression of movement in space or of objects moving, usually with a loss of equilibrium

■ Etiology/Incidence

1.   Diagnosis is made by ruling out other disease

2.   Approximately 25% of patients complaining of dizziness have vertigo

3.   Most often associated with conditions of the labyrinth or the vestibular nerve, salicylate toxicity, alcohol, postural hypotension

4.   May be a manifestation of progressive CNS disease

■ Signs and Symptoms

1.   Nausea with or without vomiting

2.   Hearing loss

3.   Tinnitus

4. Feeling of "fullness" in the ear

5. Episodic

6. Sense of rotation

7. Sense of impending faint

8. Imbalance; relieved by sitting or lying down

9. Ill-defined lightheadedness; floating, swimming

- Differential Diagnosis

    1. Middle ear disease

    2. Otitis externa

    3. Meniere's disease

    4. Vestibular neuritis

    5. Otosclerosis

    6. Multiple sclerosis

    7. Acoustic neuroma

    8. Cerebrovascular accident

- Physical Findings

    1. Since this is a diagnosis of exclusion, a complete physical examination should be performed

    2. Nystagmus when testing extraocular movements

    3. Conductive hearing loss with otitis media

    4. Changes in positional B/P associated with positional hypotension

    5. Carotid bruits associated with carotid insufficiency

- Diagnostic Tests/Findings

    1. Inspect external auditory canal and tympanic membrane

    2. Neurological and neurovascular examination

        a. Cranial nerves—5 and 7

        b. Cerebellar tests

        c. Gait testing

        d. Romberg test

        e. Motor testing

3. Serological test for syphilis to confirm luetic labyrinthitis

4. TSH to rule out hypothyroidism

5. Hematocrit to test for anemia

6. FBS to rule out diabetes mellitus

7. Audiologic evaluation

8. Hallpike Maneuver—patient examined on table with head hanging over back of table for one minute; put in upright position for one minute; observed for symptoms and nystagmus (*select patients only*)

- Management/Treatment: Management is based on symptoms

1. Bed rest is helpful

2. Antivertigo antihistamines—meclizine (Antivert) 12.5 to 25 mg tablets orally t.i.d.

3. Antiemetic for nausea and vomiting—prochlorperazine (Compazine) 5 to 10 mg every four hours orally prn

4. Do *not* perform tests for positional vertigo on older patients

5. Instruct patient on side effects of antivertigo antihistamines—dry mouth, sedation

6. Instruct patient on major side effects of antiemetic—sedation

7. Refer for persistent vertigo

Otitis Externa

- Definition: Any inflammatory process involving the skin of the auricle and lining of the external auditory canal. Commonly referred to as "Swimmer's Ear"

- Etiology/Incidence

1. Five times more common in swimmers than non-swimmers

2. More common in hot humid climates

3. Causes may be

   a. Infectious—most common; results from normal ear flora that assume pathologic charactistics with excessive wetness; secondary invasion by foreign pathogens also occurs

   b. Allergic

   c. Neurogenic

4. Involvement of both ears in 20% of cases

■ Signs and Symptoms
1. Ear pain ranging from itching to excruciating pain
2. Increased pain on movement—chewing, moving jaw
3. Itching precedes pain
4. Hearing loss occasionally (conductive)

■ Differential Diagnosis
1. Localized furuncle
2. Otitis media
3. Mastoiditis
4. Seborrhea
5. Eczema

■ Physical Findings
1. Erythema and edema of skin of auditory canal
2. Pain on manipulation of auricle, or palpation of tragus
3. Tympanic membrane usually not involved
4. No middle ear fluid
5. No swelling or pain over mastoid

■ Diagnostic Tests/Findings
1. Culture may be done if response to usual treatment is ineffective

■ Management/Treatment
1. Pharmacologic
   a. Combined antibiotic steroid preparations—cortisporin otic solution 4 drops in ear(s) three to four times a day
   b. Antifungal and antibacterial preparations—vosol otic solution
   c. Cotton gauze wick usually inserted to facilitate medication reaching site of inflammation; removed after pain and swelling have subsided
   d. Antibiotics if an organism is identified, and fever and lymphadenopathy are present
2. Warm compresses for localized external otitis

3. Use combination of white vinegar and rubbing alcohol (50/50) in both ear canals at the end of each swim and/or upon arising and at bedtime

4. Avoid swimming during acute period

5. Protect ears when swimming

6. Report symptoms as soon as possible

Acute Otitis Media

- Definition: Inflammation of the middle ear
- Etiology/Incidence
  1. Caused by bacteria
     a. *Streptococcus pneumoniae*
     b. *Hemophilus influenzae*
     c. *Branhamella catarrhalis*
  2. High risk includes
     a. Recent upper respiratory infection
     b. Cleft palate
     c. Down syndrome
     d. Allergic rhinitis
     e. Native American or Eskimo
  3. Occurs most frequently in the first two years, but can occur in adults
  4. Most frequent in winter months
- Signs and Symptoms
  1. Ear pain
  2. Otorrhea
  3. Hearing loss (conductive)
  4. Vertigo
  5. Occasional fever
  6. Intense pain, followed by acute relief (membrane rupture yields relief)
- Differential Diagnosis
  1. Otitis externa

2.   Mumps

3.   Dental abscess

4.   Ear canal furuncle

5.   Foreign body in ear canal

6.   Tonsillitis

7.   Trauma to ear

8.   Subacute mastoiditis

- Physical Findings

    1.   Otoscopic examination—red, dull, bulging tympanic membrane

    2.   Evidence of perforation with discharge may be present

    3.   Tenderness to palpation over mastoid bone

- Diagnostic Tests/Findings

    1.   Pneumatic otoscope—normal membrane motility is impeded

    2.   Impedance tympanometry may be abnormal

    3.   Aspiration of middle ear fluid for culture in immunosuppressed patients

- Management/Treatment

    1.   Pharmacologic

        a.   Antibiotics—10 day course

            (1)   Drugs of choice

                (a)   Ampicillin 250 to 500 mg orally q.i.d.

                (b)   Amoxicillin 500 mg orally t.i.d.

            (2)   Bactrim two tablets orally every 12 hours for penicillin allergic patients

        b.   If perforation occurs—cortisporin otic 4 gtts t.i.d. for 1 week

        c.   Analgesia

            (1)   ASA or acetaminophen

            (2)   Codeine 30 mg with aspirin orally every four hours as needed

    2.   Follow-up on impaired hearing—impairment should resolve in 1 to 4 weeks

    3.   Refer when

      a. Worse after several days of treatment

      b. Not improved after 10 days of antibiotic treatment

      c. Hearing loss of longer than three weeks

      d. Bulging membrane with severe pain and vertigo

   4. Stress importance of remaining on antibiotics for 10 days

Serous Otitis Media

- Definition: Fluid in the middle ear not associated with acute inflammation ("glue ear")
- Etiology/Incidence
  1. Associated with
     a. Subacute infection
     b. Allergy
     c. Barotrauma
     d. Persistent fluid following acute otitis
  2. Very common in childhood, relatively common in adults
- Signs and Symptoms
  1. Feeling of fullness in ear(s)
  2. Decreased hearing in ear(s)
- Differential Diagnosis
  1. Acute purulent otitis media
  2. Chronic otitis media
  3. Eustachian tube obstruction
  4. Conductive hearing loss
  5. Meniere's disease
- Physical Findings
  1. Retraction of tympanic membrane
  2. Air-fluid level behind membrane
  3. Conductive hearing loss
     a. Weber test will lateralize to side with conductive loss

    b. Rinne test—bone conduction is greater than air conduction

- Diagnostic Tests/Findings

    1. Pneumatic otoscopy—membrane does not move on insufflation

    2. Audiometry—decreased acuity of hearing

- Management/Treatment: Objective is to relieve eustachian tube obstruction and symptoms

    1. Pharmacologic

        a. Topical decongestants—neo-synephrine nasal spray 0.25 to 0.50% two sprays each nostril q.i.d. for three days

        b. Antihistamines for patients with history of allergy

    2. If no nasal discharge is present, patient can perform the valsalva maneuver several times per day

    3. Instruct patient not to use topical decongestants for more than three days

    4. Re-evaluate patient in 4 to 6 weeks

    5. Refer to specialist if

        a. Hearing loss lasts more than six weeks

        b. Condition occurs more than two times per year

Impaired Vision

- Definition: Decreased visual acuity

- Etiology/Incidence

    1. Most common causes are

        a. Hereditary defects in people under 20 years of age

        b. Glaucoma

        c. Diabetic retinopathy between ages 21 to 60

        d. Macular degeneration in patients over 60 years of age

    2. Legal blindness—20/200 or less in best eye with correction

    3. 500,000 legally blind people in U.S., half over 65 years of age

- Signs and Symptoms

    1. Decreased visual acuity may be sudden or gradual, bilateral or

         unilateral, intermittent

   2. Pain on moving eyes

   3. Floaters

   4. Visual field loss

- Differential Diagnosis
  1. Refractive error
  2. Cataract
  3. Macular degeneration
  4. Diabetic retinopathy
  5. Vitreous hemorrhage
  6. Retinal detachment
  7. Multiple sclerosis
  8. Visual field loss
     a. Monocular—related to disease of retina or optic nerve
     b. Bitemporal field loss—due to lesions of optic chiasm
     c. Contralateral homonymous field defects—related to cerebrovascular disease and tumors

- Physical Findings
  1. Visual acuity—using Snellen chart for each eye in turn; corrected acuity of less than 20/30 is abnormal
  2. Visual fields—use Amsler charts to detect central field abnormalities due to macular disease
  3. Pupils—observe for
     a. Absolute and relative size
     b. Reactions to light and accommodation
  4. Conjunctivae—inspect for edema, injection
  5. Cornea and lens—inspect for clarity, corneal reflex
  6. Extraocular movements

- Diagnostic Tests/Findings
  1. Direct ophthalmoscopy used to examine and detect abnormalities of
     a. Retina and retinal vessels

    b. Cornea

    c. Lens

    d. Vitreous

    e. Optic disk for swelling, size

    f. Macular lesions

  2. Tonometry measures intraocular pressure—normal is 10 to 21 mm Hg

- Management/Treatment: Depends on the disease or condition causing the symptoms

  1. Refer patient to ophthalmologist for

    a. Sudden loss of vision—with or without pain

    b. Gradual loss of vision—refractive errors

    c. Findings on PE not within normal limits

    d. Any complaints of flashing lights

  2. Encourage patients with diabetes mellitus (DM) to report visual disturbances immediately

Foreign Body (Eye)

- Definition: Objects or material in the eye, causing irritation
- Etiology/Incidence

  1. Frequently seen in primary care

  2. Most often lodge in conjunctiva or cornea

- Signs and Symptoms

  1. "Foreign body sensation"

  2. Pain

  3. Tearing

  4. Occasional decreased acuity

  5. Photophobia

  6. Red eyes

  7. Blepharospasm

- Differential Diagnosis

  1. Imbedded foreign body

    2.   Corneal abrasion

- Physical Findings
  1. Corneal foreign bodies—evident when using a hand light on an oblique angle as a dark speck against iris
  2. Tarsal conjunctiva—evert upper lid to inspect upper eye and lid
  3. "Rust ring" in affected area suggests metal

- Diagnostic Tests/Findings
  1. Diagnosis is made on inspection
  2. Fluorescein staining renders foreign bodies and abrasions more apparent

- Management/Treatment
  1. Conjunctival foreign body that is not embedded—remove with pointed corner of gauze pad lightly moistened with water
  2. Do not irrigate eye or attempt to remove a penetrating object
  3. Antibiotic ophthalmic ointment
  4. Refer
     a. Implanted foreign bodies
     b. Suspected cases of intraocular foreign bodies
     c. Changes in visual acuity
     d. Follow-up after foreign body is removed
  5. Caution patient against rubbing eye
  6. Education regarding eye safety

Corneal Abrasion

- Definition: An interruption in the epithelial surface of the cornea
- Etiology/Incidence
  1. Among most frequent eye injury
  2. Associated with trauma to eye
- Signs and Symptoms
  1. Intense pain especially as time progresses
  2. Tearing

3. Decreased visual acuity

4. Redness

5. Blepharospasm

- Differential Diagnosis: Herpes simplex keratitis

- Physical Findings: Illumination with blue light following stain with sodium fluorescein identifies lesion

- Diagnostic Tests/Findings: Fluorescein stain—yellowish green dye detects abrasions and ulcers

- Management/Treatment

  1. Assure that no foreign bodies are in eye

  2. Topical antibiotic or sulfonamide eye drops

  3. Pressure patch with lid closed tightly to decrease movement

  4. Improved in 24 hours, healed in 48 hours

  5. Remove patch in 24 hours

  6. Antibiotic or sulfonamide drops q.i.d. for 24 to 48 hrs

  7. Refer if not improved in 24 hours

  8. Steroid eyedrops are contraindicated—inhibit corneal wound healing.

  9. Ophthalmic topical anesthetics are contraindicated—may lead to further eye injury if patient tends to "rub" affected eye

Conjunctivitis

- Definition: Inflammatory condition affecting the conjunctiva, that extends over the posterior surface of the lids and up over the sclera to the cornea

- Etiology/Incidence

  1. The most common eye disease in the U.S.

  2. Most cases are due to bacteria, viruses, allergy

  3. Mode of transmission—direct contact, allergens

  4. Secretions of bacterial conjunctivitis are infectious for 24 to 48 hours

  5. "Swimming pool conjunctivitis"—associated with adenopharyngeal conjunctivitis (APC)

- Signs and Symptoms

  1. Redness and irritation without photophobia

2. Watery to purulent discharge

3. Bacterial conjunctivitis

   a. Purulent discharge

   b. Upon awakening patient finds purulent discharge often mats lids shut

   c. Mild discomfort

   d. Unilateral or bilateral

   e. Self limited—10 to 14 days, if not treated

4. Gonococcal conjunctivitis

   a. Copious purulent discharge

   b. Contact with infected genital secretion

5. Viral conjunctivitis

   a. Red palpebral conjunctiva

   b. Copious watery discharge

   c. Scanty exudate

   d. Untreated symptoms last two weeks

   e. Systemic symptoms of viral infection

6. Allergic conjunctivitis

   a. Bilateral tearing

   b. Itching

   c. Redness

   d. Stringy discharge

   e. Corneal involvement related to vernal conjunctivitis

- Differential Diagnosis

  1. Acute uveitis

  2. Acute glaucoma

  3. Corneal trauma

  4. Corneal infection

  5. Mascara or eyeliner induced (usually old product)

  6. Contaminated contact lens solutions

7. Iritis

- Physical Findings
    1. Viral conjunctivitis—preauricular adenopathy
    2. See Signs and Symptoms
- Diagnostic Tests/Findings
    1. Bacterial conjunctivitis
        a. Stain conjunctival scrapings
        b. Culture exudate
    2. Gonococcal conjunctivitis
        a. Stain smear
        b. Culture discharge
    3. No specific diagnostic tests for viral and allergic conjunctivitis
- Management/Treatment
    1. Bacterial conjunctivitis
        a. Sulfacetamide 10% ophthalmic solution t.i.d.; effective in 2 to 3 days
    2. Gonococcal conjunctivitis
        a. Frequent saline wash to eyes
        b. Topical antibiotics
        c. IV antibiotics
            (1) Aqueous penicillin
            (2) Cefotaxime
    3. Viral conjunctivitis
        a. No treatment for virus
        b. Sulfonamide to decrease secondary infection
        c. Symptomatic treatment
    4. Allergic conjunctivitis
        a. Topical vasoconstrictors
        b. Antihistamines
        c. Short term local steroid therapy

       d. Cold compresses

    5. General considerations

       a. Gonococcal conjunctivitis—ophthalmologic emergency

       b. Refer if vision impaired

       c. Discourage rubbing eyes

       d. Discourage activities that strain eyes

       e. Use separate eye cups for each eye for lavage

       f. Family members applying eyedrops to patients with bacterial conjunctivitis must wash hands carefully before and after procedure.

       g. Possible viral conjunctivitis requires preventing spread by

          (1)   Washing exposed towels in hot water

          (2)   Cleaning tonometer and office equipment carefully

       h. Frequent change of cosmetic eye products

       i. Careful cleaning and care of contact lenses

Cataracts

- Definition: Degenerative opacity of the crystalline lens
- Etiology/Incidence

    1. Most common cause of severe visual impairment in the U.S.

    2. 90% due to normal aging process

    3. Usually bilateral

    4. Occur to some degree in 70% of people above 70 years of age

    5. Causes other than aging

       a. Congenital

       b. Traumatic

       c. Inflammatory—infectious

       d. Physical—temperature, radiation

       e. Metabolic—diabetes, parathyroid, thyroid

    6. 600,000 cataract extractions performed in U.S. each year.

- Signs and Symptoms

    1. Reduced visual acuity; painless, progressive loss of vision

2. Sensitivity to light, especially on night driving

3. Reduced color discrimination

4. Decreased night vision

5. Double vision

- Differential Diagnosis

    1. Determination of the cause in younger patients—traumatic, inflammatory, physical, metabolic

    2. Glaucoma

- Physical Findings

    1. Dark defects in red reflex

    2. Large cataracts may obscure the red reflex

- Diagnostic Tests/Findings

    1. Diagnosis made on physical examination

    2. Snellen chart—test visual acuity in both eyes; degrees of loss dependent upon extended opacity

- Management/Treatment

    1. Refer all patients with cataracts

    2. Treatment is by surgical removal

        a. Indication depends on visual needs of patient

        b. Most frequent procedure—extracapsular lens extraction with implantation of posterior chamber lens in the capsular bag

        c. Visual acuity improved in 95% after surgery

    3. May follow-up post operatively—observe for complications

        a. Inflammation and infection

        b. Hemorrhage

        c. Retinal detachment

        d. Glaucoma

Glaucoma

- Definition: Eye disorder with significant increase in intraocular pressure sufficient to cause damage to the optic nerve

- Etiology/Incidence

  1. Caused by inadequate drainage of aqueous fluid in the anterior portion of the eye

  2. Primary glaucoma accounts for 95% of all patients with glaucoma in U.S.

  3. Primary glaucoma, most frequently seen in primary care, includes

     a. Open-angle

        (1) 3% of people above 75 years of age

        (2) Blacks affected younger and more frequently

        (3) Causes 15 to 20% of blindness in U.S.

        (4) Familial

     b. Angle-closure

        (1) Positive family history

        (2) Women more than men

        (3) Far less common than open-angle glaucoma

        (4) May be precipitated by mydriatics

        (5) Precipitated by anxiety, darkness, large intake of fluids

        (6) Blindness in 2 to 3 days

     c. Congenital—infant and juvenile onset

  3. Secondary glaucomas result from trauma, inflammation, and pre-existing conditions of the eye

- Signs and Symptoms

  1. Primary open-angle glaucoma—resistance to aqueous outflow

     a. Asymptomatic in early stages

     b. Occasionally see halos around lights

     c. Need for frequent change of glasses

     d. Occasional headaches

     e. Late-loss of central vision and ultimate blindness

  2. Primary angle-closure glaucoma—blockage of trabecular meshwork by peripheral iris resulting in inability of aqueous humor to be filtered

     a. Ocular pain

    b. Episodes of blurred vision

    c. Halos around lights at night

    d. Redness and congestion

- Differential Diagnosis

  1. Neurological disease

  2. Conjunctivitis

  3. Acute iritis

- Physical Findings

  1. Open-angle glaucoma

    a. Fundoscopic exam

      (1) Enlarged optic cup

      (2) Asymmetry of the two cups

      (3) Splinter hemorrhage on optic disc surface

    b. Visual field examinations—decreased ability to distinguish contrast or differential light sense

  2. Angle-closure glaucoma

    a. Anterior chamber is shallow

    b. Scarring of trabecular meshwork

    c. Corneal edema during acute attack

    d. Anterior chamber appears cloudy

- Diagnostic Tests/Findings

  1. Tonometry

    a. Pressure equal to or greater than 20 mm Hg requires further evaluation

    b. U.S. Preventive Service Task Force recommends screening tests of patients 65 and older by ophthalmologist

- Management/Treatment

  1. Depends on intraocular pressure, visual field loss, optic nerve damage

  2. Aim—control pressure to prevent optic nerve damage (below 20 mm Hg)

  3. Pharmacologic—open-angle glaucoma

      a. Miotics facilitate outflow

          (1)   Levobunolol hydrochloride (Betagan) 0.5% ophthalmic solution 1 gtt each eye b.i.d.

      b. ß-blockers reduce production of aqueous humor

          (1)   Timolol maleate (Timoptic Ophthalmic Solution) 0.25-0.50%, 1 gtt each eye b.i.d.

      c. Carbonic anhydrase inhibitors—reduce rate of formation of fluid

          (1)   Acetazolamide (Diamox)

          (2)   Methazolamide

      d. Hyperosmotics—reduce rate of formation of fluid

          (1)   Mannitol

4. Pharmacologic—acute angle-closure glaucoma

      a. Emergency treatment—parenteral acetazolamide, oral glycerol, isosorbide (in diabetics) or IV mannitol

      b. In addition topical pilocarpine and a ß-adrenergic antagonist

5. Primary acute angle-closure glaucoma may be treated with bilateral laser iridectomy

6. General considerations

      a. Ensure regular follow-up by ophthalmologist

      b. Observe for side effects of medications used in treatment

3. Instruct patient that anticholinergic drugs used systemically may cause blurred vision with close work

4. Advise patient that systemic corticosteroid use may interfere with glaucoma control of open angle glaucoma

Questions

Select the best answer

1. The common cold is best treated with

    a. Antibiotics
    b. Corticosteroides
    c. Antiviral agents
    d. Decongestants

2. Ms. Foster, age 36, is a third grade teacher, who is complaining of sore throat, non-productive cough, and a fever of 99.6 °F. Which of the following diagnostic tests is indicated?

    a. Chest radiograph
    b. AFB
    c. Throat culture
    d. Nasopharyngoscopy

3. A physical finding which differentiates influenza from a cold is

    a. Injected conjunctiva
    b. Watery eyes
    c. Clear nasal discharge
    d. Rales in lower lobes

4. Amantadine is most effective when administered

    a. Within 72 hours after initial exposure
    b. 24 to 48 hours after symptoms appear
    c. Prior to exposure to influenza B
    d. Within two hours of the onset of symptoms

5. The most effective prophylaxis against influenza is

    a. Amantadine 200 mg one time only
    b. Influenza vaccine administered after exposure
    c. Amantadine 100 mg b.i.d. for 5 days
    d. Influenza vaccine administered in the fall

6. Organisms which frequently cause pharyngitis are *Corynebacterium hemolyticum* and herpes simplex. A sign which is frequently seen with corynebacterium is

    a. Associated rhinitis
    b. Mucosal vesicles
    c. Rash
    d. "Cold sores"

7. Sore throats are common and often caused by Group A streptococci. This condition is most frequently treated with

   a. Ceftriaxone
   b. Benzathine penicillin
   c. Amantadine
   d. Erythromycin

8. Mr. Adams, age 65, presents complaining of rhinitis for the past two weeks after mowing the lawn. If his condition is allergic rhinitis, the physical findings would include

   a. Pale, swollen nasal mucosa
   b. Erythematous nasal mucosa
   c. Tender lymph nodes
   d. Polyps on the vocal cords

9. An antibiotic which is frequently effective in the treatment of sinusitis is

   a. Ceftriaxone
   b. Erythromycin
   c. Decadron
   d. Ampicillin

10. Diagnosis of group A beta-hemolytic streptococcal pharyngitis is based on

    a. Elevated WBC
    b. Presence of pharyngeal exudate
    c. Positive gram stain
    d. Positive throat culture or streptococcal antigen test

11. Mr. Edwards is suffering from tinnitus and hearing loss associated with intake of streptomycin. This type of hearing loss is

    a. Conductive
    b. Sensorineural
    c. Neuromuscular
    d. Mixed conductive and sensorineural

12. Ms. Kahn, 20 years old, presents complaining of itching eyes and nose and sneezing, which began after being exposed to dust when cleaning her attic. The initial approach to her care would be

    a. Begin skin testing
    b. Avoidance of exposure to irritant
    c. Begin immunotherapy
    d. Determine her vital capacity

13. A concern associated with the use of topical decongestent nasal sprays is

    a. Addiction
    b. Anaphylactic reaction
    c. Rhinitis medicamentosa
    d. Dehydration

14. Presbycusis is most frequently associated with aging and is a type of

    a. Hearing loss
    b. Visual impairment
    c. Neurovascular disorder
    d. Vestibular obstruction

15. Hearing impairment caused by otosclerosis is considered a

    a. Sensorineural hearing loss
    b. Condition associated with osteoarthritis
    c. Conductive hearing loss
    d. Obstructive hearing loss

16. Mr. Adams was previously diagnosed with chronic serous otitis media in the right ear. When conducting a Rinne test, you would most likely find

    a. Air conduction greater than bone conduction, bilaterally
    b. Bone conduction greater than air conduction in the right ear
    c. Bone conduction greater than air conduction in the left ear
    d. Bone conduction less than air conduction in the right ear

17. Mrs. James, age 35, presents complaining of tinnitus, nausea, and a sensation of motion. When testing extraocular movements, you would specifically observe for

    a. Lid lag
    b. Unequal pupil size
    c. Nystagmus
    d. Inability to accommodate to light

18. Ear pain, which is exacerbated by movement of the jaw, is most often associated with

    a. Otitis externa
    b. Serous otitis media
    c. Acute otitis media
    d. Meniere's disease

19. Acute otitis media in adults is frequently caused by

    a. Staphylococcus

    b. Streptococcus

    c. Fungus

    d. Pneumococcus

20. The definition of legal blindness is

    a. 20/200 in the worst eye with correction

    b. 100/200 in the best eye

    c. 20/200 in the best eye with correction

    d. 20/100 in the best eye without correction

21. Topical anesthetics should not be prescribed for patients with corneal abrasions because

    a. They inhibit tearing

    b. They may lead to iritis

    c. They increase risk of eye injury

    d. They interfere with canal of Schlem circulation

22. Ms. Cahan, a 30 year old school teacher, presents with an injected right eye, watery discharge, and a palpable preauricular lymph node. She is diagnosed with viral conjunctivitis. Which of the following symptoms might be expected on history

    a. Blurred vision

    b. Itching

    c. "Flashing lights"

    d. Sore throat

23. Management of viral conjunctivitis for Ms. Cahan should include

    a. Broad spectrum antibiotics

    b. Instruction to stay home from work until eye is clear

    c. Corticosteroid optic solution

    d. Visine OTC ophthalmic solution

24. When visualizing the red reflex in a patient with a suspected cataract, the following might be found

    a. Arteriovenous nicking

    b. Dark defects

    c. Bright red inflammatory response

    d. A "flashing" pattern on the retina

25. Upon entering a dark room, after being out in the sun, Mrs. Adams, age 45, experiences pain in her right eye and blurred vision. These symptoms are consistent with

    a. Traumatic cataract

    b. Open angle glaucoma

    c. Angle closure glaucoma

    d. Trachoma

26. Infectious mononucleosis is caused by

    a. Herpes simplex virus

    b. Herpes zoster virus

    c. Epstein-Barr virus

    d. Echovirus

27. Epistaxis is primarily treated with

    a. Rest and ice packs to the anterior segment of the nose

    b. Phenylephrine 0.25% applied to the nasal mucosa for 10 minutes

    c. Compression of the nasal alae for 10 minutes

    d. Ice pack to forehead with patient in forward leaning position

Answers

1. d
2. c
3. d
4. b
5. d
6. c
7. b
8. a
9. d
10. d
11. b
12. b
13. c
14. a
15. c
16. b
17. c
18. a
19. b
20. c
21. c
22. d
23. b
24. b
25. c
26. c
27. c

Bibliography

Abrams, W. B., & Berkow, R. (Eds.) (1990). *The Merck manual of geriatrics*. Rahway, NJ: Merck & Co.

Andreoli, T. E., Carpenter, C. J., Plum, F., & Smith, Jr., L. H. (1990). *Cecil: Essentials of medicine*. Philadelphia: W. B. Saunders

Barker, L. R., Burton, J. R., & Zieve, P. D. (Eds.). (1991). *Principles of ambulatory medicine*. Baltimore: Williams and Wilkins.

Cleaskin, L. G. (1992). Angle closure glaucoma precipitated by atropine. *Archives of Internal Medicine, 68*(796), 132-133.

Del Mar, C. (1992). Managing sore throat: A literature review. *Medical Journal of Australia, 156*(8), 572-575.

Gacek, R. R. (1992). A differential diagnosis of unilateral serous otitis media. *Laryngoscopy. 102*(4), 461-468.

Garahan, M. B. (1992). Hearing loss prevalence and management in nursing home residents. *Journal of the American Geriatric Society. 40*(2), 130-134.

Nathenson, A. L. (1992). Cataract development and removal. How to answer the questions a patient asks, *Postgraduate Medicine. 91*(5), 129-130, 133, 136-138.

Sapira, J. D. (1990). *The art and science of bedside diagnosis*. Baltimore: Urban & Schwartzenberg.

Schroeder, S., Krupp, M. A., Tierney, Jr., L. M., & McPhee, S. J. (Eds.). (1991). *Current medical diagnosis and treatment*. Norwalk, CT: Appleton & Lange.

Sibbald, B. (1991). Epidemiology of seasonal and perennial rhinitis: Clinical presentation and medical history. *Thorax. 46*(12), 895-901.

Respiratory Disorders

Madeline Turkeltaub

Pulmonary Function Testing

Proper assessment of most patients with pulmonary disease requires the use of pulmonary function testing. Knowledge of these tests is important to obtaining accurate results and relating the results to the patient's diagnosis. The most frequently used pulmonary function testing will be discussed, prior to specific respiratory problems.

- Indications for use of pulmonary function tests (PFT)
  1. Evaluation of dyspnea, cough, pulmonary dysfunction
  2. Evaluation of effectiveness of therapy
  3. Disability assessment, including evaluation of risk factors in work settings
  4. Pre-operative evaluation
  5. Re-evaluation of progress of restrictive or obstructive disease
- Types of pulmonary function tests
  1. FVC—forced vital capacity; produced by forceful expulsion from lungs after maximum inhalation
  2. FEV_1—forced expiratory volume; the volume of air expelled in the first second of FVC
  3. PEFR—peak expiratory flow rate; the maximum air flow rate on forceful expulsion after maximum inspiration
  4. TLC—total lung capacity; volume of air in the lungs after maximum inhalation
  5. FRC—functional residual capacity; air left in lungs after a normal unforced expiration
  6. RV—residual volume; air remaining in the lungs after maximum exhalation
- General relationship of PFTs to pulmonary disease
  1. Obstructive pulmonary disease is characterized by reduced air flow rates.
  2. Restrictive pulmonary disease is associated with reduced lung volumes.

Acute Bronchitis

- Definition: Inflammation of the tracheobronchial tree, usually as a sequela to an upper respiratory tract infection

- Etiology/Incidence

  1. Rhinovirus and coronavirus are associated with short and afebrile episodes of bronchitis

  2. Adenovirus, influenza, and *M. pneumoniae* cause more severe, febrile bronchitis

  3. Frequency and severity increases in cigarette smokers

- Signs and Symptoms

  1. Purulent sputum

  2. Frequent cough

  3. Fever or chills occur infrequently

  4. Headache

  5. Myalgias

  6. Lethargy

  7. Wheezing and mild dyspnea on exertion

- Differential Diagnosis

  1. Pneumonia

  2. Noninfectious causes of cough

     a. Allergens

     b. Repeated aspiration of small amounts of fluid in patients with difficulty in swallowing

  3. Pertussis

  4. Upper respiratory infection

  5. Influenza

- Physical Findings

  1. Chest and lungs

     a. Wheezing

     b. Scattered crackles

     c. Diffuse rhonchi

- Diagnostic Tests/Findings

  1. Chest radiograph—normal in acute bronchitis

2. Sputum cultures are *not* useful.

3. WBC—normal or slightly elevated

- Management/Treatment

   1. Usually *not* treated with antibiotics in otherwise healthy persons.

   2. Symptomatic relief

      a. Cough suppression for night cough—codeine preparation

      b. Expectorants

      c. Bronchodilators for wheezing

      d. Force fluids to 3,000 cc/day to liquify secretions

      e. Steam inhalations

      f. Cool mist

      g. Decrease irritants in environment

         (1) Stop smoking

         (2) Avoid pollutants

   3. Smokers must be supported in attempts to stop

   4. Condition usually resolves in 7 to 10 days

   5. Refer to M.D. if symptoms do not begin to improve in 72 hours

Chronic Bronchitis (Simple)

- Definition: A productive cough for at least 3 months of the year during at least 2 to 3 successive years

- Etiology/Incidence

   1. All forms strongly linked to cigarette smoking

   2. Some occupations, e.g., those involving dust, grain and mining associated with high incidence; also environmental pollution

   3. Chronic inflammation primary pathological mechanism

- Signs and Symptoms

   1. Earliest symptom is usually a frequent, productive cough; as severity increases patient coughs more frequently and sputum production increases

   2. Change in sputum

     a. Color

     b. Consistency

     c. Amount

  3. Dyspnea

  4. Fatigue

  5. Fever and chills

- Differential Diagnosis

  1. Pneumonia

  2. Lung cancer

  3. Cystic fibrosis in young adults

  4. Bronchiectasis

  5. Tuberculosis (TB)

- Physical Findings

  1. Lungs

     a. Percussion—resonant $->$ dull, if consolidation is present

     b. Auscultation—rales, rhonchi, wheezes

     c. Slight to marked increase in anteroposterior diameter

- Diagnostic Tests/Findings

  1. Gram stains and cultures are generally not useful.

  2. Chest radiograph—increased bronchovascular markings

  3. Spirometry—during acute infection will be decreased from patient's baseline

  4. Hematocrit and hemoglobin increased

  5. Arterial blood gases (ABGs)—decreased Pa O_2, increased Pa CO_2

  6. PPD—to rule out TB

- Management/Treatment

  1. Cigarette smoking should be stopped; other bronchial irritants removed

  2. Clear secretions

     a. Postural drainage

     b. Bronchodilators

(1) Theophylline—200 mg every 12 hours initially, then 200 to 600 mg orally every 8 to 12 hours

(2) Albuterol—metered dose inhaler, 1 to 4 puffs every 4 to 6 hours

3. Do *not* use cough suppressants

4. Short term antibiotic therapy if an organism is identified

5. Support efforts to stop smoking

6. Patient should seek professional assistance if

   a. Develops "chest cold"

   b. Increased cough, dyspnea, fatigue

Pneumonia

- Definition: Inflammation of the lower respiratory tract (terminal airways and alveolar spaces)

- Etiology/Incidence

1. 3,000,000 episodes annually in U.S.

2. Influenza pneumonia

   a. Fifth ranked cause of death in U.S.

   b. First ranked cause of death from infectious disease

   c. Most common cause of death in centenarians

3. Caused by

   a. Viruses

   b. Chlamydia

   c. Rickettsia

   d. Mycoplasma

   e. Bacteria—*S. pneumoniae* most common

   f. Protozoans

   g. Parasites

- Signs and Symptoms

1. Mycoplasma pneumonia

   a. Hacking non-productive cough

      b. Malaise

      c. Myalgia

      d. Fever without increased pulse

  2. Bacterial pneumonia

      a. Sudden onset of shaking chills

      b. Severe pleuritic pain

      c. Cough

      d. Fever

      e. Rusty or yellow sputum

  3. Viral pneumonia

      a. Non-productive cough

      b. Malaise

      c. Headache

      d. Fever

■ Differential Diagnosis

  1. Differentiated based on duration of symptoms

      a. 0 to 5 days

          (1)   Pneumococcus

          (2)   Mycoplasma

          (3)   Virus

      b. 10 days or more

          (1)   Mycobacterium

          (2)   Fungal

          (3)   Anaerobic

  2. Primary tuberculosis

  3. Lung tumor

  4. Bronchial asthma

  5. Congestive heart failure

■ Physical Findings

  1. Physical examination may be normal in early stages

2. Bacterial pneumonia

    a. Evidence of consolidation

        (1) Dullness to percussion

        (2) Bronchial breath sounds, egophony

        (3) Rales

        (4) Increased fremitus

        (5) Whispered petroliloquy

        (6) Shortness of breath

3. Crepitant rales that do not clear with cough

4. No physical findings of consolidation in viral pneumonia

- Diagnostic Tests/Findings

    1. Chest radiograph will show infiltrate (lobar consolidation) in bacterial

    2. Gram stained sputum smear

        a. May be positive for pneumococci

        b. Large gram positive cocci related to staphyloccus

        c. Small gram negative cocci related to *Haemophilus influenzae*

    3. Sputum culture—in high risk elderly who are at greater risk for non-pneumococcal pneumonia

    4. Blood cultures in more severely ill patients to identify specific organisms related to differential diagnosis

    5. Refer for thoracentesis if pleural effusion present

    6. WBC often elevated

        a. Bacterial pneumonia

            (1) 20 to 30,000/mm^3

            (2) Shift to left

        b. Non-bacterial pneumonia

            (1) Slight elevation

    7. Serum bilirubin elevation

        a. Bacterial pneumonia

        b. Most common in pneumococcal pneumonia

8. PPD to rule out tuberculosis

■ Management/Treatment

1. Antimicrobial therapy

    a. Pneumococcal pneumonia—300,000 U procaine penicillin IM one time; then, penicillin V 250 mg every 6 hours orally for 10 days

    b. Atypical pneumonia syndrome—erythromycin 250 to 500 mg q.i.d. for 14 days

2. Force fluids to 3,000 cc/day

3. Acetaminophen for fever and headache

4. Avoid cough suppressants and cigarettes

5. Follow-up chest radiograph, if no improvement in 3 to 4 days

6. Follow-up chest radiograph in 4 to 6 weeks in all patients over 40 and all smokers

7. Review fluid intake requirements

8. Educate regarding adherence to medication administration schedule

    a. Erythromycin

        (1) Take with meals

        (2) Monitor theophylline levels

        (3) Not to be taken with Seldane or Hismanal

9. Schedule to return to office in 3 to 4 days to determine progress on medication

10. Review importance of deep breathing exercises

11. Review importance of follow-up radiograph

Asthma

■ Definition: A reversible (episodic) lung disorder characterized by inflammation, edema of respiratory mucosa, excessive sputum production, and bronchospasm

■ Etiology/Incidence

1. Caused by

    a. Allergens (most commonly pollens, molds, house dust, animal danders)

b. Nonallergenic factors (infection, irritants, emotional factors)

2. Affects men and women equally; approximately 4% of the population in the U.S.

3. Chronic condition with acute exacerbations

- Signs and Symptoms

    1. Cough

    2. Wheezing

    3. Shortness of breath

    4. Chest tightness

    5. Sputum production (moderate)

    6. Exercise intolerance

    7. Conditions associated with asthma

        a. Rhinitis

        b. Sinusitis

        c. Nasal polyps

        d. Atopic dermatitis

- Differential Diagnosis

    1. Heart disease—congestive heart failure

    2. Foreign bodies in airways

    3. Chronic obstructive pulmonary disease

    4. Chronic bronchitis

    5. Pulmonary embolism

    6. Cough secondary to beta blockers or ACE inhibitors

    7. Acute attack may resemble anaphylaxis

- Physical Findings

    1. Purulent nasal and post nasal discharge, consistent with sinusitis

    2. Evidence of hyperinflation of lungs

        a. Use of accessory muscles

        b. "Pigeon chest"

    3. Quality of breath sounds

    a. Wheezing—usually expiratory

    b. Decreased intensity of breath sounds

    c. Prolonged phase of forced expiration

- Diagnostic Tests/Findings
  1. Pulmonary function tests
     a. Peak expiratory flow rate < 80% of predicted norm for gender, age, height
     b. Vital capacity reduced
  2. CBC—eosinophils are increased in asthma related to an allergic response
  3. Sputum examination positive for eosinophilia
  4. Nasal secretion stain positive for eosinophilia
  5. Determination of allergic component by skin testing or in vitro methods
  6. Bronchoprovocation with methacholine, histamine, or exercise challenge induces symptoms
  7. Pulsus paradoxus—an exaggerated fall in systolic blood pressure during inspiration

- Management/Treatment
  1. Monitor measures of lung function, using peak flow meter
     a. Establish patient's "personal best" and treat based on percent of personal best. The "personal best" is the highest PEFR measurement after a period of maximum therapy
        (1) 80 to 100%—maintain on treatment as prescribed
        (2) 50 to 80%—acute exacerbation; adjust maintenance program
        (3) Below 50%—medical alert identification; bronchodilator
  2. Medications
     a. Anti-inflammatory agents
        (1) Corticosteroids—most effective
           (a) Inhaled corticosteroids, e.g.,
               1) Beclomethasone
               2) Triamcinolone
               3) Flunisolide

        (b)   Oral corticosteroids—in treatment of exacerbations of asthma

     (2)   Cromolyn sodium—decreases airway narrowing after exercise

  b. Bronchodilators—relax bronchial smooth muscle

     (1)   Beta-adrenergic agonists—inhaled preferred

     (2)   Methylxanthines—theophylline, if other drugs not effective

  c. Anticholinergics—reduce vagal tone to airways

3. Environmental measures to decrease irritants

  a. Avoid outdoor allergens

  b. Eliminate indoor allergens

4. Educating the patient—key components

  a. Signs and symptoms to report

  b. Controlling asthma triggers and planning avoidance strategies

  c. Correct use of inhalers

  d. Use of peak flow meter

5. Indications for referral

  a. Newly diagnosed patients

  b. Elderly patients

  c. Lack of response to therapy

6. Indications for hospitalization

  a. Pulsus paradoxus

  b. Cardiovascular-system disease (CVS)

  c. Nonresponse to emergency treatment

  d. Persistently low PEFR

  e. Respiratory acidosis

7. Review use of peak flow meter at home

8. Review adverse effects of oral steroids, including need to taper dose

9. Review adverse effects of inhaled corticosteroids

a. Oropharyngeal candidiasis

b. Dysphonia

10. Advise patient receiving theophylline to report conditions that reduce or interfere with elimination of theophylline

a. Fever

b. Liver disease

c. Use of antibiotics—erythromycin

11. Develop written action plans to help the patient co-manage asthma exacerbations

12. Include patient's family in treatment plan

13. Review use of metered dose inhalers

14. ASA is contraindicated in patients with asthma

15. Stress management

Chronic Obstructive Pulmonary Disease (COPD)

- Definition: Progressive respiratory disease syndrome associated with varying combinations of chronic bronchitis, asthma and emphysema.

- Etiology/Incidence

  1. Affects 8 to 9 million people in U.S.

  2. Affects more males than females, but prevalence in women is rising rapidly

  3. 10% of smokers develop COPD

  4. Heredity and age increase risk

  5. Occupational exposure to irritants

  6. Peak age

      a. Chronic bronchitis—45 to 65 years of age

      b. Emphysema—65 to 75 years of age

- Signs and Symptoms

  1. Emphysema (Pink Puffer)

      a. Early stage—mild dyspnea, little cough, fatigue

      b. Later stage—severe dyspnea, at times through pursed lips; thin, barrel chest

c. Flushed

d. Clear, mucoid sputum

2. Chronic bronchitis (Blue Bloater)

a. Mild

(1) Morning cough productive of clear sputum

(2) Dyspnea on exertion (DOE)

(3) Copious mucus production, causing nocturnal wakenings

b. Severe

(1) Cyanosis

(2) Edema

(3) Cardiomegaly

(4) Recurrent respiratory failure

(5) Development of mucopurulent sputum

■ Differential Diagnosis

1. Asthma

2. Congestive heart failure

3. Tuberculosis (TB)

4. Acute bronchitis

■ Physical Findings

1. Emphysema

a. Thin

b. Hypertrophied accessory muscles of respiration

c. Increased chest diameter (barrel chest)

d. Lungs

(1) Hyperresonance

(2) Diminished breath sounds

2. Chronic bronchitis

a. Obese

b. Central cyanosis

c. Lungs—wheezes, rhonchi

d. Heart—enlarged

- Diagnostic Tests/Findings

  1. Forced expiratory volume greater than 3 seconds in COPD (both emphysema and chronic bronchitis

  2. Decreased vital capacity and expiratory flow rates in COPD

  3. Increased respiratory volume and total lung capacity in emphysema

  4. 15 to 20% increase in expiratory flow after bronchodilator in COPD

  5. Arterial blood gases indicate hypoxemia

  6. Polycythemia in advanced stages of chronic bronchitis

  7. Chest radiograph—increased markings in chronic bronchitis

  8. ECG may disclose right ventricular hypertrophy in severe chronic bronchitis

  9. Respiratory acidosis occurs in chronic bronchitis

  10. PPD—to rule out tuberculosis

- Management/Treatment

  1. Refer all patients with COPD to M.D. until stable

  2. Avoid irritants

     a. Smoking (major irritant)

     b. Air pollutants

     c. ASA and beta-blockers

     d. Temperature extremes

  3. Sputum liquification

     a. Adequate hydration—force fluids to 3,000 cc/day

     b. Humidifier in home

  4. Bronchodilators—metaproterenol, terbutaline, albuterol

  5. Chest physiotherapy and postural drainage

  6. Oxygen therapy to achieve a PaO_2 of greater than 55 mm Hg (usually 1 to 3 L/min)

  7. Education regarding factors which contribute to upper respiratory

infection

8. Support smoking cessation efforts

9. Respiratory rehabilitation, including deep breathing exercises with pursed lip exhalation

10. Review signs and symptoms of respiratory infection and CHF

11. One out of four with COPD develop peptic ulcer at some time; therefore, review signs and symptoms

12. Instructions on coughing effectively—prior to coughing, take a deep breath

Tuberculosis

- Definition: Chronic bacterial infectious disease; usually involves lungs, but can occur in lymph nodes, bones, kidneys and meninges and can be disseminated throughout the body. Primary pulmonary tuberculosis will be the focus of this section.

- Etiology/Incidence

    1. Cause is mycobacteria of "tuberculosis complex," primarily *Mycobacterium tuberculosis*

    2. Usually spread by airborne droplet nuclei

    3. 25,000 cases per year in U.S.; expected to increase as a complication of AIDS

    4. Estimated that approximately 10 million people in the U.S. are infected

    5. High risk populations include

        a. HIV infected individuals

        b. Close contacts of infected patients

        c. Low income populations

        d. Alcoholics and IV drug users

        e. Residents of long-term care facilities

        f. Refugees from Asia and Central America

        g. Correctional institution frequenters

- Signs and Symptoms

    1. Fatigue

    2. Weight loss

3. Fever

4. Night sweats

5. Cough productive of purulent sputum

6. Hemoptysis with advancing disease

7. Pleuritic chest pain

- Differential Diagnosis

    1. Pneumonia

    2. Bronchogenic cancer

    3. Pleurisy

    4. Histoplasmosis

- Physical Findings

    1. Appear chronically ill

    2. Weak and cachectic

    3. Chest

        a. Auscultation—apical rales, following cough or normal

        b. Palpation—increased tactile fremitus over consolidated areas

        c. Percussion—dull

- Diagnostic Tests/Findings

    1. Chest radiograph—pulmonary infiltrates with hilar adenopathy

    2. PPD

        a. Positive with active disease or prior exposure

        b. BCG is a variable, but PPD should be done

        c. AIDS patients may have diminished reactivity

    3. PPD interpretation

        a. A reaction of 5 mm is considered positive in patients with

            (1) Recent close contact with infected person

            (2) Evidence of inactive disease

            (3) HIV infected

        b. A reaction of 10 mm is considered positive in the following

            (1) Medical risk patients, such as diabetes mellitus, cancer and

end stage renal disease

    (2)   Immigrants from Asia, Africa, Latin America

    (3)   Medically underserved, low income populations

    (4)   High risk minorities

    (5)   Residents of nursing homes and prisons

  c. A reaction of 15 mm is considered positive for all populations

4.   Sputum, gastric/tracheal culture

  a. Essential to confirm diagnosis of TB

  b. Takes 3 to 6 weeks for results to be obtained

■ Management/Treatment

1.   Medication (for sensitive organisms)

   a. Isoniazid (INH) daily—5 mg/kg up to 300 mg per day for 2 months, together with

   b. Rifampin daily—10 mg/kg up to 600 mg per day for 2 months

  c. Pyrazinamide—15 to 30 mg/kg up to 2 grams per day for 2 months

  d. Follow a, b, c with 4 months of daily or twice weekly INH and rifampin

2.   Medication (for resistant bacilli) in addition to above, until sensitivities to drugs are known

  a. If INH resistance suspected, ethambutol added first 2 months—15 to 20 mg/kg for 2 months, or

  b. Pyrazinamide—15 to 30 mg/kg for 2 months, or

  c. Streptomycin—15 mg/kg IM

3.   Contact tracing

4.   BCG vaccine may be recommended for skin test negative individuals who have repeated exposure

5.   Refer patients with positive skin tests and follow-up after treatment is initiated

6.   Almost all properly treated patients are cured

7.   Reportable disease—report to state and local health departments

8.   Stress importance of compliance with medication regimen

9.   Review symptoms of drug toxicity

    a. INH—peripheral neuropathy, hepatitis, hypersensitivity

    b. Rifampin—orange discoloration of secretions and urine; nausea and vomiting

    c. Pyrazinamide—hepatotixicity, hyperuricemia

10. Stress importance of nutritious diet and education regarding selection of foods

Lung Cancer

- Definition: Primary malignant neoplasm of the lung; cell types involved include squamous cell, adenocarcinoma, large cell carcinoma, and small cell carcinoma.

- Etiology/Incidence

  1. Lung cancer is the leading cause of death of men and women in the U.S.

  2. Males 2.5 times more frequent than females

  3. Most common in the 50 to 60 years old

  4. Occurrence is directly proportional to the number of cigarettes smoked per day

  5. Cigarette smoke in combination with other environmental pollutants (e.g., asbestos) influence increased incidence

- Signs and Symptoms: Depend on the area of metastasis, involvement of nodes or other organs. The focus is on the signs and symptoms most frequently seen in primary care.

  1. Symptoms due to primary tumor

     a. "Smoker's cough"—most common early symptom

     b. Weight loss

     c. Dyspnea—related to obstruction of major bronchus

     d. Hemoptysis—20% of all patients with hemoptysis have lung cancer

     e. Wheezing

     f. Fever

     g. Chest pain—related to extension beyond parenchyma

- Differential Diagnosis

  1. Pneumonia

2. Lung abscess

3. Bronchitis

4. Tuberculosis (TB)

- Physical Findings

    1. Physical examination may not reveal significant changes, unless a major bronchus is obstructed.

    2. Visible or palpable lymph nodes in supraclavicular fossae

- Diagnostic Test/Findings

    1. Chest radiograph

        a. Negative in 15% of patients with lung cancer

        b. Not diagnostic in itself, but indicates need for additional investigation

        c. Manifestations—enlarging mass, infiltrate, atelectasis, cavitation, or pleural effusion

    2. Laboratory

        a. CBC

        b. Liver function tests

        c. Serum electrolytes and calcium

    3. Definitive diagnosis requires cytologic or histologic evidence.

    4. Sputum for cytology—positive in 40 to 50% of patients

    5. Bronchoscopy with biopsy

- Management/Treatment

    1. Surgery—25% of patients with lung cancer are candidates for surgery

    2. Chemotherapy

    3. Radiation therapy—generally palliative

    4. Refer to M.D. as soon as lung cancer is suspected

    5. Encourage patient to stop smoking

    6. Decrease exposure to pollutants

    7. Report change in symptoms, for example, hemoptysis

    8. Instruction on side effects of chemotherapy/radiation; assistance in

managing side effects

9. Diet high in nutrients

10. Pain control

Questions

Select the best answer

1. Which of the following characteristics is common to Mycoplasma pneumonia?

   a. Seizures due to extreme temperature elevation
   b. Respiratory rate increase of 40 to 80 per minute
   c. Increased fever without increased pulse rate
   d. Severe chills preceding onset of other symptoms

2. A 55 year old patient, with frequent cough productive of thick yellow mucus, presents for evaluation. Thick yellow exudate is consistent with

   a. Viral pneumonia
   b. Bacterial pneumonia
   c. Hypostatic pneumonia
   d. Mycoplasma pneumonia

3. All of the following signs and symptoms are associated with emphysema, except

   a. Purse-lipped breathing
   b. Barrel shaped chest
   c. Usually thin in appearance
   d. Continuous cough with copious sputum

4. The purpose of beclomethasone in the treatment of asthma is

   a. Anti-inflammatory
   b. Diuretic
   c. Antitussive
   d. Decongestant

5. A condition associated with acute asthma may be

   a. Bronchopneumonia
   b. Rhinitis
   c. Epiglottitis
   d. Infectious mononucleosis

6. John Greene, age 63, presents with increased shortness of breath over the past week and a previous diagnosis of emphysema. Pulmonary function studies on Mr. Greene would most likely demonstrate

   a. Decreased forced expiratory volume, increased total lung capacity, increased residual volume
   b. Increased forced expiratory volume; decreased total lung capacity, increased

residual volume

 c. Decreased forced expiratory volume, decreased total lung capacity, decreased residual volume

 d. Increased forced expiratory volume, increased total capacity, decreased residual volume

7. In teaching Mr. Greene to cough, it is important to emphasize that he

 a. Take a deep breath and cough
 b. Actively cough at the end of full expiration
 c. Cough after taking medication
 d. Take a moderately deep breath, exhale and then cough

8. A teaching concern for Mr. Greene is his understanding about the avoidance of respiratory irritants. Select the single most important cause of respiratory irritation

 a. Inhaling dust or fumes
 b. Breathing cold air
 c. Cigarette smoke
 d. Allergens

9. Which of the following is definitively diagnostic of acute bronchitis?

 a. Chest radiograph
 b. WBC
 c. Sputum culture
 d. None of the above

10. When initially treating acute bronchitis, you would be least likely to order

 a. Antibiotics
 b. Expectorants
 c. Bronchodilators
 d. Antitussives at night

11. The area of consolidation most frequently associated with bacterial pneumonia is

 a. Bronchial
 b. Lobar
 c. Central
 d. Pleural

12. All of the following provide evidence of consolidation, except

 a. Increased fremitus
 b. Whispered petroliloquy
 c. Dullness on percussion
 d. Resonance on percussion

13. Pulsus paradoxus is most frequently associated with

    a. Pneumonia
    b. Asthma
    c. Bronchitis
    d. Emphysema

14. Following physical examination on Mr. Amos, you suspect bacterial pneumonia. A change that would be anticipated in the WBC is

    a. Shift to the right
    b. No change
    c. Shift to the left
    d. Slight elevation

15. Occasionally, a serum bilirubin elevation will be seen in a patient with pneumonia. The organism most commonly associated with this finding is

    a. Chlamydia
    b. Mycoplasma
    c. Pneumococci
    d. Rickettsia

16. Mr. Somer, age 46, smokes 1 pack of cigarettes per day. He was treated for pneumonia and has returned 4 weeks later for a follow-up visit. At this time it would be appropriate to

    a. Discontinue the antibiotics
    b. Obtain a chest radiograph
    c. Repeat the WBC
    d. Order a CAT scan

17. Pulsus paradoxus is

    a. An increase in diastolic blood pressure on expiration
    b. A decrease in systolic blood pressure on inspiration
    c. A decrease in systolic blood pressure on exhalation
    d. An increase in systolic blood pressure on inspiration

18. Asthma affects what percentage of people in the United States?

    a. 25%
    b. 50%
    c. 10%
    d. 4%

19. You are obtaining a peak expiratory flow rate on a patient suspected of asthma. You should provide the following instruction

    a. Take a deep breath and blow out as hard and fast as you can with your lips around the mouthpiece.

b. Take a normal breath and use the monitor to measure exhalation

c. Slowly exhale after maximal inhalation

d. Take a deep breath and blow into the meter for one second

20. Examination of nasal secretions and sputum of an asthmatic will typically yield

a. Clue cells

b. Bacteria

c. Viral particles

d. Eosinophilia

21. The purpose of a methacholine challenge for a patient with asthma is to

a. Improve symptoms

b. Provide bronchodilation

c. Reproduce symptoms and confirm diagnosis

d. Confirm that the airway obstruction is not reversible

22. Mr. Chuong, who recently emigrated from Viet Nam, presents with fatigue, night sweats, and anorexia. You suspect tuberculosis and administer a PPD skin test. In this patient, the size of a positive reaction would be

a. 5 mm

b. 10 mm

c. 15 mm

d. 20 mm

23. When the diagnosis of tuberculosis is confirmed, it is required that

a. The results are reported to the county and state health departments

b. The patient is treated within 24 hours of diagnosis

c. All contacts are notified by the patient

d. The patient stop working

24. A major reason for the increase in the incidence of tuberculosis in the U.S. is

a. An increase in the elderly population

b. Decreased effectiveness of medication

c. Increase in the number of HIV infected individuals

d. Increase in population below the poverty level

25. Mr. Chuong is found to have active tuberculosis. He weighs 220 pounds and is to start on a regimen of Isoniazid, Rifampin, and Streptomycin. The maximum daily dose of Isoniazid to be prescribed is

a. 300 mg

b. 500 mg

c. 1 gm

    d. 100 mg

26. The majority of patients with tuberculosis can be cured. The greatest barrier to the success of treatment is

    a. Inadequate diagnostic testing
    b. Ineffective medication
    c. High risk family history
    d. Non-compliance

27. The diagnosis of tuberculosis is not confirmed until culture results are returned. Treatment until that point is presumptive. Culture results are generally available in

    a. 2 to 3 days
    b. 2 to 3 weeks
    c. 24 hours
    d. 3 to 6 weeks

28. Risk factors for lung cancer include all of the following, except

    a. Gender—male
    b. Age—50 to 60 years of age
    c. Cigarette smoking
    d. Co-existing asthma

29. Definitive diagnosis of lung cancer is dependent upon

    a. Sputum culture
    b. Elevated liver enzymes
    c. Chest radiograph
    d. Histologic evidence

30. Beclomethasone is an example of

    a. Decongestant
    b. Inhaled corticosteroids
    c. Antihistamine
    d. Antitussive

Answers

1. c
2. b
3. d
4. a
5. b
6. a
7. a
8. c
9. d
10. a
11. b
12. d
13. b
14. c
15. c
16. b
17. b
18. d
19. a
20. d
21. c
22. b
23. a
24. c
25. a
26. d
27. d
28. d
29. d
30. b

Bibliography

Abrams, W. B., & Berkow, R. (Eds.). (1990). *The Merck manual of geriatrics*. Rahway, NJ: Merck & Co., Inc.

Andreoli, T. E., Carpenter, C. J., Plum, F., & Smith, Jr., L. H. (1990). *Cecil: Essentials of medicine*. Philadelphia: W. B. Saunders.

Barker, L. R., Burton, J. R., & Zieve, P. D. (Eds.). (1991). *Principles of ambulatory medicine*. Baltimore: Williams & Wilkins.

Core curriculum on tuberculosis. (1991). Atlanta: Centers for Disease Control.

Goldstein, T. S. (1991). *Geriatric orthopedics*. Rockville, MD: Aspen Publishers.

Guidelines for the diagnosis and management of asthma (1991). (Publication No. 91-3042A). Bethesda, MD: National Institutes of Health.

Hofford, J. M. (1992). Metered dose inhaler therapy for asthma, bronchitis and emphysema. *Journal of Family Practice. 34*(4), 485-492.

Jones, K. (1992). Late onset asthma. *The Practitioner, 236*(1520), 1047-1050.

Pearson, R. (1991). Nurses in the management of asthma. *The Practitioner, 235*(1509), 947-8, 951.

Ruder, K. P. (1990). Peak flow meters: Are they monitoring tools or training devices? *Journal of Asthma, 27*(4), 219-27.

Sapira, J. D. (1990). *The art and science of bedside diagnosis*. Baltimore: Urban & Schwartzenberg.

Schroeder, S., Krupp, M. A., Tierney, Jr., L. M., & McPhee, S. J. (Eds.). (1991). *Current medical diagnosis and treatment*. Norwalk, CT: Appleton & Lange.

Cardiovascular Disorders

Marilyn W. Edmunds

Hypertension

■ Definition: A persistent elevation of systolic blood pressure (SBP) and/or diastolic blood pressure (DBP) at or above the normal parameters of 140 SBP and 90 DBP on at least 3 consecutive readings (National Heart, Lung and Blood Institute [NHLB] 1993)

1. Classification of blood pressure for adults age 18 years and older (NHLB, 1993, p.4)

Category	Systolic (mm Hg)	Diastolic (mm Hg)
Normal	under 130	under 85
High Normal	130-139	85-89
Hypertension*		
Stage 1 (Mild)	140-159	90-99
Stage 2 (Moderate)	160-179	100-109
Stage 3 (Severe)	180-209	110-119
Stage 4 (Very Severe)	210 and above	120 and above

"When systolic and diastolic pressures fall into different categories, the higher category should be selected to classify the individual's blood pressure status. For instance, 160/92mm Hg should be classified as Stage 2, and 180/120mm Hg should be classified as Stage 4" (NHLB, 1993, p. 4)

2. Isolated systolic hypertension (ISH) is systolic blood pressure 140 mm Hg or higher and DBP less than 90 mm Hg

3. *Based on an average of 2 or more readings taken at each of two or more visits following an initial screening. (NHLB, 1993, p. 4)

■ Etiology/Incidence

1. Idiopathic, essential, or primary hypertension has no demonstrable underlying cause; approximately 95% of all patients have primary hypertension

2. Approximately 1 to 3% of hypertension may be produced as part of another disease process. The most common types of this secondary hypertension include

   a. Renovascular or kidney disease

      (1) Glomerulonephritis and pyelonephritis

      (2)   Renal artery stenosis—renal bruit may be present

  b. Coarctation of the aorta—blood pressure may differ between arms or between upper and lower extremities

  c. Endocrine disease, including

      (1)   Cushing's syndrome

      (2)   Primary aldosteronism—nocturia

      (3)   Pheochromocytoma—paroxysmal or persistent hypertension

      (4)   Diabetes mellitus

      (5)   Hypercalcemia

  d. Toxemia of pregnancy

  e. Miscellaneous causes

      (1)   Drugs—oral contraceptives, MAO inhibitors, steroids

      (2)   Collagen vascular disease

      (3)   Increased intravascular volume

      (4)   Burns

      (5)   Chronic alcoholism

      (6)   Smoking

3. The most prevalent cardiovascular disorder in the U.S. affecting over 60 million Americans (Wyngaarden, Smith, Bennett, 1992)

  a. Approximately 84% of individuals who have hypertension have been diagnosed, 13% of these individuals are receiving treatment, and only 55% of those receiving treatment have blood pressure under control (NHLB, 1993)

  b. Prevalence of hypertension increases with age

  c. Black population more commonly affected than white

  d. In young adulthood and middle age, prevalence is greater in men than women; thereafter, the reverse is true

4. Other risk factors which may lead to hypertension include

  a. Obesity

  b. Heredity

  c. Increased salt intake

- Signs and Symptoms
  1. Often there are no symptoms except high blood pressure
  2. The following symptoms may be present
     a. Throbbing occipital headache, worse in the morning
     b. Dizziness
     c. Blurred vision
     d. Nocturia
     e. Dyspnea
     f. Chest pain
     g. Epistaxis
     h. Swelling of lower extremities
- Differential Diagnosis: While most cases of hypertension are idiopathic, any disease producing secondary hypertension must be ruled out
- Physical Findings
  1. Usually none
  2. Occasionally, the following may be present depending upon status and degree of hypertension
     a. Hypertensive arteriosclerotic retinopathy
        (1) Grade I
           (a) Increased A:V ratio (normal 3:4 or 5:6)
           (b) Mild AV nicking
        (2) Grade II
           (a) Increased A:V ratio, (e.g., 1:4)
           (b) Moderate AV nicking
           (c) Copper wire appearance of arterioles
        (3) Grade III
           (a) Increased A:V ratio
           (b) Prominent AV nicking
           (c) Silver wire appearance of arterioles
           (d) Flame hemorrhages in fundus

(e) Occasional soft exudates from retinal infarcts

(4) Grade IV

(a) Increased A:V ratio

(b) Marked AV nicking

(c) Silver wire appearance of arterioles

(d) Blurring of optic disc margins revealing optic disc edema

(e) Flame hemorrhages, especially around disc

(f) Numerous soft exudates and macular exudates with a star pattern

b. S_4 gallop—low pitched heart sound in mitral area immediately before S_1

c. Abdominal bruit—seen in renal artery stenosis

d. Dependent edema

e. Displacement of PMI downward and laterally with left ventricular hypertrophy

f. Harsh soft systolic murmur at the apex—murmer of mitral regurgitation

■ Diagnostic Tests/Findings

1. Baseline studies for all patients

a. Urinalysis—to exclude proteinuria and hematuria

b. Serum electrolytes, fasting blood glucose, BUN, creatinine, CBC, calcium, phosphorus, uric acid, cholesterol (total and high density lipoprotein) and triglycerides (evaluating pre-treatment status)

c. Electrocardiogram—evaluate for arrhythmias, bundle branch block, left ventricular hypertrophy

d. PA and lateral chest radiograph—cardiomegaly

2. Selected studies to rule out causes of secondary hypertension

a. Coarctation of aorta—Aortogram

b. Aldosteronism—plasma aldosterone level

c. Cushings—a.m. and p.m. cortisol level; 24-hour urine for total catecholamines, metanephrine and vanillylmandelic acid (VMA)

      d. Renovascular disease—rapid sequence IVP

      e. Thyroid disease—T4, TSH

      f. Renal artery stenosis—renal arteriogram, renal scan, radionuclide study of kidney

      g. Structural problems or tumors—CT scan and digital subtraction angiography

  3. Useful tests in selected patients to assess cardiovascular status

      a. Urinary microalbumin determination

      b. Echocardiography

      c. Plasma renin/urinary sodium determination

- Management/Treatment

  1. Step-care Strategies (NHLB, 1993)

      a. Step One—Lifestyle modifications with non-pharmacologic approaches

        (1) Salt restriction—less than 6g of sodium chloride

        (2) Weight reduction goal is within 15% of desirable weight

        (3) Regular aerobic physical activity

           (a) Current recommendations for BP and cardiovascular risk reduction indicates maintaining 70 to 80% of maximal heart rate (MHR) for 20 to 30 minutes 3 times per week

           (b) MHR—subtract age from 220

        (4) Muscle relaxation, biofeedback and stress management

        (5) Moderation of alcohol intake

        (6) Potassium-rich diet

        (7) Smoking cessation

      b. Step Two—Continue lifestyle modifications and add a diuretic or beta blocker

        (1) Diuretics

           (a) Carbonic anhydrase inhibitors

           (b) Loop diuretics—bumetanide, ethacrynic acid, furosemide; side effects same as for thiazides except no

hypercalcemia

(c) Potassium sparing—amiloride HCl, spironolactone, triamterene; side effects are hyperkalemia

(d) Thiazides—bendroflumethiazide, benzthiazide, chlorothiazide, chlorothalidone, cyclothiazide, hydrochlorothiazide, hydroflumethiazide, methyclothiazide, metolazone, polythiazide, quinethazone, trichlormethiazide; side effects are hypokalemia, hypomagnesemia, glucose intolerance, hyponatremia, hyperuricemia, hypercalcemia, hyperglycemia, hypertriglyceridemia, hypercholesterolemia; sexual dysfunction

(2) Beta blockers

(a) Alpha-adrenergic—prazosin, terazosin, doxazosin

(b) Beta-adrenergic—propranolol, metoprolol, nadolol, atenolol, timolol, pindolol, acebutolol

(c) Alpha and beta adrenergic— labetalol

(d) Side effects—bradycardia, fatigue, insomnia, CHF, cardiac conduction abnormalities, hypoglycemia, hypertriglyceridemia, decreased HDL cholesterol; may exacerbate bronchospasm, peripheral vascular constriction

c. Step Three—If blood pressure does not decrease, increase drug dosage or substitute another drug or add a second agent from a different class

(1) Calcium channel blockers— nifedipine, diltiazem, verapamil, nicardipine; side effects are headache, dizziness, peripheral edema, tachycardia, gingival hyperplasia, hypotension

(2) Angiotensin-converting enzyme inhibitors—captopril, enalapril, lisinopril; side effects are cough, rash, hyperkalemia

(3) Sympatholytic agents— clonidine, methyldopa, guanethidine; side effects are drowsiness, sedation, dry mouth, fatigue, orthostatic dizziness

(4) Vasodilators—hydralazine, minoxidil; side effects are positive antinuclear antibody (ANA); hypertrichosis (rare)

  d. Step Four—If a blood pressure does not decrease, add a second or third drug and/or diuretic if not already prescribed

  e. Some medications are more effective in some races and in the presence of other diseases than others (Barker, Burton, & Zieve, 1991, p. 775)

   (1) Diuretics should be the first drug of choice in black population

   (2) ACE inhibitors may be helpful in diabetics

■ General Considerations

 1. Teach all patients critical facts about high blood pressure (HBP)

  a. Untreated HBP leads to increased risk of disabling illness or premature death

  b. Patients often initially asymptomatic

  c. Treatment reduces risk

  d. Treatment continues for life

  e. Use American Heart Association pamphlets in teaching

 2. Prescribe drugs that can be taken daily or b.i.d.

 3. Teach about common drug side effects

 4. Have patient state how they are taking medications each visit; bring medicine bottles to appointments

 5. See patients every 2 to 3 months initially, and then supervise on regular basis

 6. Facilitate patient compliance when possible through ease in making telephone calls, renewal of prescriptions, helping with transportation, etc.

 7. Involve family members in teaching

  a. Have them take BP at home and bring record to appointments

  b. Have group meetings with patient and family

Coronary Artery Disease—Angina Pectoris

■ Definition

 1. Chronic stable (classic exertional angina)—a clinical syndrome characterized by periods of precordial pressure or discomfort usually

secondary to exertion and relieved by rest or sublingual nitroglycerin

2. Unstable—angina that has begun to intensify; typical chest discomfort and dyspnea may occur at rest or at night while patient is in recumbent position

3. Prinzmetal's angina—variant form of unstable angina; chest discomfort characteristically occurs at rest or awakens patient from sleep; may be explosive in onset, severe, and frightening; may be accompanied by palpitations or severe shortness of breath

- Etiology/Incidence

  1. Caused by coronary artery obstruction which results in inadequate supply of oxygenated blood to meet myocardial oxygen needs

  2. Risk factors for coronary artery disease include

     a. Hypertension

     b. Diabetes mellitus

     c. Tobacco use

     d. Hyperlipidemia

     e. Family history of coronary artery disease

     f. Oral contraceptives

     g. Personality type A

     h. Diet

     i. Sedentary living

  3. Afflicts over 3 million persons in U.S.

- Signs and Symptoms

  1. Chest discomfort—midline and substernal chest pressure with radiation, burning, tightness, fullness, squeezing, smothering

  2. Attacks may vary in frequency from several/day to symptom-free intervals of weeks/months

  3. Stable usually precipitated by physical activity, persists no more than a few minutes, and subsides with rest; angina worsened when exercise follows a meal and is exaggerated in cold weather; unstable and Prinzmetal's episodes may occur at rest or at night

  4. Pain often so unique patients can document date/time of first pain

- Differential Diagnosis

  1. Gastroesophageal reflux, peptic ulcer disease, cholecystitis
  2. Pericarditis, myocardial infarction
  3. Pulmonary embolism
  4. Costochondritis
  5. Anxiety states
  6. Aortic disection
  7. Muscle spasm
  8. Spontaneous pneumothorax
  9. Exertional bronchospasm secondary to asthmatic bronchitis

- Physical Findings

  1. Often no findings between, and even during, attacks
  2. General appearance may reveal risk factors associated with atherosclerosis
  3. Palpation may reveal thickened or absent peripheral arteries, signs of cardiac enlargement, and abnormal contraction of cardiac impulse
  4. Fundi may reveal arteriovenous nicking
  5. Arterial bruits may be present
  6. During an attack, one or more of the following may be present

     a. Increased heart rate and BP
     b. S_3, S_4 present in about 50% of patients; S_3 may represent left ventricular failure or volume overload; S_4 reflects atrial contraction into a noncompliant ventricle as in HBP, cardiomyopathy, coronary artery disease
     c. Systolic bulge at or near apex (especially in left, lateral decubitus position)
     d. Paradoxical splitting of S_2 (due to delay in aortic valve closure due to increase in contractility of left ventricle)
     e. Mid-to-late-systolic, mitral regurgitant murmurs related to ischemic-induced mitral papillary muscle dysfunction

- Diagnostic Tests/Findings

  1. Electrocardiogram—often normal; during episode of angina, horizontal or down-sloping depression of ST segment, T-wave peaking or

inversion may occur

2. Exercise ECG—evidence of ischemic or ECG changes, angina or other limiting symptoms considered a clinically positive response

3. Radionuclide studies—exercise tests that identify the ischemic myocardial zone; can be expensive; may not be necessary

4. Coronary arteriography—indicated with severe symptoms or unstable angina; other evidence of myocardial ischemia; patients with recurrent chest pain of unknown etiology to determine extent of disease

■ Management/Treatment

1. Identification of underlying disease, usually atherosclerosis

2. Non-drug therapy

   a. Dietary management of cholesterol and saturated fat intake

   b. Risk factor modification instructions

   c. Smoking cessation instructions

   d. Patient education about etiology, medications, when to seek emergency help

2. Drug therapy

   a. Nitrates

      (1) (Short acting sublingual nitroglycerin)—for acute or prophylactic use; 0.15 to 0.6 mg dissolved under tongue or in buccal pouch at first sign of attack; may be repeated every five minutes in a 15 minute period; need medical attention if no relief

      (2) Long acting

         (a) Oral, e.g., isosorbide; pentaerythritol tetranitrate

         (b) Cutaneous nitroglycerin

   b. Beta blockers

   c. Calcium channel blockers

   d. Low-dose enteric coated aspirin—81 to 325 mg daily; (studies have shown decreased incidence of M.I. in men; effects under study in women)

3. Surgery—coronary arterial bypass surgery is highly effective in select patients

■ General Considerations

1. Refer for initial diagnosis of angina and for any change in character of angina pain

2. Document consultation with physician in records throughout care of patient

3. Counseling regarding serious and unpredictable nature of disorder

4. Education regarding care and use of nitroglycerine and when to seek emergency treatment

   a. Keep sublingual (SL) medication in dark colored glass container

   b. Remove cotton packing—absorbs nitroglycerine

   c. Store in refrigerator

   d. Renew medication every six months—it deteriorates

   e. Review carefully procedure for applying paste or patches and administration of sublingual

   f. Side effects, e.g., headache, postural dizziness, sweating

   g. Instructions in prophylactic use prior to activities which might cause an attack

Myocardial Infarction (M.I.)

■ Definition: Ischemic myocardial necrosis resulting from reduction in blood supply to a portion of the myocardium

■ Etiology/Incidence

1. Most infarctions caused by thrombotic occlusion related to severe coronary atherosclerosis; instability of atherosclerotic plaques with hemorrhage and plaque rupture leading to acute thrombotic occlusion is common

2. Other causes include coronary emboli, thrombotic coronary artery disease, coronary vasculitis, coronary vasospasm, congenital anomalies, trauma

3. Risk factors for infarction include

   a. Hypertension

   b. Diabetes mellitus

   c. Smoking

    d. Truncal obesity

    e. Increased LDL and decreased HDL

    f. Genetic predisposition

  4. In the U.S. approximately 1.5 million M.I.s occur each year; no significant change in numbers since early 1970s (Pasternak & Braunwald, 1994)

- Signs and Symptoms

  1. Prolonged chest discomfort with increasing intensity that may radiate into jaw, left arm, or scapular area

  2. Associated symptoms—pallor, respiratory distress, diaphoresis, nausea, restlessness, feeling of apprehension, denial

- Differential Diagnosis

  1. Pericarditis, pleurodynia

  2. Pulmonary embolism or infarction

  3. Esophagitis or esophageal spasm

  4. Peptic ulcer disease

  5. Gall bladder disease

  6. Pancreatitis

  7. Dissecting aortic aneurysm

  8. Musculoskeletal or chest wall pain

- Physical Findings

  1. Arrhythmia is common

  2. Blood pressure may be initially elevated or hypotension may develop

  3. Fundoscopic examination—may show atherosclerotic vascular disease

  4. Presence of 4th heart sound almost universal

  5. May be a soft systolic blowing apical murmur

  6. Pericardial rub

  7. Rales/rhonchi if congestive failure is present

  8. Low-grade fever usually during first 48 hours

  9. Hepatojugular reflux—may be elicited when hepatomegaly is not marked

- Diagnostic Tests/Findings
  1. Sequential electrocardiograms
     a. ST segment elevation/depression
        (1) ST elevation, followed by T-wave inversion, then Q-wave development (reliable indicator)
        (2) ST depression followed by persistent T-wave changes without Q-wave development
  2. Nonspecific ECG changes include intraventricular conduction delays; signs of atrial infarction with changes in P-wave activity; ventricular and supraventricular arrhythmias, etc.
  3. Myocardial enzymes/isoenzymes
     a. CK-MB (myocardial component of creatine kinase—cornerstone of diagnosis)
        (1) Elevations above normal within 4 hours
        (2) Peak in 16 to 24 hours; return to baseline in 3 to 4 days
     b. Lactic dehydrogenase (LDH)
        (1) Rises within 24 to 48 hours; peaks in 3 to 4 days; returns to normal 14 days after M.I.
        (2) Normal LDH_1/LDH_2 is $< 0.6-0.7$. If ratio becomes > 1, suspect recent M.I. (more sensitive and specific than total LDH level)
     c. Serum aminotransferase enzymes AST and ALT (previously SGOT and SGPT)—utilized for many years, but no longer because of lack of tissue specificity
  4. White blood cell count—may be normal initially; generally increases within 2 hours and persists for 3 to 7 days; often reaches levels at 12,000 to 15,000
  5. Other specialized studies
     a. Thallium 201 scan—M.I. reveals a "cold spot" within a few hours
     b. 2-D echocardiography/Doppler studies
        (1) Detection of abnormal wall motion
        (2) Gives estimation of overall ventricular performance
     c. Coronary angiography

          (1)   Locate lesion or lesions; assess severity

          (2)   Presence of collateral circulation

          (3)   Left ventricular function

■ Management/Treatment

1. Immediate hospitalization and cardiology referral (50% of deaths from M.I. occur within 3 to 4 hours of onset; therefore, initial management is critical)

2. Oxygen

3. Analgesics

4. Treatment of associated symptoms or complications

    a. Arrhythmias

    b. Congestive failure

■ General Considerations

1. Refer patients suspected of infarction

2. Nurse practitioners often see patients on follow-up after hospitalization

3. Pharmacotherapy to reduce pain, prevent reoccurrence

    a. Sedatives

    b. Nitrates

    c. Calcium channel blockers

    d. Beta-blockers

    e. Low-dose enteric-coated aspirin—81 mg to 325 mg daily

    f. Anticoagulation therapy

    g. Diuretic therapy

4. Cardiac rehabilitation program important for recovery

    a. Education—specifics of disease, risk reduction, medication use, indications for surgery

    b. Exercise

    c. Risk factor reduction—smoking cessation programs, weight reduction

5. Preparation for surgery

    a. Coronary artery bypass graft

b. Percutaneous transluminal coronary artery angioplasty

c. Anticipatory education

Congestive Heart Failure (CHF)

■ Definition

1. A syndrome with a variety of etiologies that affect the mechanical action of the heart leading to an inadequate supply of blood to meet metabolic requirements of the body

2. Types of heart failure (differences between types may be less clear as heart failure progresses)

   a. Acute versus chronic

      (1) Acute—abrupt onset, in a previously well patient, following an acute M.I. or valve rupture

      (2) Chronic—develops or progresses slowly as in mutivalvular disease or dilated cardiomyopathy

   b. Right-sided versus left-sided (controversial distinction since both mechanisms present in most cases of heart failure) (Braunwald, 1994)

      (1) Riget-sided—caused by valvular pulmonic stenosis, pulmonary hypertension and left ventricular failure; edema, congestive hepatomegaly, systemic venous distention present

      (2) Left-sided—secondary to high incidence of cardiac disorders which overload or damage left ventricle; breathlessness, orthopnea, paroxysmal nocturnal dyspnea common symptoms

   c. Backward versus forward (has limited clinical usefulness; been replaced with more specific ventricular filling pressures and cardiac output) (Smith, 1992)

      (1) Backward—elevated cardiac filling pressures

      (2) Forward—decreased cardiac output and inadequate organ perfusion

   d. High-output versus low-output (distinguishes clinical manifestations rather than causes)

      (1) High-output—occurs in patients with heart failure and hyperthyroidism, anemia, pregnancy

(2) Low-output—secondary to ischemic heart disease, hypertension, dilated cardiomyopathy, valvular disease

e. Systolic versus diastolic

(1) Systolic—inability to contract normally and expel adequate blood; results in weakness, fatigue, decreased exercise tolerance

(2) Diastolic—inability to relax and fill normally; caused by increased resistance to ventricular inflow, reduced capacity, impaired relaxation

(3) New technology demonstrates that CHF often occurs with reduced left ventricular systolic function. However, up to 40% of patients may have normal left ventricular systolic function, but abnormal left ventricular diastolic function

■ Etiology/Incidence

1. May be caused by cardiac myopathies-abnormality in heart muscle

2. May result from extra myocardial abnormalities such as coronary atherosclerosis; abnormalities of heart valves or rheumatic process

3. May also be a result of excess load on normal heart as in hypertensive crisis, rupture of an aortic valve cusp or massive pulmonary embolism

4. Other causes may be infection, anemia, thyrotoxicosis, arrhythmias; physical, dietary, fluid, environmental and emotional excesses in those with existing heart disease

5. Most common DRG throughout U.S. for patients 65 years of age and above (Smith, 1992)

■ Signs and Symptoms

1. Great variability—no distress to extreme distress and depends upon cause

2. Fatigue on exertion

3. Dyspnea with mild exertion

4. Decreased exercise tolerance

5. Paroxysmal nocturnal dyspnea

6. Wheezing, cough

7. Weight gain, ankle swelling

8. Nocturia, oliguria

9. Cyanosis or pallor

10. Orthopnea (later manifestation)

11. Cerebral symptoms, e.g., confusion, memory impairment in the elderly

- Differential Diagnosis

  1. Pneumonia

  2. Chronic Obstructive Pulmonary Disease (COPD)

  3. Bronchial asthma

  4. Pulmonary embolism

- Physical Findings—may vary, depending upon degree of failure

  1. Jugular venous distention

  2. S_3 heart sound—low pitched sound heard with bell at mitral area after S_2 in diastole—sounds like "Kentucky"

  3. Murmurs

  4. Cardiomegaly

  5. Cyanosis/pallor

  6. Peripheral edema

  7. Weight gain

  8. Shortness of breath, tachypnea, wheezing

  9. Hepatomegaly/ascites

  10. Tachycardia; narrow pulse pressure, pulsus alterans (sign of severe failure)

  11. Altered mental status

  12. Bilateral basilar rales

- Diagnostic Tests/Findings

  1. No specific test to determine CHF; focus testing on determining causes of CHF

     a. CBC

     b. Liver function studies

     c. Cardiac enzymes—rule out M.I.

     d. Urinalysis

e. Chest radiograph

    (1) Cardiomegaly

    (2) Increased vascular markings—characteristic of pulmonary edema

    (3) Kerley B lines—reflect chronic elevation of left atrial pressure and represents chronic thickening of intralobular septa

f. 2-D echocardiography and Doppler study (selected patients)

    (1) Evaluate left ventricular systolic and diastolic function

    (2) Detect abnormalities of cardiac valves

    (3) Wall motion abnormalities

    (4) Presence of pericardial effusion, intracardiac thrombi, and tumors

g. Coronary radionuclide angiography/biopsy (selected patients)

    (1) Determine left ventricular systolic and diastolic function

    (2) Evaluate degree of coronary artery disease

    (3) Determine etiology or cardiomyopathy

h. MRI—evaluates regional myocardial function

- Management/Treatment

  1. Physician referral for acute failure

    a. Treatment of primary underlying cause which may include medical and/or surgical problems, e.g., surgical correction of congenital anomalies or valvular lesions; treatment of hypertension

    b. Removal of precipitating causes, e.g., fluid overload, renal failure, hepatic failure, thyrotoxicosis, respiratory insufficiency, pulmonary embolism

  2. General management

    a. Improve pump action of failing heart

      (1) Drug therapy with cardiac glycosides, sympathomimetic drugs, other positive inotropic drugs

      (2) Decrease work load of heart with rest (physical and emotional); vasodilator drugs; treatment of obesity

        (3)   Control of retention of salt and water with diuretics, decreased sodium intake

    3.   Chronicity of problem requires therapeutic relationship with patient to allow for sensitivity to changes in status

Peripheral Vascular Disorders

Thrombophlebitis

- Definition

    1.   Superficial thrombophlebitis—venous thrombus formation with accompanying inflammation of venous wall; involves saphenous veins and tributaries

    2.   Deep vein thrombophlebitis involves development of venous thrombi in the deep vessels in the presence of inflammatory changes in the vessel wall before or after clot formation; involves posterior tibial, other deep calf veins, popliteal, pelvic

- Etiology/Incidence

    1.   Venous stasis—occurs in postoperative period, postpartum; with varicosities; prolonged bedrest

    2.   Hypercoagulability—malignant tumors, blood dyscrasias, oral contraceptives

    3.   Injury to venous wall—injection of irritating substances, indwelling catheters, thromboangiitis obliterans

    4.   Deep vein thrombosis—a common disorder; more common in women; all races affected equally; increases with advancing age

    5.   Superficial thrombophlebitis—most common in those with varicose veins; frequent after pregnancy

- Signs and Symptoms

    1.   Superficial thrombophlebitis

        a. Begins with sudden onset of pain

        b. Localized heat, erythema, tenderness over affected vein

        c. Mild temperature elevation may be present

    2.   Deep vein thrombophlebitis

        a. May be asymptomatic or present with pain, tenderness, swelling, skin discoloration, warmth over involved area

b. Pain in the involved area at rest, or only during exercise with swelling distal to obstructed veins, are usual symptoms

- Differential Diagnosis
  1. Superficial thrombophlebitis
     a. Rupture of calf muscles
     b. Severe muscle cramp
     c. Cellulitis
  2. Deep vein thrombophlebitis
     a. Ruptured popliteal (Baker's cyst)
     b. Lumbar disc problems
     c. Lymphedema

- Physical Findings
  1. Superficial thrombophlebitis
     a. Palpation of red tender cord
     b. Erythema, tenderness, warmth may be present at vein site
  2. Deep vein thrombophlebitis
     a. Edema or pitting of malleolar fossa may be present
     b. May be difference in circumference of calf of both legs
     c. Temperature of skin may be increased
     d. Tenderness on palpation
     e. Positive Homan's sign (considered an unreliable diagnostic sign by some authorities)

- Diagnostic Tests/Findings
  1. Impedance plethysmography—detects alterations in blood volume of extremities; abnormal finding is slow outflow
  2. Doppler ultrasound—detects venous obstruction
  3. "Duplex" ultrasonography—excellent specificity and sensitivity for deep vein thrombosis above the knee
  4. Venography—one of the most accurate means for diagnosis of deep vein thrombosis

■ Management/Treatment

1. Superficial thrombophlebitis

   a. Anticoagulation therapy not necessary

   b. Elevation of the extremity

   c. Warm compresses over involved veins

   d. Nonsteroidal anti-inflammatory drugs, e.g., indomethacin

   e. Smoking cessation program

   f. Discontinue oral contraceptives, all estrogen and progesterone preparations

2. Deep vein thrombophlebitis—above knee more serious than below knee

   a. Physician referral

   b. Goal of therapy is to prevent pulmonary embolism and chronic venous insufficiency

   c. Antithrombotic therapy, e.g., heparin, warfarin

   d. Thrombolysis with streptokinase or urokinase

   e. Discontinue oral contraceptives and all estrogen contraceptives and progesterone preparations

   f. Bedrest and elevation of affected extremity

   g. Analgesics for pain should not include aspirin or other compounds that interfere with platelet function

   h. Ambulation with elastic stockings usually allowed after local signs of inflammation have subsided

   i. Anticoagulation therapy may be indicated for several weeks to months to prevent recurrence

■ Prophylaxis

1. Modification of behavior often reduces recurrence

2. Patient education essential

   a. Proper use of compression stockings

   b. Avoid crossing legs at the knees

   c. Avoid prolonged sitting or standing in motionless, dependent position

    d. Medications and possible adverse reactions

    e. Avoidance of contraceptives, estrogen and progesterone with recurrent thrombophlebitis

    f. Hazards of smoking

    g. Need to avoid constrictive girdles/garters

    h. Balanced program of rest and exercise

Arteriosclerosis Obliterans

- Definition: Segmental arteriosclerotic narrowing or obstruction of the lumen of the arteries supplying the limbs
- Etiology/Incidence
  1. Usually caused by atherosclerosis
  2. Most common cause of arterial obstructive disease of extremities
  3. Usually occurs between ages of 50 and 70
  4. Men affected more often; high incidence in diabetics
  5. Most commonly affected vessel is superficial femoral artery
- Signs and Symptoms
  1. Intermittent claudication (initial symptom)—pain, ache, fatigue with walking, which is relieved by rest
  2. With progression "rest pain" occurs
- Differential Diagnosis
  1. Arterial embolism
  2. Thrombophlebitis
  3. Arthritis
  4. Lumbar disc disorders
- Physical Findings
  1. Reduced or absent pulses distal to obstruction
  2. Bruits may be audible over aorta or branches
  3. Severity increase will show a cold, numb area; skin may be dry and scaly with poor nail and hair growth; pallor or cyanosis; dependent rubor of affected extremity

4. As ischemia worsens, ulceration may occur

■ Diagnostic Tests/Findings

1. Doppler ultrasonography—stenosis and occlusion identified

2. Ankle/brachial index—.5 to .9 indicates significant disease

3. Treadmill testing—assessment of functional limitations, ankle/brachial ratio and presence of coronary artery disease

4. Arteriography—will provide details of location and extent of occlusion

■ Management/Treatment

1. Encourage walking 60 minutes per day, if possible; when pain occurs, stop walking; resume when pain disappears

2. Eliminate all forms of tobacco

3. Maintain skin integrity of affected limbs

4. Treat hyperlipidemia

5. Control diabetes mellitus, if present

6. No evidence that vasodilative drugs are effective

7. Thromboendarectomy

8. Percutaneous transluminal angioplasty

9. Bypass operation with vein graft

10. Amputation to arrest advancing gangrene

11. Weight control

■ General Considerations

1. Patients often have reduced mobility due to chronic problems and may be reluctant to attempt exercise

2. May have concomitant health problems which make intervention difficult

Chronic Venous Insufficiency

■ Definition: Impaired venous return caused by destruction of deep venous valves; may lead to varicose veins

■ Etiology/Incidence

1. Defective valves

2. Secondary to sustained elevations of venous pressure from obstruction

3. Inherent weakness in vein walls

4. Pressure on pelvic veins during pregnancy or obesity

5. Secondary to deep vein thrombophlebitis

6. More common in women than men

7. Familial history has some effect

8. Increased with periods of prolonged standing

9. Seven million Americans affected; more than 500,000 individuals have stasis ulcers

- Signs and Symptoms
    1. Many patients may be asymtomatic in early stages
    2. Aching of lower extremities relieved by elevation of affected leg or use of compression hosiery
    3. Symptoms may worsen during menstrual period
    4. Swelling, especially after prolonged standing
    5. Lower extremity night cramps

- Differential Diagnosis
    1. Lumbar nerve root irritation
    2. Osteoarthritis of hip or knee
    3. Arterial insufficiency
    4. Peripheral neuritis

- Physical Findings
    1. Visibly dilated and tortuous superficial veins (varicose veins)
    2. Other findings which may be present
        a. Stasis leg ulcers — usually occur above medial malleolus
        b. Trophic changes with brownish discoloration of skin
        c. Dermatitis

- Diagnostic Tests and Findings: Trendelenburg test done to determine if saphenofemoral junction is incompetent

■ Management/Treatment

1. Lightweight compression hosiery for mildly symptomatic condition and heavier elastic stockings for more advanced cases

2. Frequent periods of rest with elevation of limbs when possible

3. Avoid sitting or standing for long periods of time

4. Avoid restrictive clothing, girdles, garters

5. Weight reduction if appropriate

6. Treatment of stasis ulcers with hydrocolloid dressings; dome paste boot, etc.

7. Ligation and stripping of saphenous veins

8. Injection therapy (sclerotherapy)

■ General Considerations

1. Instructions on application of dressings

2. Review medications, skin and foot care

3. Referral for severe infections and stasis ulcers

4. Referral for surgical debridement if necessary

5. Concomitant health problems may make interventions difficult

Questions

Select the best answer.

1. Mr. Sam Jones, a 45-year-old black male, comes to see you for follow-up of an elevated blood pressure of 148/112 recorded at a local health fair. You take his blood pressure and find it to be 150/110. Based on this information you would

   a. Start patient today on hydrochlorothiazide, 500 mg every day
   b. Ask patient to return later in the week for another blood pressure evaluation
   c. Perform a complete history and physical examination today
   d. Order screening laboratory work today

2. On her quarterly visit for evaluation of her hypertension, Mrs. Hazel Brown, a 57-year-old female reports that she has been having lots of headaches. The type of headache often reported by hypertensive patients is

   a. Throbbing occipital headache, worse in the morning
   b. Unilateral temporal headache with eye tearing
   c. Pounding temporal headache, worse in the evening
   d. Feeling of pressure over eyes and forehead, worse when patient leans forward

3. You meet a group of patients for a discussion on health and diet. You have been told that one of the patients in the room has high blood pressure. In the room there are 5 patients. Based on your knowledge of risk factors for hypertension, which one of the following patients is the most likely to have hypertension?

   a. 52 year old Japanese immigrant
   b. 28 year old female ski instructor
   c. Obese 64 year old black male with diabetes
   d. 66 year old caucasian retired football coach

4. While most cases of hypertension are idiopathic, several conditions that may cause secondary hypertension include

   a. Renal artery stenosis, repeated urinary tract infections
   b. Grave's disease, venous stasis
   c. Pheochromocytoma, Cushing's syndrome, primary hyperaldosteronism
   d. Toxemia/leukemia

5. Patients who are newly diagnosed with hypertension and present with nocturia should be evaluated for

   a. Glomerulonephritis causing diuresis
   b. Primary hyperaldosteronism leading to lack of concentrating ability of kidney

    c. Renal artery stenosis causing dilatation of loop of Henle

    d. Toxemia of pregnancy producing radical diuresis

6. Evaluation of the optic fundus gives evidence of end organ condition in hypertensive patients and is an effective method of evaluating patient compliance or response to therapy. When you evaluate Mr. Rosenbaum, a 68-year-old professor who has been treated with hydrochlorothiazide for the last 3 years, you discover well marginated optic disc, 1:4 A:V ratio with moderate nicking of the superior temporal arteries, copper wire appearance of artery, and one soft exudate in the macular area. Blood pressure is 160/98. Based on this information, you would conclude

    a. Patient has progressive and normal changes in optic fundus for his age and disease process

    b. Patient has signs of malignant hypertension

    c. Patient should be suspected of having diabetes in addition to his hypertension

    d. Patient has signs of progressive hypertensive end organ damage despite antihypertensive therapy

7. Mild hypertension is defined as

    a. Diastolic BP 85 to 89 mm Hg.

    b. Diastolic BP 90 to 99 mm Hg.

    c. Diastolic BP 100 to 109 mm Hg.

    d. Diastolic BP greater than 119

8. Abdominal bruit auscultated on physical examination on a hypertensive patient might indicate

    a. Renovascular disease

    b. Glomerulonephritis

    c. Renal artery stenosis

    d. Abdominal aneurysm

9. The stepped-care regimen for treating hypertension begins with use of

    a. Nonpharmacologic therapies

    b. Use of a diuretic

    c. Use of a Beta blocker and a calcium antagonist

    d. Use of an ACE inhihibitor

10. Common side effects associated with beta blockers include

    a. Hyponatremia

    b. Bradycardia

    c. Hyperkalemia

    d. Orthostatic dizziness

11. Major findings commonly present in congestive heart failure include

    a. Weight gain, shortness of breath, S_3 heart sound
    b. Confusion, weight loss, arrhythmia
    c. Lung consolidation on chest radiograph, temperature elevation, excitability
    d. ECG changes, weight gain, hypotension, positive Homan's sign

12. Basic therapeutic regimen in congestive heart failure includes

    a. Digitalis
    b. Diuretics
    c. Antiarrhythmias
    d. Digitalis and diuretics

13. Describe the heart sound that is most commonly found in congestive heart failure

    a. Soft diastolic sound heard best with the bell at the mitral area immediately before S_1
    b. Soft diastolic sound heard best with the bell at the tricuspid area immediately before S_1
    c. Soft diastolic sound heard best with the bell at the mitral area immediately after S_2
    d. Soft diastolic sound heard best with the diaphgram at the mitral area immediately after S_2

14. Instructions concerning nitroglycerine include

    a. Keep medication in plastic container
    b. Keep medication in pill box padded with cotton and carry in pocket for emergency use
    c. Discard medicine and get new nitroglycerine pills every 6 months
    d. Store medication in a dry, well lighted cabinet at room temperatures

15. Differential diagnosis for coronary artery disease include

    a. Gastrointestinal disorders
    b. Emphysema
    c. Bronchitis
    d. Pancreatitis

16. Electrocardiogram in angina may reveal

    a. T-wave depression
    b. New Q-wave development
    c. Transient loss of R-wave
    d. Horizontal or down sloping depression of ST segment

17. Which of the following conditions has shown no change in occurrence over the

last several years?

   a. Congestive heart failure
   b. Hypertension
   c. Coronary artery disease
   d. Myocardial infarction

18. The key diagnostic events that would lead you to believe that the patient was having a myocardial infarction include

   a. Pain occurs with rest and not just with exercise
   b. Pain is associated with symptoms of tachycardia, flushing, stupor
   c. Prolonged chest discomfort with increasing intensity which may radiate into jaw or left arm
   d. Stabbing chest pain associated with extreme hypertension and belching

19. Which of the following is not usually seen following acute myocardial infarction?

   a. S_4 heart sound
   b. Pericardial rub
   c. Low-grade fever
   d. Murphy's inspiratory arrest with deep breath

20. Serial cardiac enzymes and CBCs assist in the diagnosis of myocardial infarction. One of the most specific blood tests to document M.I. is

   a. SGOT
   b. CK-MB
   c. Isoenzyme LDH 1 and 2
   d. CBC

21. Precipitating causes of thrombophlebitis

   a. Extensive weight-bearing exercise
   b. Use of heating pads to provide warmth
   c. Pregnancy
   d. Idiopathic thrombocytopenia

22. 32-year-old Jean Taylor works as a cashier at a local market. She presents with sudden onset of right calf pain, localized heat, erythema and tenderness to palpation. The area appears swollen. Based on this presentation, the diagnosis is probably

   a. Deep vein thrombophlebitis
   b. Superficial vein thrombophlebitis
   c. Ruptured Achilles tendon
   d. Arterial embolism

23. What one factor reported by Mrs. Taylor is most likely related to her current symptoms?

    a. I do not smoke
    b. I sit down a lot at work
    c. I have varicose veins
    d. I am taking oral contraceptive pills

24. Vasodilators have been used with questionable effectiveness in treating

    a. Arteriosclerosis obliterans
    b. Deep vein thrombophlebitis
    c. Chronic venous insufficiency
    d. Superficial vein thrombophlebitis

25. Varicose veins is a diagnosis made primarily by obtaining a history of

    a. Acute pain in buttocks when walking rapidly
    b. Aching lower extremities after prolonged standing, swelling of feet
    c. Sudden onset of pain in calf of leg, swelling
    d. Legs very pale at night; holds them over side of bed to reduce pain

Answers

1. c
2. a
3. c
4. c
5. b
6. d
7. b
8. c
9. a
10. b
11. a
12. d
13. c
14. c
15. a
16. d
17. d
18. c
19. d
20. b
21. c
22. b
23. d
24. a
25. b

Bibliography

American Heart Association. (1989). *Heart facts*. Dallas: American Heart Association.

American Heart Association. (1991). *Risk factors and coronary disease: A statement for physicians*. Dallas: American Heart Association.

Barker, L. R., Burton J. R., & Zieve, P. D. (1991) *Principles of ambulatory medicine* (3rd ed.). Baltimore: Williams & Wilkins.

Braunwald, E. (1994). Heart failure. In K. J. Isselbacher, E. Braunwald, J. Wilson, J. Martin, A. Fauci & D. L. Kasper (Eds.). *Harrison's principles of internal medicine* (pp. 998-1009) (13th ed.). NY: McGraw-Hill.

Hirtt, W. R., & Regensteiner, J. G. (1993). Nonsurgical management of peripheral arterial disease. *Hospital Practice, 2*, 60-82.

Jennison, S. H., & Miller, L. W. (1993). What to try while congestive heart patients are still ambulatory. *Postgraduate Medicine, 94*(5), 69-84.

Lewis, S., & Timmis, A. (1989). The management of heart failure. *Comprehensive Therapy. 15*, 27-31.

Littenberg, B., Garber, A. M., & Sox, H. (1990). Screening for hypertension. *Annals of Internal Medicine. 112*, 192-202.

Mills, R. M., Jr. (1993). Congestive heart failure. *Postgraduate medicine, 94*(4), 49-51.

Moser, M. C. (1993). The JNC report on detection, evaluation, and treatment of high blood pressure: A critique. *Primary Cardiology, 19*(2), 66-72.

National Heart, Lung, and Blood Institute. (1993). *The fifth report of the Joint National Committee on Detection, Evaluation, and Treatment of High Blood Pressure*, (DHHS) (NIH Publication No. 93-1088). Bethesda, MD: National Institutes of Health.

Olin, B. R. (Ed). (1993). *Facts and comparisons*. St. Louis: J. B. Lippincott Company.

Pasternak, R. C., & Braunwald, E. (1994). Acute myocardial infarction. In K. J. Isselbacher, E. Braunwald, J. Wilson, J. Martin, A. Fauci & D. L. Kasper (Eds). *Harrison's principles of internal medicine* (pp. 1066-1077) (13th ed.). NY: McGraw-Hill.

Schultheis, A. (1990). Hypercholesterolemia: Prevention, detection, and management. *The Nurse Practitioner, 15*, 40-56.

Smith, T. W. (1992). Heart failure. In J. B. Wyngaarden, L. H. Smith, Jr., & J. C.

Bennett (Eds.). *Cecil textbook of medicine*, (pp. 187-207), (19th ed.). Philadelphia: W. B. Saunders.

Sonnenblick, E. H., & LeJemtel, T. H., (1993). Heart failure: Its progression and its therapy. *Hospital Practice, 11*, 121-130.

Taylor, A. J., & Bergin, J. D., (1993). Noninvasive assessment of systolic and diastolic function. *Postgraduate Medicine, 94*(4), 55-70.

United States Preventive Services Task Force. (1989). *Guide to clinical preventive services*. Baltimore: Williams & Wilkins.

United States Public Health Service. (1993). *Advance report of final mortality statistics*. Hyattsville, Maryland. (DHHS Pub No. (PH5) 88-1120).

Wyngaarden, J. B., Smith, L. H. Jr., & Bennett, J. C. (Eds.). (1992). *Cecil textbook of medicine*. (19th ed.). Philadelphia: W. B. Saunders.

Hematological and Oncological Disorders

Sister Maria Salerno

Common Anemias

Anemia describes a symptom of abnormally low red blood cell count, quality of hemoglobin, and/or volume of packed cells. The World Health Organization defines it in terms of peripheral blood hemoglobin < 13.0 grams(g) [hematocrit < 42%] for men and < 12.0 grams [hematocrit < 36%] in women. Anemias are classified on the basis of red cell morphology (microcytic, normocytic, or macrocytic) and amount of pigment they contain (hypochromic, normochromic), or the etiology.

Microcytic Anemias (MCV < 80μ³)

Iron Deficiency Anemia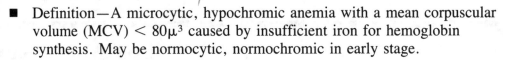

- Definition—A microcytic, hypochromic anemia with a mean corpuscular volume (MCV) < 80μ³ caused by insufficient iron for hemoglobin synthesis. May be normocytic, normochromic in early stage.

- Etiology/Incidence
  1. Inadequate iron intake (< 1 to 2 mg/day), e.g., infants on milk only diets, persons on vegetarian diets, alchoholics, pregnant women or adolescents whose demand is increased
  2. Impaired absorption of iron, e.g., after gastrectomy, in Celiac disease
  3. Slow, persistent blood loss, e.g., menorrhagia, gastritis, aspirin ingestion, polyps, GI neoplasms, peptic ulcer disease, esophageal varices, hemorrhoids. In adult males and postmenopausal females acute or chronic hemorrhage is most common cause
  4. One of the most common anemias throughout the world; particularly prevalent in women of childbearing age; estimated 20% of adult women, 50% of pregnant women, and 3% of adult males in the U.S. have iron deficiency

- Signs and Symptoms
  1. Depend on
     a. Rate at which anemia develops
     b. Age of the individual
     c. Individual's compensatory mechanisms
     d. Activity level

    e. Underlying disease state

    f. Severity of the anemia

  2. General Signs and Symptoms

    a. Easily fatigued

    b. Dyspnea on exertion

    c. Dizziness

    d. Listlessness

    e. Pallor (conjunctiva, nail beds, mucous membranes)

    f. Faintness

    g. Weakness

    h. Headaches

    i. Tachycardia

    j. Wide pulse pressure

    k. Heart murmurs

    l. Myocardial hypertrophy

    m. Angina

    n. Anorexia

    o. Pica

■ Differential Diagnosis

  1. Thalassemia

  2. Sideroblastic anemia

  3. Anemia of chronic disease

  4. Lead poisoning

■ Physical Findings

  1. General Appearance—pale, lethargic or no overt signs if anemia is mild

  2. Vital signs—pulse and respirations may be increased in moderate to severe anemia; in severe cases postural hypotension may be evident

  3. Integumentary—pallor and dryness of skin and mucous membranes; brittle, flattened, ridged, concave, or spoon shaped nails (koilonychia); brittle, fine hair

  4. HEENT—atrophy of the papillae of the tongue-smooth, shiny, beefy-

red appearance; angular stomatitis or cheilitis; pale conjunctiva and gums

5. Cardiovascular—tachycardia, mild cardiac enlargement; in severe anemias, functional systolic murmurs

6. Abdominal—may be some hepatic enlargement

7. Neurological—usually within normal limits; in severe anemia confusion may be evident

- Diagnostic Tests/Findings

1. See Table I and II for laboratory tests used in diagnosis of common anemias

2. Routine CBC (with peripheral smear)

    a. Hemoglobin—< 14 g/dl in males; < 12 g/dl in females

    b. Hct—< 42% in males; < 36% in females

    c. Low MCV (microcytic) and MCHC (hypochromic)

    d. Low erythrocyte count (RBC)

    e. Increased red cell distribution width (RDW)

    f. Serum Iron—low < 50 mg/ml (oral contraceptives may cause false elevation)

3. Iron status determinants—total iron binding capacity (TIBC) is considered the most sensitive and most specific for iron deficiency; serum ferritin and bone marrow studies are done if the diagnosis is unclear and/or there is a lack of response to a three week therapeutic trial

    a. High total iron binding capacity (TIBC)—usually normal or low in anemia of chronic disease (ACD)

    b. Low serum ferritin < 12 μg/L—infection, chronic disease, and liver disease may raise ferritin levels and mask coexisting iron deficiency; in these cases a serum ferritin level, < 30 μg/L is consistent with iron deficiency

    c. Low serum iron saturation—(< 20%)

    d. Bone marrow studies

        (1) Show depletion of iron (on staining), normocytic hyperplasia

        (2) Usually not part of initial work up

4. Bilirubin—normal

Table 1
Common Laboratory Tests Used in Diagnosing Anemia

Hematocrit (Hct)	Relative amount of plasma to total red blood cell mass; measure of RBC concentration. Normal: 40-54% males; 38-47% females
Hemoglobin (Hgb)	Basic screening test for anemia. Main component of erythrocytes. Vehicle for transport of O_2 & CO_2 Normal: 13.5-18 g/100 ml males; 12.0-15 g/100 ml females
Red Blood Cell Count (RBC)	Measure of number of Hgb carrying red blood cells (RBCs; erythrocytes). Needed to calculate other RBC indices
Mean Corpuscular Volume (MCV)	Mathematical measure of average RBC size. Expressed in micro cubic millimeters. Value classifies cells as microcytic, normocytic, macrocytic. Normal: 80-100 μ^3
Mean Corpuscular Hgb (MCH)	Mathematical measure of hemoglobin concentration of average RBC. Expressed in picograms. Calculated by dividing Hgb in grams by number of RBCs. Allows for classification of RBCs as hypochromic, normochromic. Normal 27-31 pg
Mean Corpuscular Hgb Concentration (MCHC)	Mathematical measure of concentration of Hgb in grams per 100 ml of RBCs Normal 32-36 g/dl or 32%-36%
Red Cell Distribution width (RDW)	Mathematical coefficient of width variation in red cell size. As RDW increases indicates greater variation in cell size
Serum Iron	Concentration of iron bound to transferrin. Varies conversely with TIBC Normal: 50-150 μg/dl in adults
Total Iron Binding Capacity (TIBC)	Measures amount of iron that transferrin can still bind. Varies conversely with serum iron. Normal: 250-450 μg/dl in adults
Bilirubin (indirect)	Fractionation of total bilirubin. Reflects breakdown of hemoglobin. Elevated levels indicate hemolysis
Coombs Indirect	Detects free antibodies in patient's serum and certain RBC antigens
Peripheral Blood Smear	Smear of whole blood stained with Wright's stain. Variations in cell morphology and staining characteristics important to diagnosis of hematologic conditions
Bone Marrow Aspiration	Marrow aspirated for microscopic examination. Done when anemia not obviously due to iron deficiency. Iliac crest preferred to sternum site

NOTE: Laboratory values differ in different labs. Check normals in laboratory where tests are conducted

Table 2
Select Morphological and Etiologic Categories
of Anemia and Related Laboratory Findings

	Macrocytic (MCV > 100)		Microcytic (MCV < 80)		Normocytic (MCV 80-100)
	B₁₂ Deficiency	*Folate Deficiency*	*Iron Deficiency*	*Thalessemia*	*Anemia of Chronic Disease*
Reticulocyte Ct	low	low	low	normal/sl. high	normal/low
MCH	normal	normal	low	low	normal
Fe	high	high	normal/low	normal/sl. high	low-high
TIBC	normal	normal	high	normal	normal/low
Bilirubin	sl. high	sl. high	normal	high	normal
Ferritin	high	high	low	normal	normal/high
B₁₂	low	normal	normal	normal	normal
Folate	normal	low	normal	normal/low	normal/low

■ Management/Treatment

1. Diagnostic

   a. Once diagnosis is established underlying cause must be identified and if possible, corrected. Bleeding must be suspected in the absence of clearly identifiable nutritional intake deficiency or increased body need

   b. Search for infection, trauma, neoplasm, GI disorders

   c. Stool guaiac, bilirubin, and additional studies may be needed to establish etiology

2. Therapeutic

   a. Oral Iron replacement

      (1) Oral is safer and much less expensive than IM or IV

      (2) Begin 6 month trial of ferrous sulfate tablets, 300-325 mg three times a day after meals

      (3) Determine effectiveness of iron replacement therapy during the first two weeks of therapy, (increased reticulocyte count)

      (4) Refer those on oral iron replacement therapy to a physician if 2 g/100 ml increase in Hgb is not seen in 3 to 4 weeks. In uncomplicated iron deficiency a 1 g a week increase is

expected

b. Parenteral iron is indicated if patient can not tolerate or absorb oral iron or if iron loss exceeds oral replacement. IM or IV Iron Dextran is used

    (1) More expensive

    (2) Associated with significant side effects

        (a) Anaphylaxis

        (b) Phlebitis

        (c) Regional adenopathy

        (d) Serum-sickness type reaction

        (e) Staining of IM injection sites

    (3) Dose based on the patient's weight

- General Considerations

1. Obtain physician consultation on any patient with

    a. Hct $<$ 25 %/dl

    b. Positive stool guaiac or history of unexplained bleeding

    c. Familial history of anemia

    d. Suspected underlying inflammatory, infectious, or malignant disease

    e. Failure to respond to iron supplementation

2. Education

    a. Cause of iron deficiency and treatment plan

    b. Purpose, dosage, side effect, toxic effects of iron replacement

        (1) Side effects of nausea, GI irritation, constipation, and diarrhea, and black stools

        (2) Food and fluid taken concurrently may interfere with absorption but may be warranted to alleviate gastric distress

        (3) Taking with orange juice will enhance absorption

        (4) Milk and antacids will interfere with absorption

        (5) Monitor and discuss with patients concurrent use of over the counter medications. Some products such as urine and stool deodorizers often used by elderly with incontinence problems

can lead to iron overdose and heart failure

(6) Therapy should continue for 6 or more months to replenish tissue stores

c. Medication should be kept out of the reach of children as iron overdose can be fatal to them

d. Nutrition—foods high in iron include organ and lean meats, egg yolk, shellfish, apricots, peaches, prunes, grapes, raisins, green leafy vegetables, iron fortified breads and cereals

e. Activity—frequent rest periods as needed

Thalassemia

- Definition—Thalassemia is a group of geneticly inherited syndromes of abnormal hemoglobin synthesis

- Etiology/Incidence

1. Inherited, autosomal recessive disorder that results in an impaired synthesis of either the alpha or beta chain of adult hemoglobin. Four genes control alpha chain production, two control beta chain production

2. Second most common cause of microcytic anemia

    a. Alpha Thalassemia more common in Blacks and Chinese, Vietnamese, Cambodians, and Laotians

    b. Beta Thalassemia more common in those of Mediterranean descent (Italians, Greeks, some Arabs and Sephardic Jews)

- Signs and Symptoms—The severity of the anemia can range from mild to severe depending on the number of hemoglobin controlling genes involved. Forms seen in adults include

1. Alpha trait (carrier state) (1 of 4 alpha chain-forming genes affected)— usually asymptomatic

2. Alpha-Thalassemia Minor (2 of 4 alpha chain-forming genes affected) and Beta-Thalassemia minor (heterozygous form)—both are usually asymptomatic and have mild presentations with mild to moderate microcytic, hypochromic anemia, enlarged liver and spleen, bronze coloring of the skin, and bone marrow hyperplasia

3. Beta Thalassemia Major (homozygous form affecting both beta chain-forming genes) also called Cooley's Anemia—severe anemia with significant cardiovascular burden; high output congestive failure is

common; fractures related to bone marrow expansion; retarded growth and maturation; in addition to general signs and symptoms presented in section on Iron Deficiency Anemia

4. Hemoglobin H disease (3 of 4 alpha hemoglobin chain-forming genes affected)—occurs predominantly in Chinese; moderate to severe microcytic anemia with splenomegaly

- Differential Diagnosis

  1. Iron deficiency anemia

  2. Sideroblastic anemia

  3. Anemia of chronic disease

  4. Lead poisoning—not common in adults unless occupation related

- Physical Findings—for the most part physical findings will be within normal limits unless the more severe forms of thalassemia are encountered

  1. General Appearance—pallor or bronze appearance; mild listlessness

  2. Abdominal—enlarged liver, enlarged spleen

  3. Cardiovascular—tachycardia, widened pulse pressure, systolic murmur if anemia is moderate or severe

  4. Respiratory—may have increased respiration rate

  5. Musculoskeletal—some bone deformity of the face (chipmunk deformity) related to expansion of bones caused by hyperplastic marrow

  6. Neurologic—within normal limits

- Diagnostic Tests/Findings

  1. Decreased Hgb

  2. MCV low

  3. Serum iron normal or increased

  4. TIBC normal

  5. Ferritin normal or increased

  6. RDW normal

  7. Reticulocyte count may be normal or increased

  8. Hemoglobin electrophoresis— demonstrates decreased alpha or beta hemoglobin chains

9. Peripheral smear will show microcytosis, variable hypochromia, target cells (thin, fragile RBCs), basophilic stippling

10. Skull and skeletal radiographs—widened marrow spaces in skull and long bones; osteoporosis

- Management/Treatment

1. No specific treatment for mild to moderate forms

2. Iron supplementation contraindicated in all thalassemias since iron overload can result

- General Considerations

1. Those with suspected or diagnosed severe forms should be referred to a hematologist for treatment which often includes transfusions and chelation therapy to avoid fatal iron overload (hemochromatosis)

2. Refer for genetic counseling

3. Stress overall good nutrition without additional iron supplementation

4. Discuss signs and symptoms of iron overload

   a. Weakness/lassitude

   b. Loss of body hair

   c. Weight loss

   d. Palmar erythema

   e. Gynecomastia

   f. Loss of libido

   g. Abdominal pain

   h. Thinning, darkening skin

   i. Pain and or stiffness in joints

   j. Blurred vision or other symptoms related to onset of diabetes

   k. Shortness of breath

   l. Swelling in ankles

Macrocytic Anemias (MCV > 100μ³

Pernicious Anemia

- Definition—A megaloblastic, macrocytic, normochromic anemia caused by a deficiency of intrinsic factor produced by the stomach which results in malabsorption of vitamin B_{12} necessary for DNA synthesis and maturation of RBCs

- Etiology/Incidence
  1. Possibly due to an autoimmune reaction involving the gastric parietal cell that results in nonproduction of intrinsic factor and atrophy of gastric mucosa
  2. Can also occur secondary to other factors which lead to decreased production of intrinsic factor or decreased absorption of B_{12}
     a. Loss of parietal cells post-gastrectomy
     b. Overgrowth of intestinal organisms
     c. Ileal resection or abnormalities
     d. Fish tape worm
     e. Congenital enzyme deficiencies
  3. Common in Caucasians of Northern European descent
  4. Both sexes equally affected
  5. Most present around age 60; can occur in individuals in their 20s
  6. Increased incidence in those with other immunologic disease

- Signs and Symptoms
  1. Weakness
  2. Sore tongue or glossitis
  3. Peripheral paresthesia—numbness, burning, tingling
  4. Palpitations
  5. Dizziness
  6. Swelling of legs
  7. Anorexia
  8. Diarrhea

9. Mucositis

10. Dementia and spinal cord degeneration in advanced stages

- Differential Diagnosis

    1. Folate deficiency

    2. Anemia of liver disease

    3. Mylodysplastic syndromes

- Physical Findings

    1. Vital signs—temperature may be slightly elevated, wide pulse pressure, pulse and respirations may be elevated if anemia is severe

    2. General Appearance—premature aging; premature graying of hair

    3. HEENT—smooth beefy red tongue; sclera and skin may be slightly icteric

    4. Cardiovascular—systolic flow murmur, tachycardia, and cardiomegaly if anemia is severe

    5. Abdomen—hepatomegaly and splenomegaly may be evident

    6. Neurological—deep tendon reflexes increased or decreased; diminished position sense; poor or absent vibratory sense in lower extremities; ataxia; poor finger-nose coordination; positive Romberg and Babinski; mental status changes ranging from mild forgetfulness and irritability to psychotic behavior

- Diagnostic Tests/Findings

    1. Hgb and Hct—decreased

    2. RBCs—decreased

    3. Reticulocytes—normal or low

    4. MCV—increased $> 100 \ \mu^3$

    5. MCHC—normal

    6. Serum B_{12}—decreased < 0.1 mcg/ml

    7. Increased LDH

    8. Serum folate and/or RBC level—normal or decreased

    9. Serum bilirubin—increased

    10. Urinalysis—increased urobilinogen

- Management/Treatment

    1. B_{12} (cyanocobalamin) 100 micrograms IM daily for 1 week; decrease frequency and administer a total of 2,000 micrograms during the first six weeks of therapy; maintenance treatment requires lifelong administration of 100 micrograms IM monthly

    2. Follow up elderly, and clients with cardiovascular symptoms 48 hours after initiating therapy. Rapid increase in RBC production can lead to hypervolemia in these patients

    3. Consider concomitant iron supplementation during first month of therapy. Rapid blood cell regeneration increases iron requirements and can lead to iron deficiency

- General Considerations

    1. Diagnostic—consult with physician regarding

        a. Clients who have other immunologic diseases

        b. Clients having a history of oral B_{12} replacement

        c. Clients who are suspected of having pernicious anemia for further testing which may include

            (1) GI radiographic studies

            (2) Gastric analysis—absence of free hydrochloric acid after histamine or pentagastrin injection

            (3) Bone marrow aspiration— hyperplastic, megaloblastic marrow

            (4) Schilling test (tests absorption of radiolabeled vitamin B_{12} both with and without administration of intrinsic factor on basis of 24 hour urine excretion) to distinguish between primary and secondary causes

    2. Education

        a. Teach the client about the etiology and nature of the disease

        b. Discuss the need for lifelong B_{12} replacement by injection

        c. Provide client with information on side effects of B_{12} injections

            (1) Pain and burning at injection site

            (2) Peripheral vascular thrombosis

            (3) Transient diarrhea

    d. Teach client or family member to administer injections or refer to home care agency to provide injections

    e. Teach comfort and safety measures to clients with neurological involvement (can be arrested but not reversed with treatment)

3. Follow Up—check initial hematologic response in 4 to 6 weeks; then every 6 months for Hct and stool for occult blood; incidence of gastric cancer increased in persons with pernicious anemia

Folic Acid Deficiency Anemia

- Definition—a macrocytic, normochromic, megaloblastic anemia caused by a deficiency of folic acid needed for DNA synthesis, RBC maturation, and maintenance of gastric mucosa

- Etiology /Incidence

    1. Inadequate intake may be relative to malabsorption syndrome or increased demand as in pregnancy and infancy; body stores depleted more rapidly than B_{12}

    2. Drugs that may cause decreased folic acid levels include oral contraceptives, phenytoin, antimalarials, estrogen, chloramphenicol, phenobarbital

    3. Found in all races and in all age groups

    4. More common than pernicious anemia especially in alcoholics and other chronically malnourished persons

- Signs and Symptoms

    1. Similar to those of B_{12} deficiency but more severe; neurological signs are absent

    2. General Signs and Symptoms

        a. Easily fatigued

        b. Dyspnea on exertion

        c. Dizziness

        d. Listlessness

        e. Pallor (conjunctiva, nail beds, mucous membranes)

        f. Faintness

        g. Weakness

      h. Headaches

      i. Tachycardia

      j. Wide pulse pressure

      k. Heart murmurs

      l. Myocardial hypertrophy

      m. Angina

      n. Anorexia

      o. Pica

■ Differential Diagnosis

    1. Pernicious anemia

    2. Other causes of macrocytic anemia

    3. Anemia of liver disease

    4. Mylodysplastic syndromes

■ Physical Findings— similar to those found in most anemias

    1. General Appearance—pale, lethargic or no overt signs if anemia is mild

    2. Vital signs—pulse and respirations may be increased in moderate to severe anemia; in severe cases postural hypotension may be evident

    3. Integumentary—pallor and dryness of skin and mucous membranes; brittle nails; brittle, fine hair

    4. HEENT—glossitis, angular stomatitis or cheilitis; pale conjunctiva and gums

    5. Cardiovascular—tachycardia; mild cardiac enlargement; functional systolic murmurs in severe anemias

    6. Abdominal—may be some hepatic enlargement

    7. Neurological—usually within normal limits

■ Diagnostic Tests/Findings

    1. Hct—decreased

    2. Reticulocyte count—normal or decreased

    3. MCV—elevated

    4. MCHC—normal

5. Serum folate and/or RBC level decreased

6. Schilling test—normal

7. Serum B_{12}—normal

■ Management/Treatment

1. Folate 1 mg orally or parenterally per day

   a. Duration of treatment dependent on etiology of deficiency

   b. Up to 5 mg per day may be used if deficiency is related to malabsorption, (e.g., Sprue)

   c. Large doses of folic acid will correct hematologic abnormalities of B_{12} deficiency but not arrest neurologic abnormalities

2. When possible elimination of the underlying cause

■ General Considerations

1. Diagnostic—consult with physician regarding clients with suspected folate deficiency for differential diagnosis of concurrent B_{12} deficiency and treatment

2. Education—especially important for women of childbearing age as deficiency during first trimester is associated with neural tube defects in the fetus

   a. Nature and cause of anemia

   b. Need for and purpose of therapeutic replacement

   c. Teach dietary sources of folic acid which include asparagus, bananas, fish, green leafy vegetables, peanut butter, oatmeal, red beans, beef liver, wheat bran

      (1) Encourage daily intake from these foods

      (2) Instructions in preparation as overcooking can destroy folic acid

      (3) Provide client with list of foods high in folic acid

   d. Need for frequent rest periods until anemia is corrected

   e. Importance of good oral hygiene

3. Follow Up

   a. Check initial hematologic response with Hct and reticulocyte count in 4 to 6 weeks

(1) Reticulocyte count should begin to increase within 2 to 3 days after therapy is begun and should peak in 5 to 7 days

(2) Hct begins to rise after the second week

b. Individuals with a good response can be followed every 6 to 12 months if they must continue therapy

Normocytic Anemias (MCV 80-100 μ^3)

■ Hypoproliferative—reticulocyte count normal or decreased $< 3\%$ secondary to decreased bone marrow production

■ Hyperproliferative—reticulocyte count increased $> 3\%$ secondary to increased hemolysis or bleeding

Anemia of Chronic Disease (ACD)

■ Definition: A chronic, normochromic, normocytic, hypoproliferative anemia associated with chronic inflammatory disease, e.g., systemic lupus, rheumatoid arthritis; infection, e.g., bacterial endocarditis, tuberculosis, AIDS, Crohn's disease, and some malignancies; *often progresses to a hypochromic anemia*

■ Etiology/Incidence

1. The etiology is not fully understood but involves decreased erythrocyte life span; ineffective erythropoiesis; and disturbances of the iron cycle

2. The most common cause of hypoproliferative, normocytic anemia

3. Exact incidence unknown, however association with so many other disorders probably ranks it second to iron deficiency in incidence

■ Sign and Symptoms

1. General symptoms common to all anemias such as fatigue, weakness, exertional dyspnea, lightheadedness, and anorexia

2. Usually fewer and milder than most other anemias

3. Other signs and symptoms are usually related to the specific underlying disease and may be more overt than those of anemia

■ Differential Diagnosis

1. Aplastic anemia

2. Pure red blood cell aplasia

3. Infiltration marrow diseases

4. Exclude reversible causes

- Physical Findings

    1. General Appearance—may appear thin, pale, toxic

    2. Vital Signs—increased pulse and respirations

    3. Skin—may be pale, jaundiced, moist

    4. HEENT—sclera may be icteric, tongue may be coated

    5. Cardiovascular—cardiomegaly, tachycardia, systolic murmurs

    6. Abdomen—splenomegaly, hepatomegaly

- Diagnostic Tests/Findings

    1. Hct—low

    2. Hgb—low if < 9g/dl consider other causes

    3. MCV—normal or slightly low

    4. Serum iron—low

    5. TIBC—normal or low

    6. Serum ferritin—normal or increased

    7. Percentage of iron saturation (FE/TIBC)— 30% or more rules out iron deficiency

- Management/Treatment

    a. Treatment of associated disease

    b. Adequate nutritional intake; use of B_{12}, folic acid, and liver extract have not been effective in treatment of this type anemia

    c. Adequate rest

- General Considerations

    1. Diagnostic—consult with physician regarding clients with suspected anemia of chronic disease for further testing (bone marrow biopsy), and treatment of underlying disorder

    2. Education—patient education will most likely be centered on etiology and treatment of the underlying chronic disease and its relationship to anemia

    3. Follow-up—will depend on identified etiology

Sickle Cell Anemia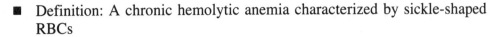

- Definition: A chronic hemolytic anemia characterized by sickle-shaped RBCs

- Etiology/Incidence

    1. Autosomal recessive genetic disorder; individual is homozygous for hemoglobins (Hb SS)

    2. Abnormal hemoglobin (Hb S) develops in place of hemoglobin A (Hb A)

    3. Some individuals may have *sickle cell trait* (heterozygous with about 1/4 of their hemoglobin in abnormal S form and remainder as normal A

    4. Mutation that causes Hb S to develop involves one amino acid; one valine amino acid is substituted for a glutamic acid

    5. Prevalent in black persons of African or Afro-American ancestry; also found at a lower frequency in persons of Mediterranean ancestry

- Signs and Symptoms

    1. Sickle Cell Trait

        a. Essentially asymptomatic

        b. Symptoms from vaso-occlusion occur only in cases of severe hypoxia

    2. Sickle Cell Anemia

        a. Manifestations due to anemia and vaso-occlusive events and to secondary end-organ damage

        b. Vaso-occlusive crises

            (1) Due to an increased rate of sickling

            (2) Precipitating factors include conditions that cause hypoxia or deoxygenation of the RBCs, e.g., viral or bacterial infections, high altitudes, emotional or physical stress, surgery, blood loss, dehydration; occasionally crisis occurs spontaneously

            (3) Episodes characterized by sudden onset of excruciating pain in back, chest, or extremities

            (4) Occasionally a low-grade fever may occur 1 to 2 days following attack

            (5) Pain may last from a few hours to a few days

       (6)   Severe abdominal pain with vomiting may be present

- Differential Diagnosis
  1. Acute pulmonary infarction without sickle ß thalassemia
  2. Acute hepatitis
  3. Choledocholithiasis
  4. Cholecystitis

- Physical Findings
  1. During vaso-occlusive crises, there may be no external findings such as heat, swelling or tenderness over the affected bones; if bone infarction occurs close to a joint, an effusion can develop
  2. Chronic findings
     a. Skin ulcers
     b. Detached retina secondary to hemorrhage of new blood vessel formation in eye
     c. Degenerative arthritis
     d. Mild sclera icterus
     e. Increased susceptibility to infection

- Diagnostic Tests/Findings
  1. Peripheral smear
     a. Sickle Cell Trait—normal
     b. Sickle Cell Anemia—partially or completely sickled cells
  2. Sickle Cell preparation
     a. Sickle Cell Trait—sickle cells
     b. Sickle Cell Anemia—sickle cells
  3. Sickledex
     a. Sickle Cell Trait—positive
     b. Sickle Cell Anemia—positive
  4. Hemoglobin Electrophoresis
     a. Sickle Cell Trait—Hb S and Hb A
     b. Sickle Cell Anemia—Hb S

- Management/Treatment
  1. Physician referral for suspected cases/physician consultation
  2. Cornerstone of therapy consists of supportive measures
     a. Large volumes of IV fluids
     b. Analgesics to control pain
     c. Antibiotics to treat associated bacterial infection including prophylactic antibiotics
     d. Oxygen to treat hypoxemia
- General Considerations
  1. Patient education
     a. Basis of disease and reasons for supportive care
     b. Instructions in methods to avoid crises
     c. Education on pain control
  2. Prevention
     a. Genetic counseling of identified heterozygotes (sickle cell trait)
     b. Prenatal diagnostic services for pregnancies at risk for sickle cell anemia

Leukemia

- Definition: Neoplasms derived from hematopoietic cells that develop in bone marrow prior to dissemination to blood, spleen, lymph nodes and tissue (Scheinberg & Golde, 1994)
- Etiology/Incidence
  1. In most cases no known cause can be found
  2. Possible causes which have been identified include
     a. Exposure to ionizing radiation and certain chemicals, e.g., benzene, prior exposure to alkylating agents
     b. Genetic and congenital factors
  3. Incidence of all leukemias is approximately 13 per 100,000/per year
  4. More frequent in males than females
- General features of the four common forms of leukemia are shown in Table 3

- Differential Diagnosis
    1. Viral induced cytopenia, lymphadenopathy
    2. Immune or drug-induced cytopenia
    3. Aplastic anemia
- Diagnostic Tests/Findings. See Table 3
    1. CBC/differential—subnormal RBCs, neutrophils and occasionally subnormal platelets
    2. Sedimentation rate—elevated
    3. Reticulocyte count— < 0.5
    4. Bone marrow studies—confirmatory for final diagnosis
    5. Chest radiograph—identification of mediastinal mass
    6. Ultrasound or CT—organamegly
- Management/Treatment
    1. Physician referral for suspected cases
        a. Goal of treatment is remission
        b. Chemotherapy
        c. Bone marrow transplantation
    2. Assistance in meeting psychosocial needs
    3. Assistance for patient and families in adjusting to chronic effects of illness, e.g., dependence, withdrawal, changes in role responsibilities, alterations in body image

Table 3
Comparison of Most Common Types of Leukemia

Type	Age of Onset	Signs & Symptoms Physical Findings	Diagnostic Tests/Findings	Prognosis
Acute Lymphocytic	Childhood More gradual rise in frequency in later life	Fever; pallor; bleeding; anorexia; fatigue; generalized lymphadenopathy and several other manifestations	WBC—H, L, or N RBC, Hgb, Hct-L platelets-L Bone marrow- lymphoblasts	Good response to treatment
Acute Myelogenous	Increase with age; 50% under age of 50	Fatigue; weakness; headache; mouth sores; bleeding; fever; sternal tenderness; occasional lymphadenopathy	RBCs, Hgb, Hct-L Platelet ct— very low WBC—H to L Myeloblasts—many	Remission rates range from 50 to 85%; patients > 50 years are less likely to achieve remission
Chronic Lymphocytic	Middle and old age	May be asymptomatic; may have fatigue anorexia, weight loss, dyspnea on exertion; splenomegaly; lymphadenopathy; hepatomegaly	Hallmark is sustained absolute lymphocy- tosis 40,000-150,000/μl; Bone marrow— increased lymphocytes	Median survival— approximately 10 yrs
Chronic Myelogenous	Occurs most often at median age of 45	may be asymptomatic; or insidious onset of nonspecific symptoms, e.g., fatigue, weakness, anorexia, weight loss, fever	RBCs, Hgb, Hct-L Platelet count— H early, L later; WBC-H; leukocytosis with immature granulocytes WBC—usually about 200,000/μl in sympto- matic pt; Bone marrow— Ph[1] chromosome presence is significant	Median survival is 3 to 4 years after clinical onset

L = low; N = normal; H = high

- Patient Education

    1. Importance of compliance with chemotherapy regimens; side effects and management

    2. Disease process and rationale for treatment

    3. Adaptation to any physical limitations

Non-Hodgkin's Lymphoma

- Definition: Heterogenous group of lymphocytic malignancies with absence of giant Reed-Sternberg cells characteristic of Hodgkin's Disease

- Etiology/Incidence

1. Etiology unclear; animal studies have suggested a viral etiology
2. Other factors associated with increased incidence includes
   a. Ionizing radiation
   b. Hereditary predisposition
   c. Congenital or acquired immunodeficiency
   d. Exposure to pesticides
3. Approximately 40,000 new cases occur each year in the U.S., and appear to be increasing (Freedman & Nadler, 1994)
4. Most common neoplasm between ages of 20 and 40; with increased incidence of AIDS, number of cases has sharply increased

- Signs and Symptoms
  1. More than 2/3 of patients present with persistent painless peripheral lymphadenopathy
  2. Some patients may present with persistent cough and chest discomfort (mediastinal involvement)
  3. If abdominal contents involved, chronic pain, abdominal fullness, early satiety or viscus obstruction may be presenting symptoms
  4. Diffuse disease may present with skin lesions, testicular masses

- Differential Diagnosis
  1. Infectious mononucleosis
  2. Cytomegalovirus infection
  3. Human immunodeficiency virus involvement
  4. Toxoplasmosis
  5. Other malignant tumors
  6. Cat-scratch disease
  7. Tuberculosis
  8. Syphilis
  9. Sarcoidosis

- Physical Findings
  1. Painless peripheral lymphadenopathy may be initial finding
  2. May present with abdominal mass, massive splenomegaly

3. Early systemic findings usuallly absent

■ Diagnostic Tests/Findings

1. Requires skilled interpretation of adequate tumor tissue to determine tumor architecture and cell type

2. B cell and T cell typing—complements pathologic interpretation

3. Bone marrow biopsy—pathologic confirmation of disease process

4. Staging procedures conducted once diagnosis established—no perfect classification system exists; various types include the Rappaport classification, Luke and Collins classification, the International Panel Working Formulation (NCI), Ann Arbor staging system

■ Management/Treatment
(Based on grade and extent of disease)

1. Radiotherapy

2. Chemotherapy

3. Bone marrow transplantation

4. Newer modalities include MAbs alone and combined with radionuclides or toxins to produce cytotoxic effects; cytokines, e.g., interferons, tumor necrosis factor and interleukin 2 are currently under study

■ General Considerations

1. Prognosis not usually as good as with Hodgkin's disease.

2. Both family and patient require supportive therapy during diagnosis and treatment stages

3. Education and necessity of drug compliance important factor

4. Increased susceptibility to infection

Hodgkin's Disease

■ Definition: Malignant disorder with lymphoreticular proliferation

■ Etiology/Incidence

1. Cause is unknown

2. Approximately 8,000 new cases are diagnosed each year in the U.S.

3. Average age is 32 years; peaks at 15 to 35 years and again after age 50

4. More common in males

- Signs and Symptoms
    1. Most patients present with a painless, enlarging mass, most often in the neck or occasionally in axilla or inguinal region; often the only manifestation at time of diagnosis
    2. Older patients may present with
        a. Fatigue
        b. Weight loss
        c. Persistent fever and/or night sweats
    3. Pruritis—may be mild and localized, but may be progressive; rarely occurs in the absence of fever
    4. An unexplained symptom is immediate pain in diseased areas after consuming alcoholic beverages
- Differential Diagnosis
    1. Infectious mononucleosis
    2. Toxoplasmosis
    3. Cytomegalic inclusion disease
    4. Non-Hodgkin's lymphoma
    5. Leukemia
    6. Bronchogenic carcinoma
    7. Sarcoidosis
- Physical Findings
    1. Initial findings are usually enlargement of cervical, axillary, or inguinal lymph nodes (movable, nontender)
    2. Other findings may include hepatomegaly and splenomegaly; usually not present unless the disease is advanced
- Diagnostic Tests/Findings
    1. Presence of characteristic Reed-Sternberg giant cell on biopsy of lymph node tissue or other sites (needle aspiration not sufficient)
    2. WBC—polymorphonuclear leukocytosis may be present
    3. CBC—hypochromic, microcytic anemia in advanced disease
    4. Low serum iron, low iron binding capacity
    5. Chest radiologic examinations—to determine medistinal involvement

- Management/Treatment
  1. Physician referral for suspected cases
     a. Radiotherapy
     b. Chemotherapy
     c. Autologous bone marrow transplant for chemotherapy failures
  2. For treatment to be precise, Hodgkin's disease needs to be staged which involves determining the extent and involvement of the disease
- General Consideratiolns
  1. Psychosocial considerations for patient and family
  2. Since prognosis is usually good, patients need to be helped to deal with the disease realistically even though it is a malignant disorder
  3. Once patient is in remission, ongoing maintenance treatment is usually not needed; patients need to be instructed in the importance of returning for follow-up visits
  4. Patient education
     a. Gonadal side effects of treatment
     b. Consideration of sperm banking for males
     c. Risk of secondary malignancy

Questions

Select the best answer

A 50 year old male of Italian descent comes in for a routine work related health assessment. He has no complaints. His history and physical examination are unremarkable. A routine CBC indicates
Hgb 11.2 g/100 ml MCV 72mm^3, WBC 5.7 x 10^3,
Hct 35%, MCH 25

1. Based on this information how would his anemia be classified?
   a. Normocytic, normochromic
   b. Microcytic, hypochromic
   c. Macrocytic, hypochromic
   d. Microcytic, normochromic
   e. Macrocytic, normochromic

2. Which aspect of this patient's history would provide the least useful information for diagnostic decision making?

   a. Diet (including alcohol use)
   b. Social history
   c. Family history
   d. Medical history

You find that this patient has a diet with regular intake of lean red meats, vegetables, and fruits and he denies alchohol use except once or twice a year. He does use Maalox almost daily for indigestion. He says that weak blood runs in his family, although he has never had this problem. He has no surgical history and has never been treated for any medical problems except high cholesterol which was treated with diet and exercise

3. This information helps rule out which of the following as cause for his anemia

   a. Folate deficiency
   b. Inadequate dietary intake
   c. GI bleeding
   d. Malabsorption of vitamins and minerals

4. This patient's lack of abnormal physical signs and symptoms

   a. Probably indicate a lab error in the blood work
   b. Is not unusual given the degree of his anemia
   c. Is not unusual in a patient of this age
   d. May be masked by use of Maalox

5. Your next step would be to

    a. Order B_{12} and folate serum levels
    b. Order serum iron and TIBC
    c. Obtain a urine culture
    d. Order a Schilling test

6. What other test would be essential at this point?

    a. Stool Guaiac
    b. GI Series
    c. Bilirubin
    d. Liver functions tests

7. Which is the most likely etiology of the type of anemia exhibited in this patient?

    a. B_{12} or folate deficiency
    b. Chronic disease
    c. Dehydration
    d. GI bleeding

8. If you obtain a negative stool guaiac in a male patient with a microcytic, hypochromic anemia who has a low serum iron and a high TIBC, you would

    a. Begin ferrous sulfate 300 mg orally t.i.d.
    b. Order a Schilling test
    c. Repeat the stool guaiac
    d. Refer to a hematologist

Mrs. M. is a 30 year old graduate student from Morocco with a family and personal history of "weak blood" who presents with a complaint of abdominal pain, increasing fatigue, and weight loss. She has never needed treatment for her blood problem but has been supplementing her usually well balanced diet with high potency vitamin and mineral supplements because of the increased stress of graduate studies in a foreign country. A routine CBC indicates a mild microcytic, hypochromic anemia.

9. It is likely that this patient's "weak blood" is

    a. Thalassemia Minor
    b. Thalassemia Major
    c. Related to an unidentified chronic disease
    d. Related to an iron deficiency from gastrointestinal bleeding

10. You need to consider which of the folowing as a strong etiology for her current symptoms?

    a. Iron deficiency

   b. Folate deficiency
   c. Peptic ulcer
   d. Iron overload

11. If further blood studies indicate a decreased TIBC and increased serum iron your next step shoud be which of the following?

   a. Tell Mrs. M. to discontinue her vitamin/mineral supplements and refer her for hematologic consult
   b. Refer her for genetic counseling
   c. Refer for hemoglobin electrophoresis
   d. Begin chelation therapy and refer for a GI consult

Ms. Z is a 26 year old, black female who comes in complaining of fatigue, shortness of breath, and lightheadedness. Her history reveals no significant medical problems but several years of fad dieting without vitamin supplementation. Physical findings are unremarkable except for pallor of the mucous membranes, tachycardia, and a systolic flow murmur

12. Your next step would be to

   a. Start on B_{12} injections
   b. Order a CBC, reticulocyte count
   c. Order a TIBC and serum iron
   d. Start on multivitamins with iron

13. Further testing of Ms. Z. reveals a low reticulocyte count and macrocytic cells. Your next step should be to

   a. Start B_{12} injections
   b. Order serum iron and TIBC
   c. Order RBC-folate and B_{12} levels
   d. Order a Schilling test

14. Which of the following would help in your differential diagnosis

   a. Patient's history of ice pica
   b. Patient's use of oral contraceptives
   c. A confirmed diagnosis of sickle cell trait
   d. Family history of iron deficiency

15. The anemias most often associated with pregnancy are

   a. Folic acid and iron deficiency
   b. Folic acid deficiency and Thalassemia
   c. Iron deficiency and Thalassemia
   d. Thalassemia and B_{12} deficiency

16. Neural tube defects in the fetus have been primarily associated with which type deficiency in the mother?

    a. Iron
    b. Folic Acid
    c. Vitamin B_{12}
    e. Vitamin E

17. Most common causes of megaloblastic, macrocytic anemia are

    a. Folate and or B_{12} deficiency
    b. Chronic disease
    c. Iron deficiency and infection
    d. Hemolysis of blood cells

18. Patients with iron deficiency anemia should be instructed that

    a. Return of normal blood values will occur within a week of oral iron supplementation
    b. Iron supplements will need to be taken for the rest of their life
    c. Taking iron preparations with milk will enhance absorption
    d. Iron preparation may be taken with meals

19. Elderly persons with pernicious anemia should

    a. Be instructed to increase their dietary intake of food high in B_{12}
    b. Be told they will not need to return for follow-up for at least a month after initiation of treatment
    c. Be told that oral B_{12} is safer and less expensive than parenteral replacement
    d. Be told that diarrhea can be a transient side effect of B_{12} injections

20. Which of the following would be included in diet rich in iron?

    a. Peaches, eggs, beef
    b. Cereals, kale, cheese
    c. Red beans, enriched breads, squash
    d. Legumes, green beans, eggs

21. A woman taking folic acid supplements for Folic Acid Deficiency will need to know that

    a. It will take several months before she will feel better
    b. Folic acid should not be taken with meals and may cause diarrhea
    c. Iron supplements are contraindicated while one is on folic acid
    d. Oral contraceptives, pregnancy and lactation increase dietary requirements for folic acid

22. In alcoholics with anemia

    a. Pernicious anemia is more common than folic acid deficiency
    b. Iron deficiency, folic acid deficiency may coexist
    c. The alcohol interferes with iron absorption
    d. All of the preceding

23. Hypoproliferative normocytic anemia

    a. Is marked by a normal or decreased reticulocyte count
    b. Is usually secondary to hemolysis or bleeding
    c. Is relatively rare and usually only associated with malignancies
    d. Is only associated with chronic infections

24. In normocytic anemia of chronic disease

    a. Treatment is purely symptomatic
    b. Long term supplementation of folic acid and B_{12} is needed
    c. Treatment is focused on the associated disease
    d. Serum iron and TIBC are the most specific and sensitive diagnostic tests

25. Which of the following is true of anemia of chronic disease?

    a. A Hgb of < 9 g/dl confirms the diagnosis
    b. Symptoms associated with the anemia may be masked by the symptoms of the underlying disease
    c. Is manifested by more severe signs than most of the other common anemias
    d. Is never associated with reversible causes

26. Sickle Cell Anemia is caused by

    a. Replacement of hemoglobin A with hemoglobin CS
    b. Transposition of glutamic acid on hemoglobin A molecule
    c. Abnormal hemoglobin S in place of hemoglobin A
    d. Sickle cell trait

27. The most sensitive test for the diagnosis of sickle cell anemia/sickle cell trait is

    a. Sickle cell preparation
    b. Peripheral smear
    c. Sickledex
    d. Hemoglobin electrophoresis

28. Chronic myelogonous leukemia usually presents with the following

    a. Increased platelets and leukocytosis
    b. Presence of Reed-Sternberg cells in bone marrow aspirate

c. Ph[1] chromosome in bone marrow

d. With typical fatigue, weakness, anorexia and frequent nosebleeds

29. A 32 year-old male presents in the office with concerns about a lump in the area of his collar bone. He states that someone told him that it might be a sign of some kind of cancer. Your best response at this time would be to

a. Examine him and tell him to come back in two weeks to be reevaluated

b. Inquire whether he has any cats which might cause Cat Scratch fever

c. Work him up for a possibility of infectious mononucleosis

d. Examine him with referral to physician for possible Hodgkin's disease work-up

30. Diagnosis of Hodgkin's disease is based upon

a. Presenting symptoms of fatigue, weight loss and pruritis associated with night sweats

b. Presence of Ph[1] chromosome in lymphoid tissue

c. Extensive lymphadenopathy with elevated WBC count

d. Presence of Reed-Sternberg cells in lymph node tissue

Answers

1. b
2. b
3. b
4. b
5. b
6. a
7. d
8. c
9. a
10. d
11. a
12. b
13. c
14. b
15. a
16. b
17. a
18. d
19. d
20. a
21. d
22. b
23. a
24. c
25. b
26. c
27. d
28. c
29. d
30. d

Bibliography

Brown, B. (1993). *Hematology: Principles and procedures* (6th ed.). Philadelphia: Lea and Febigen.

Brown, R. (1991). Determining the cause of anemias: General approach with emphasis on microcytic hypochromic anemia. *Postgraduate Medicine*, 89(6), 161-170.

Bunn, H. F. (1994). Disorders of hemoglobin. In K. J. Isselbacher, E. Braunwald, J. Wilson, J. Martin, A. Fauci & D. L. Kasper (Eds.). *Harrison's principles of internal medicine* (pp. 1734-1741) (13th ed.). NY: McGraw-Hill.

Bushnell, F. (1992). A guide to primary care of iron deficiency anemia. *Nurse Practitioner*, 17(11), 68, 71-74.

Colon-Otero, G., Menke, D., & Hook, C. (1992). A practical approach to the differential diagnosis and evaluation of the adult patient with macrocytic anemia. *Medical Clinics of North America*, 76(3), 581-597.

Fairbanks, V. (1991) Laboratory testing for Iron status. *Hospital Practice*, 26 (suppl. 3), 17-24.

Freedman, A. S., & Nadler, L. M. (1994). Malignant lymphomas. In K. J. Isselbacher, E. Braunwald, J. Wilson, J. Martin, A. Fauci & D. L. Kasper (Eds.). *Harrison's principles of internal medicine* (pp. 1774-1788) (13th ed.). NY: McGraw-Hill.

Johnson, J. M., Leidal, B., & Littler, J. E. (1990). Anemia. In J. E. Littler & T. Momany (Eds.), *The family practice handbook* (pp. 165-171). Chicago: Year Book Medical Publishers.

Massey, A. (1992). Microcytic anemia. *Medical Clinics of North America*, 76 (3), 549-566.

Parker-Cohen, P., & McCance, K. (1990). Alterations of erythrocyte function. In K. McCane & S. Huether (Eds.), *Pathophysiology: The biological basis for disease in adults and children* (pp.784-799). St. Louis: C. V. Mosby.

Portlock, C. S. (1992). Non-Hodgkin's lymphomas. In J. B. Wyngaarden, L. H. Smith, Jr., & J. C. Bennett (Eds.). *Cecil textbook of medicine*, (pp. 951-955), (19th ed.). Philadelphia: W. B. Saunders.

Scheinberg, D., & Golde, D. W. (1994). The leukemias. In K. J. Isselbacher, E.

Braunwald, J. Wilson, J. Martin, A. Fauci & D. L. Kasper (Eds.). *Harrison's principles of internal medicine* (pp. 1764-1774) (13th ed.). NY: McGraw-Hill.

Snyder, C. S. (1990). Hematologic Disorders. In *Manual of geriatric nursing* (pp.357-388). Glenview, IL: Scott, Foresman/Little Brown Higher Education.

Welborn, I., & Meyers, F. (1991). A three-point approach to anemia. *Postgraduate Medicine*, 89, 179-183,186.

Wesler, B., Moore, A., & Tepler, J. (1990). Hematology. In T. E. Andreoli, C. C. Carpenter, F. Plum, & L. H. Smith (Eds.), *Cecil essentials of medicine* (2nd ed.), (pp.342-402). Philadelphia: W. B. Saunders.

Gastrointestinal Disorders

Sister Maria Salerno

Peptic Ulcer Disease (PUD)

- Definition: Ulceration of the GI mucosa in areas bathed by acid pepsin; stomach, duodenum, and esophagus are common sites

- Etiology/Incidence

  1. Involves an imbalance between mucosal protective factors and corrosive effects of acid and pepsin which may include

     a. Hypersecretion of the gastric mucosa

     b. Increased parietal cell mass

     c. Increased secretion of gastrin and hydrochloric acid

     d. Increased gastric emptying time

     e. Recent research indicates infection with *Helicobacter pylori*, formerly known as *Campylobacter pylori*, appears to be a requisite factor

  2. Precipitating or aggravating factors include

     a. Steroidal and nonsteroidal anti-inflammatory drug therapy, particularly aspirin

     b. Physiologic stress—severe trauma, burns, shock

     c. Psychological stress

     d. Alcohol and nicotine use

     e. Presence of alcoholic liver cirrhosis, chronic pancreatitis, chronic lung disease, hyperparathyroidism, rheumatoid arthritis

  3. Thought to affect about 10% of the adult population

     a. Duodenal

        (1) 80% are duodenal

        (2) Higher incidence in males

        (3) 80% recur in year following initial healing

        (4) Incidence decreasing in the U.S.

        (5) Familial disposition-more frequent in persons with Type O blood

     b. Gastric

        (1) Occur with about the same incidence in males and female

        (2) About 5% are malignant

    (3)   Common in the 5th and 6th decades of life

- Signs and Symptoms

  1. Intermittent epigastric pain—gnawing, burning, boring, nagging

  2. Pain begins 1 to 3 hours after eating, frequently awakens person at night

  3. Pain relieved by food or antacids

  4. Food sometimes aggravates pain of gastric ulcer

  5. Weight loss frequent in persons with gastric ulcer

  6. Dyspepsia (bloating, nausea, anorexia, excessive flatulence)

- Differential Diagnosis

  1. History of typical pain-food-relief pattern is most important criterion for diagnosis of duodenal ulcer

  2. History not helpful in distinguishing gastric from duodenal

  3. Rule out other causes of epigastric pain

     a. Pancreatitis

     b. Biliary tract disease

     c. Neoplasms

     d. Liver disease

     e. Gastritis

     f. Pneumonia

     g. Functional problems

     h. Cardiovascular disease

- Physical Findings: Usually limited to epigastric tenderness

- Diagnostic Tests/Findings

  1. Barium radiograph of the upper GI tract will detect 90% of peptic ulcers

     a. Diagnose atypical cases

     b. Typical presentations with failure to respond to treatment in 3 to 4 weeks; and cases of recurrence

     c. Differentiate gastric from duodenal

     d. Differentiate between malignant and nonmalignant gastric ulcers

   e. Document healing

2. Endoscopy

   a. More expensive, but also more sensitive and specific than barium radiographs; becoming test of choice in many settings

   b. Indicated if clinical symptoms persist despite negative barium studies

   c. To rule out malignancy in gastric ulcers

   d. To locate bleeding site in those with diagnosed or suspected blood loss

3. Stool for occult blood—positive if bleeding is present

4. CBC

   a. Hgb and Hct may be decreased

   b. With chronic slow bleeding— hypochromic, microcytic anemia is likely

   c. If bleeding is acute—normocytic, normochromic anemia

5. Gastric analysis with culture for *H. pylori*—positive in 90% with duodenal ulcer and 75% of those with gastic ulcer

■ Management/Treatment

1. Goals

   a. Relief of symptoms

   b. Healing

   c. Prevention of recurrence

2. Nonpharmacological

   a. Stop smoking

   b. Avoid ASA and nonsteroidal anti-inflammatory drugs

   c. Reduce stress

   d. Reduce use of alcohol and caffeine (conflicting data, but still recommended until healing is documented)

3. Pharmacological

   a. H_2 receptor antagonists

      (1) Cimetidine (Tagamet)—300 mg orally t.i.d. with meals and

at bedtime for 4 to 6 weeks (more recent studies indicate similar healing with 400 mg b.i.d. or 800 mg at bedtime)

(a) May be given IV in inpatient settings

(b) Side effects
  (i) Frequently associated with acute confusional states in elderly or very ill patients.
  (ii) Muscular pain; mild, transient diarrhea; impotence; gynecomastia; leukopenia; mildly elevated creatinine and transaminase levels are rarer and tend to be seen only with long-term use

(c) Interferes with metabolism of benzodiazapines, lidocaine, metronidazole, phenytoin, theophylline, and warfarin and their blood levels are increased

(d) Should not be taken within an hour of taking antacids

(2) Ranitidine (Zantac)—150 mg orally b.i.d. or 300 mg orally at bedtime, inactive PUD; 150 mg orally at bedtime for maintenance

(a) Also available for IV use

(b) Side effects—rise in transaminase levels (SGPT); dizziness; tachycardia; malaise; constipation; diarrhea; rash; and rarely confusion

(c) No significant drug interactions

(d) May cause false-positive protein on urinary dip-stick analysis

(3) Famotidine (Pepcid)—20 mg orally twice a day or 40 mg at bedtime

(a) Appears to be as efficacious as Rantidine

(b) Safety profile not as clearly defined as Rantidine

b. Antacids

(1) Should give dose equivalent to 80 to 100 mEq acid neutralizing capacity; for most, 30 to 40 ml given 1 and 3 hours after each meal; see Table 1 for comparison of various antacid preparations

(2) Primarily aluminum, calcium, or magnesium containing agents; sodium bicarbonate very short acting and systemic

absorption can cause alkalosis (not recommended)

- (3) Length of effect dependent on gastric emptying time; 30 minutes on an empty stomach, longer when taken with meals

- (4) Side effects
    - (a) Diarrhea with magnesium hydroxide based agents
    - (b) Constipation with aluminum hydroxide containing agents
    - (c) Hypophosphatemia in aluminum containing agents due to aluminum phosphate binding and decreased GI absorption
    - (d) Osteopenia with long-term use of agents containing aluminum
    - (e) Rebound acid secretion and hypercalcemia with calcium containing agents

- (5) Drug interactions
    - (a) Most inhibit absorption of tetracyclines and should not be used concurrently with them
    - (b) Interfere with effectiveness of oral contraceptives

c. Anticholinergics

- (1) Rarely used in contemporary treatment and only with advice of physician
- (2) Primarily for relief of refractory pain
- (3) High dosage with severe side effects required to achieve antisecretory effect

d. Sucralfate (mucosal protectant)—1 gm orally q.i.d. on an empty stomach

- (1) No significant side effects
- (2) Drug Interaction
    - (a) Decreases absorption of digoxin, tetracycline, phenytoin, and cimetidine
    - (b) Antacids interfere with effectiveness and should not be given within 1 hour of sucralfate administration

e. Treatment with antacids, H_2 receptor antagonists, or sucralfate results in 90 to 95% cure rate in 8 to 12 weeks. Frequently recurring duodenal ulcers are treated with maintenance doses of sucralfate and/or H_2 receptor antagonists

f. "Triple treatment" to eradicate *H. pylori*, especially for recurrent ulcers

    (1) Colloidal bismuth subcitrate 30 cc q.i.d. *with* Metronidazole 200 to 500 mg t.i.d. *plus* Amoxicillin 250 to 500 mg q.i.d. or tetracycline 500 mg q.i.d.

    (2) Given for 2 to 3 weeks

    (3) Concomitant use of H_2 blocker

- General Considerations

  1. Consult with physician regarding

    a. Additional diagnostic studies for persons with suspected underlying disease or failure to respond to treatment in 2 to 4 weeks

    b. Persons with concurrent weight loss

    c. Persons with indications of peritonitis (rigidity, rebound tenderness, fever)

  2. Refer to physicians persons with confirmed or suspected complications

    a. Bleeding occurs in about 10 to 15% of persons with PUD

      (1) Immediate medical emergency with possible surgical intervention required

      (2) Signs and symptoms— heartburn, belching, epigastric discomfort, vomiting of bright red or coffee ground liquid

      (3) Sudden relief of epigastric pain may be related to bleeding as blood acts as an acid buffer

      (4) Diarrhea may also be evident; blood is a cathartic

    b. Perforation occurs in about 5 to 10% of persons with duodenal and 2 to 5% of those with gastric ulcers

      (1) Surgery is the indicated treatment

      (2) Signs and symptoms include acute pain, fever, leukocytosis, hypotension, peritoneal irritation

      (3) Peritoneal irritation is evidenced by abdominal rigidity, guarding, rebound tenderness, decreased or absent bowel sounds

      c. Gastric Outlet (Pyloric) Obstruction is seen in less than 5% of all patients diagnosed with PUD and is most often associated with duodenal ulceration

        (1)   Surgical intervention may be indicated

        (2)   Signs and symptoms include worsening pain; vomiting of undigested food; dehydration; hypokalemia; and metabolic alkalosis

3.   Patient Education

    a. Disease and therapeutic management

    b. Purpose, dosage, side effects of medications

    c. Diet

        (1)   No evidence to support need for bland diet or small frequent meals

        (2)   Encourage avoidance of known gastric acid stimulants, e.g., coffee, cola, and other caffeine containing beverages

        (3)   Avoidance of any foods or beverages which aggravate symptoms

        (4)   Avoid eating within 3 hours of bedtime to avoid nocturnal stimulation of acid secretion

    d. Stress reduction

    e. Need to report to health care provider lack of response to medications, rectal bleeding, weight loss, increased weakness or dizziness, increasing pain

4.   Follow up

    a. In 2 to 4 weeks to check on

        (1)   Symptom response to medications

        (2)   GI bleeding

        (3)   Side or toxic effects of medications

    b. For those with gastric ulcers document healing with Upper GI barium radiograph or endoscopy: in 6 weeks for small ulcers; 12 weeks for large; imperative in gastric ulcers; unnecessary in uncomplicated duodenal

Table 1
Antacids

Content Comments	Brand Name	Dose required for 80-100 mEq of acid neutralizing effect per dose	mEq of sodium per dose
Low Buffering Capacity			
$CaCO_3$ Rebound hyperacidity	Tums Alka II Chooz	8-10 tablets	0.5-0.6
$Al(OH)_3$ Constipating; high sodium	Amphogel	60-75 ml	1.2-1.5
$Al(OH)_3$ & $Mg(OH)_3$ Only for esophageal reflux.	Gaviscon	94-118 ml	10.6-13.2
Moderate Buffering Capacity			
$Al(OH)_3$ & $Mg(OH)_3$ Low Sodium	Gelusil Mylanta Maalox Plus Riopan	35-44 ml 32-40 m. 30-38 ml 30-38 ml	0.23-0.29 0.20-0.25 0.36-0.45 0.08-0.1
High Buffering Capacity			
$Al(OH)_3$ & $Mg(OH)_3$ Liquid more effective than tablets.	Gelusil II Maalox TC Mylanta II	17-21 ml 14-18 ml 16-20 ml	0.2-0.25 0.1-0.13 0.16-0.2

Note: Sodium Bicarbonate, Alka Seltzer have a very short duration of action; acid rebound, systemic alkalosis are problems.

Gastroesophageal reflux disease

- Definition: Reflux of stomach and duodenal contents into the esophagus leading to a spectrum of clinical manifestations predominated by inflammation of the esophagus; classified with gastric and duodenal ulcers as a peptic ulcer disease

- Etiology/Incidence

    1. Most often related to inappropriate relaxation of the lower esophageal sphincter (LES) which allows reflux of gastric acid and pepsin into the distal esophagus

    2. Narcotics, benzodiazepines, calcium channel blockers, alcohol, nicotine, chocolate, and peppermint cause LES relaxation

    3. Inflammation can also be caused by ingestion of caustic agents such as lye, or infectious agents such as candida, herpes simplex, or cytomegalovirus which directly attacks esophageal mucosa

4. Infectious agents most often noted in immunosupressed individuals, e.g., persons with AIDS, diabetes, and persons receiving chemotherapy

5. Incidence not known, however, a daily prevalence rate of heartburn, the major symptom of esophagitis, has been estimated to be 17–65% in a normal adult population

- Signs and Symptoms

1. Retrosternal aching or burning occurring 30 to 60 minutes after eating; associated with large meals, and aggravated by lying down or bending over

2. Chest heaviness, pressure radiating to neck or jaw, or shoulders

3. Regurgitation of fluid or food particles

4. Nocturnal aspiration

5. Recurrent pneumonia or bronchospasm

6. Pain or difficulty swallowing

7. Iron deficiency anemia

- Differential Diagnosis

1. Myocardial infarction/Angina

2. Esophageal spasm

3. Cholelithiasis

4. Neoplasms

5. Mediastinal inflammation

6. Conditions leading to gastric dysmotility, e.g., scleroderma, diabetes

7. Infections (CMV, herpes, candida)

- Physical Findings: Generally insignificant

- Diagnostic Tests/Findings

1. Usually only needed in atypical or severe cases

2. Barium radiograph of upper GI tract

    a. To rule out neoplasm or other acid-peptic disease indicated in patients with

        (1) Dysphagia

       (2)   Painful swallowing

       (3)   Significant weight loss

       (4)   Occult blood loss

   b. Usually normal, but may show inflammation, ulcer, or stricture

3.   Endoscopy is becoming more routine than barium radiography in most settings and is indicated in same instances as barium radiography; may show visible mucosal damage which can be confirmed by biopsy. In cases of caustic ingestion or suspected infectious etiology endoscopy is usually first diagnostic test

4.   Bernstein Acid Perfusion—rarely needed with classic history. Requires alternating infusion of 0.1 N hydrochloric acid and normal saline into the esophagus. Positive reproduction of symptoms with the hydrochloric acid infusion and not the saline is usual in esophageal reflux

5.   Esophageal motility and 24 hour esophageal pH tests are more specialized and reserved for atypical cases; consult with or refer patient to gastroenterologist

- Management/Treatment

1.   Implement general measures

   a. Weight reduction if obese

   b. Elevation of head of bed

   c. Avoid large meals and carbonated beverages particularly 3 hours prior to going to bed; no indication that fruit juices aggravate the problem

   d. Limit fats and carbohydrates

   e. Avoid straining at stool

   f. Avoid agents that decrease LES tone— nicotine, alcohol, chocolate, caffeine, theophylline, calcium channel blockers, anticholinergics

   g. Antacids—(See Table 1)

       (1)   Mainstay of therapy

       (2)   80 to 100 mEq of neutralizing activity (30 cc for most agents) after meals and at bedtime.

       (3)   Liquid preferred to tablet forms

2. If general measures are ineffective add H_2 antagonist—cimetidine or ranitidine in same dosages as in Peptic Ulcer Disease

3. If these generally conservative measures are ineffective consult with physician regarding further testing and use of more aggressive therapy which might include

   a. Use of agents to increase LES tone

      (1) Metoclopramide 10 mg orally 30 minutes before meals and at bedtime; dopamine antagonist increases sphincter tone and increases gastric motility; severe CNS side effects in about 33% of those who receive it necessitating discontinuance

      (2) Bethanechol 25 mg orally 30 minutes before meals and at bedtime; cholinergic agent contraindicated in persons with asthma, ischemic heart disease, or urinary retention

   b. Surgical intervention—reserved for patients with stricture, bleeding, pulmonary aspiration, or severe refractory symptoms

- General Considerations

  1. Consult with physician regarding persons

     a. With atypical presentation

     b. Refractory to simple treatment

     c. With dysphagia and or weight loss in addition to heartburn

  2. Education

     a. Mechanism of esophageal reflux and goals of management

     b. Aggravating factors

     c. Correction of misconceptions regarding causes (hiatal hernia seldom a cause) and treatment

     d. Proper use, dosage, side effects of pharmacologic agents

Cholecystitis

- Definition: Acute or chronic inflammation of the gallbladder.

- Etiology/Incidence

  1. About 90% related to presence of pigmented or cholesterol calculi which can vary in diameter from 1 mm to 1 to 4 cm; when a stone becomes impacted in the cystic duct, inflammation develops behind

the obstruction; if not relieved, pressure builds up in the gallbladder and leads to distension, ischemic changes, gangrene, and perforation with subsequent abscess formation and less frequently generalized peritonitis

2. Occurs subsequent to bile stasis, bacterial infection, or ischemia

3. Most common form of gallbladder disease; affects more than 15 million Americans

4. Advanced age, being female, and being obese are all risk factors

5. Pregnancy, sedentary lifestyle, and low fiber diets also associated with the development of cholecystitis

- Signs and Symptoms

  1. Episodic occurrences of postprandial fullness, heartburn, nausea, flatulence, regurgitation of bitter fluid, vomiting often precipitated by a large or fatty meal.

  2. Anorexia (Inability to finish an average size meal).

  3. Recurrent episodes of biliary colic — sudden appearance of severe pain in the epigastrium or right hypochondrium which subsides relatively slowly (12 to 18 hours)

     a. Tenderness of the same area may persist for days

     b. Accompanied by vomiting in 75% of the cases

  4. Constant aching pain or pressure in the right upper quadrant or epigastrium that radiates to the back or right shoulder

- Differential Diagnosis

  1. Perforated peptic ulcer

  2. Acute pancreatitis

  3. Appendicitis

  4. Salpingitis

  5. Diverticulitis

  6. Perforated hepatic carcinoma

  7. Liver abscess

  8. Hepatitis

  9. Pneumonia with right sided pleurisy

  10. Myocardial infarction

■ Physical Findings

1. General appearance—unremarkable between attacks; ill appearance during attack

2. Vital signs—mild temperature elevation, tachycardia, and increased respiratory rate during acute attack

3. Integument—mild jaundice occurs in about 20% of cases

4. Abdomen—guarding, rebound tenderness in right hypochondrium; palpable, tender sausage shaped mass in RUQ during acute attack in 20 to 30% of cases

5. Positive Murphy's sign—inspiratory arrest secondary to extreme tenderness when subhepatic area is palpated during deep inspiration

■ Diagnostic Tests/Findings

1. CBC—mild leukocytosis with increased bands (shift to the left)

2. ECG—normal, important in ruling out myocardial infarction as cause of symptoms

3. Chest radiograph—normal, important in ruling out pneumonia as cause of symptoms

4. Flat plate radiograph of abdomen—gallstones

5. Ultrasound (study of choice)—gallstones, thickened gallbladder wall

6. Technetium T_c99_m PIPIDA (HIDA) scan—cystic duct occlusion and non-visualized gallbladder

7. Alkaline phosphatase—elevated

8. Serum amylase—elevated

9. Serum aspartate aminotransferase (AST, formerly termed SGOT) and serum alanine aminotransferase (ALT, formerly SGPT) may be transiently elevated

10. Bilirubin—mildly increased

■ Management/Treatment

1. Elective cholecystectomy recommended for

   a. Symptomatic patients with radiologic or ultrasound evidence of gallbladder disease

   b. Those at high risk for complications such as those with

      (1) A calcified gall bladder

      (2)   Gallstones > 2 cm in diameter

      (3)   Diabetes

2.   Conservative treatment for those who are asymptomatic

  a. If on clofibrate (an antilipemic) or oral contraceptives stop or decrease dosage

  b. Avoid foods that seem to precipitate symptoms, otherwise no need to alter diet or restrict fats

  c. Anticholinergics not helpful

  d. Treat dyspeptic symptoms with antacids (25 to 50% of patients will respond)

  e. Some patients may be put on a trial of chenodiol 750 mg orally per day

     (1) Best results are obtained in patients with small floating cholesterol stones

     (2) Contraindicated in patients with inflammatory bowel disease or peptic ulcer disease

     (3) Approximately 50% recurrence rate within 5 years after treatment

     (4) Side effects— hepatotoxicity, diarrhea, and increased LDL cholesterol

     (5) Expensive

3.   Lithotripsy or destruction of stones with extracorporeal shock waves has limited application at present

- General Considerations

1.   Refer all persons with suspected cholecystitis to physician for further evaluation, possible hospitalization, and possible surgery

2.   Patient education

  a. Disease course, expected outcomes, and treatment

  b. Changes in symptoms which necessitate contact of health professional, e.g., change in pain pattern or pain accompanied by fever, chills

  c. Teach purpose, dosage, side effects of medications

  d. Nutrition

(1) If fatty foods seem to precipitate symptoms a low-fat diet may be helpful

(2) Some research has shown that increased fiber in the diet reduces incidence of gallstone formation

(3) If obese, a reducing diet is indicated; avoid rapid weight loss and fad diets which may actually increase risk of gallstone formation and precipitate acute symptoms

e. Encourage regular physical exercise; sedentary life style is associated with stone formation as well as obesity

3. Follow-up annually and for acute attacks

4. Complications include empyema, gangrene, and perforation

Appendicitis

- Definition: Inflammation of the vermiform appendix
- Etiology/Incidence
  1. Obstruction of the appendix with hardened feces (fecalith), stricture, inflammation, foreign body, or neoplasm
  2. Occurs in all age groups, but more common in males between 10 and 30 years of age
  3. Higher mortality rate due to complications in children, adolescents, and person over 55 years of age
  4. One of the leading causes for abdominal surgery
- Signs and Symptoms
  1. Acute onset of periumbilical or epigastric pain which ranges from mildly diffuse to severe
  2. Anorexia, nausea, and vomiting (usually subsequent to pain onset)
  3. Shifting of pain to right lower quadrant (McBurney's point) after several hours; aggravated by walking or coughing
  4. Occasional radiation of pain into the testicles
  5. Spasm of abdominal muscles
  6. Constipation usual; diarrhea rarer
  7. Elderly clients may present with mild symptoms of unexplained weakness, anorexia, tachycardia, and abdominal distention with little pain

8. After 24 hours may progress to perforation with sudden cessation of pain and subsequent peritonitis manifested by

   a. Abdominal rigidity

   b. Generalized abdominal tenderness

   c. High fever

   d. Vomiting

   e. Dehydration

   f. Decreased bowel sounds

   g. Shock

- Differential Diagnosis

  1. Gastroenteritis

  2. Pneumonia

  3. Ruptured ovarian cyst

  4. Tubal pregnancy

  5. Acute cholecystitis

  6. Neoplastic perforation of the colon

  7. Renal calculi

  8. Pyelonephritis of the right kidney

- Physical Findings

  1. General appearance—may or may not appear ill

  2. Vital signs—fever 100 to 102 °F.

  3. Slight tachycardia related to pain and fever

  4. Abdominal—point and rebound tenderness in RLQ; decreased or absent bowel sounds

  5. Positive psoas and obturator signs

  6. Rectal exam—tenderness in the right perirectal area

  7. Musculoskeletal—abdominal pain (RLQ) with hip extension and with straight leg raise

- Diagnostic Tests/Findings

  1. CBC with differential—leukocytosis with increased band cells (shift

to the left); in the elderly shift may be present without leukocytosis

2. Radiograph of the abdomen may show fecalith

- Management/Treatment: All persons with suspected or diagnosed appendicitis should be immediately referred to a physician for hospitalization and surgery. Appendicitis that has progressed to perforation or peritonitis will be associated with longer morbidity and higher mortality

Diverticulitis

- Definition: Inflammation of one or more diverticula in the bowel wall with microperforation and abscess formation in the pericolic fat
- Etiology/Incidence
  1. Inflammatory process similar to etiologic agents in appendicitis
  2. Occurs in about 33% of persons with diverticula (estimated to be 5 to 10% of the adult population)
     a. Incidence increases from 40 years on
     b. More frequent in females than males
     c. Higher incidence in persons with low fiber dietary habits
     d. Diverticula found most often in the sigmoid colon but may occur anywhere in the GI tract
  3. Free perforation with signs of peritonitis is rare
- Signs and Symptoms
  1. Acute left lower quadrant pain—steady and severe lasting for several days or crampy and intermittent
  2. Constipation more usual than diarrhea
  3. Pain increased with defecation
  4. Flatulence
  5. Nausea
  6. Low grade fever
- Differential Diagnosis
  1. Appendicitis
  2. Carcinoma of the colon
- Physical Findings
  1. Vital Signs—mild fever, tachycardia

2. Abdomen—guarding, rebound tenderness, rigidity especially over LLQ; if abscess has formed, a tender palpable mass may be noted

3. Rectal examination—tender painful mass may be present

- Diagnostic Tests/Findings
  1. CBC—slight leukocytosis
  2. Sed Rate—elevated
  3. Stool guaiac—positive in about 25% of cases
  4. Urine—normal unless bladder rectal fistula present
  5. Barium enema will confirm presence of diverticulosis and help rule out other etiologies, however not indicated during acute phase
  6. Proctoscopic examination—negative
  7. Sigmoidoscopy—inflamed mucosa

- Management/Treatment: For most patients with mild disease outpatient treatment will be indicated and include
  1. Clear liquids for 1 to 2 days followed by a bland diet once symptoms have subsided
  2. Medications with one of the following
     a. Ampicillin 500 mg orally every 6 hours
     b. Tetracycline 500 mg orally every 6 hours
     c. Amoxicillin/clavulanate potassium (Augmentin) 500 mg every six hours
     d. A combination of ampicillin and an aminoglycoside is common
  3. Bedrest to promote colon rest recommended until symptoms subside

- General Considerations
  1. Consult with physician regarding client management and additional testing
  2. Patients with severe disease require hospitalization, antibiotics, bowel rest, and IV hydration
  3. Patient education
     a. Etiology/Incidence and usual clinical course of the disease and rationale for recommended treatment
     b. Instruction on recommended dietary guidelines

(1) After acute phase, high fiber diet to include foods such as bran, whole grains, cereals, raw, cooked or died fruit, raw vegetables, cooked high residue vegetables

(2) High fiber diet may cause bloating and flatulence during the first two weeks of use; this resolves with continued high fiber intake

c. Avoid laxatives, enemas, and antidiarrheal agents

d. Report fever, bleeding, increasing pain to health care provider immediately

e. Bulk forming agents such as psyllium hydrophilic muciloid (Fiberall, Metamucil) and use of stool softeners such as colace may help prevent frequent recurrence

4. Follow up—return visit or phone follow-up in 24 to 48 hours to verify relief with initiating therapy; and then again after completion of antibiotic therapy

Viral Hepatitis

■ Definition: Inflammation of the liver

■ Etiology/Incidence

1. Type A (Infectious)

a. Infection with hepatitis A virus (HAV), a small RNA enterovirus

(1) Spread primarily by fecal-oral route; also parenterally

(2) Found in infected water, food, shellfish

(3) Intimate contact and poor sanitation and personal hygiene seem to be contributing factors

(4) Incubation period 2 to 6 weeks

(5) Infectivity—2 to 3 weeks in late incubation and early clinical phase

b. Common in crowded situations such as low income housing, school, military, and prison dormitories. Can occur in any age group; common in immigrants from under developed countries, school age children, and young adults.

(1) Self limiting in > 99% of cases

(2) No carrier state or chronic infection

      (3)   Severity increases with age

      (4)   In U.S. seroprevalence of Anti HAV in adults indicates 40 to 50% have had the disease.

2.   Type B (Serum)

   a. Infection with hepatitis B virus (HBV), a DNA virus with core and surface components

      (1) HB_sAg (Hepatitis B surface antigen) found in serum, saliva, semen, stool, and urine

      (2)   Core contains HB_cAg (Hepatitis B core antigen) and when present, HB_eAg (Hepatitis e antigen). HB_eAg associated with high virus titer and high infectivity

      (3)   Incubation period 6 weeks to 6 months

      (4)   Transmission by blood, by blood products, and sometimes by other body fluids, such as saliva and semen

      (5)   Mother-infant transmission if mother infected during 3rd trimester

      (6)   Approximately 10% of infected individuals become chronic carriers

   b. Common in drug addicts, homosexual males, and densely populated urban neighborhoods; higher risk individuals include persons exposed to needle punctures and blood products such as IV drug abusers; those on hemodialysis, requiring blood transfusions, or IV chemotherapy; and health care personnel such as nurses, laboratory workers, surgeons, and hemodialysis personnel

      (1)   Considered to be a sexually transmitted disease

      (2)   Seroprevalence by any marker in the U.S

          (a) General population—3 to 14%

          (b) Blacks—14%

          (c) Whites—3%

          (d) IV drug abusers—60 to 80%

          (e) Gay men—35 to 80%

          (f) Unvaccinated health care workers with frequent blood exposure—15 to 30%

3. HDV (Hepatitis Delta Virus) incomplete RNA virus

    a. Requires antecedent or simultaneous HBV infection

    b. Common in IV drug users and recipients of multiple transfusions

    c. Concomitant infection usually results in more severe manifestations than HBV alone

    e. Immunity to HBV protects against HDV

4. Type C (Parenteral Non-A, Non-B)

    a. Infection with Hepatitis C Virus (HCV), an RNA virus.

        (1) Incubation variable—5 to 10 weeks

        (2) Chronic liver disease develops in 10 to 40%

        (3) Related to development of hepatocellular carcinoma in 10%

    b. Leading cause of post transfusion hepatitis

    c. High risk population—hospital personnel, male homosexuals, and those receiving multiple transfusions

5. Type E (Enteral or Epidemic Non-A, Non-B)

    a. Infection with Hepatitis E Virus (HEV), a single stranded RNA virus

        (1) Viral particles found in stool of infected persons

        (2) Does not progress to chronic liver disease

        (3) Incubation—2 to 9 weeks

        (4) Usually mild disease in adults > 15 yrs

        (5) Mortality as high as 10 to 20% in pregnant woman

    b. Rare in the U.S.

- Signs and Symptoms: Clinical manifestations for all types are similar and can vary from a minor flu-like illness to fatal liver failure.

1. HAV may present with nonspecific or "flu" syndrome

2. HBV clinical course more variable than HAV and associated with extrahepatic manifestations, e.g., urticaria, other rashes, arthritis

3. HCV acute illness variable and subsides spontaneously

4. Prodromal phase or preicteric phase (lasts approximately 2 weeks)

    a. Fatigue, malaise

    b. Anorexia

    c. Nausea/vomiting

    d. Headache

    e. Hyperalgia

    f. Cough, coryza, pharyngitis

    g. Changes in taste with aversion to alcohol and smoking

    h. Right upper abdominal pain

    i. Weight loss of 2 to 4 kg

  2. Active or icteric phase (lasts 2 to 6 weeks)

    a. Jaundice—sclera and skin (never manifested in some patients)

    b. Dark urine

    c. Clay-colored stools; often precedes jaundice

    d. Enlarged tender liver

    e. Pruritus, urticarial rash more often associated with HBV

  3. Post-icteric or Recovery Phase

    a. Resolving jaundice, increasing sense of well-being, and decrease in symptomatology

    b. Chronic active hepatitis in those with HBV may begin at this point and is manifested by persistence of symptoms

- Differential Diagnosis

  1. Infectious mononucleosis

  2. Choledocholithiasis

  3. Hepatotoxic drugs, e.g., chloramphenicol, acetaminophen, methyldopa

  4. Carcinoma of the head of the pancreas

  5. Alcoholic cirrhosis

  6. History and serological tests assist in differentiating type; Type C (parenteral Non-A, Non-B) identification still relies primarily on exclusion of other types

- Physical Findings

  1. General Appearance—mildly ill to generally debilitated

2. Vital Signs—mild fever

3. Integumentary—slight jaundice; rash

4. HEENT—yellow sclera, lymphadenopathy

5. Abdomen—enlarged, tender liver; splenomegaly (in about 10% of cases); normal bowel sounds

- Diagnostic Tests/Findings

  1. CBC with differential—WBC-low to normal

  2. Urinalysis—proteinuria; bilirubinuria

  3. Abnormal liver function tests

     a. Elevated AST (formerly SGOT), ALT (formerly SGPT) typically 500 to 2000 IU/L

     a. Rise 7 to 10 days before jaundice

     b. Begin to fall shortly after onset of jaundice

     c. Degree of increase does not necessarily parallel disease severity

     d. LDH, serum bilirubin, alkaline phosphatase, prothrombin time normal or slightly increased

  4. Serology tests—refer to Table 2

Table 2
Serology Tests for Viral Hepatitis

IgM antibody to HAV—appears during acute or early convalescent phase and disappears in about 8 weeks; implies recent infection with HAV
IgG antibody to HAV implies previous infection with HAV; confers immunity
HB$_S$Ag (Hepatitis B surface antigen)—positive throughout the active phase of illness; first test to obtain if acute HBV infection is suspected; will remain positive in asymptomatic carriers and in chronic hepatitis
Anti-HB$_S$ (Antibody specific to HB$_S$Ag [Hepatitis B surface antigen]); positive indication of non-infectious state and recovery, and immunity; appears after HB$_S$Ag disappears
Anti-HB$_C$ (Antibody to HB$_C$Ag [Hepatitis B core antigen]); present at onset of acute illness; remains present for years, and is found in asymptomatic carriers; in many patients there is a period (window) between the disappearance of HB$_S$Ag and the appearance of Anti HB$_S$ Antibody, usually during late stages of acute phase or early convalescence; during this period, Anti-HB$_C$ will be the only serological marker of the infection
Anti-HDV (Antibody to Hepatitis D)—Marker of co- or superinfection by hepatitis D in persons with Hepatitis B; appears late and is short lived
HB$_e$Ag (Protein derived from HBV core)—indicates circulating HBV and highly infectious sera
Anti-HB$_e$ (Antibody to HB$_e$Ag)—appears weeks-months after HB$_e$Ag and HBV are no longer detecable in blood; presence indicates substantially less infectious sera
Anti-HCV (Antibody to HCV)— appears in 6 months after infection

- Management/Treatment
    1. Consult with physician regarding patient management
    2. Approach is primarily supportive in uncomplicated cases
        a. Activity/Rest
            (1) Rest recommended during active phase
            (2) Resumption of full activities during the recovery period does not appear to prolong illness, cause relapse or development of chronic disease
            (3) Avoidance of activity that might cause trauma to liver or spleen
        b. Adequate fluid and dietary intake
            (1) 3,000 to 4,000 ml fluid per day; high carbohydrate fluids such as fruit juices, carbonated beverages are encouraged but not always well tolerated
            (2) Foods high in protein, carbohydrates, and calories
            (3) Low fat diet not shown to be beneficial
            (4) Most important to eat whatever is tolerated
        c. Antiemetics may be prescribed 30 minutes before meals to control nausea and vomiting; rectal administration may be better tolerated than oral
        d. Patients with elevated PT may be given vitamin K
        e. Symptomatic relief of pruritus with colloidal baths, soaps, and lotions
        f. Avoid alcohol and other drugs detoxified or metabolized by the liver
        g. Avoid birth control pills and C-17 alpha alkyl-substituted androgenic steroids during acute phase; may increase bilirubin levels
- General Considerations
    1. Refer for possible hospitalization and further testing
        a. Complicated cases
        b. Severely ill patients

     c. Persons with signs of fulminating hepatitis or encephalitis

     d. Dehydrated persons

     e. Those with a PT > 15 seconds

     f. Those suspected of having another underlying disease process

2. Newly diagnosed cases reported to health department

3. Patient Education

     a. Disease course and expected outcomes

     b. Verify any drug use including over the counter medications and vitamin supplements with the physician until completely recovered

     c. Maintain proper hygiene; proper hand-washing, disposal of all body wastes

        (1) Should not donate blood

        (2) Close personal contacts, family members, and sexual contacts should be evaluated for active disease and may receive immune serum globulin for passive immunity (not useful once disease is clinically evident)

4. Follow up

     a. Follow weekly for the first 2 to 3 weeks; monthly thereafter if symptoms subside and liver function tests improving

     b. Closer follow-up in those > 40 years of age.

5. Complications

     a. HBV infection tends to be longer and more severe than HAV

     b. Carrier states and chronic hepatitis are associated with HBV, but not with HAV

     c. Fulminant liver failure occurs in less than 1% of those with HAV and in about 5% of those with HBV

     d. Chronic hepatitis can be associated with hepatic cancer

     e. Of those patients with Hepatitis C, 50% will develop chronic hepatitis

6. Prophylaxis—see Table 3

Table 3
Adult Prophylaxis for Viral Hepatitis

Time of Exposure	Agent	Dose	Time
PREEXPOSURE			
Hepatitis A Travel to endemic areas; tropical and underdeveloped countries Less than 3 months	Immune Serum Globulin	0.02 ml/kg	once
More than 3 months		0.02 ml/kg	q 4-6 mo
For workers with nonhuman primates	Immune Serum Globulin	0.06 ml/kg	q 4-6 mo
Hepatitis B Recommended for health care personnel especially laboratory personnel; surgeons; dialysis personnel. Also recommended for adolescents in areas with high incidence of HBV, drug abuse, STDs, teen pregnancies and for homosexually active men	HB vaccine X 3	1 ml IM	usually given in 3 doses; 2nd & 3rd given approximately 1 mo & 6 mo after the 1st dose; need all 3 doses for adequate protection
POST EXPOSURE			
Hepatitis A Close contacts; Family members; Sexual partners	Immune Serum Globlulin	0.02 ml/kg	once not more than 2 weeks post exposure
Hepatitis B Percutaneious needle stick or mucosal exposure if unvaccinated and source HB$_S$AG +	HB Immune Globulin & HB Vaccine X 3	0.06 ml/kg 1 ml Im	Within 24-48 hours of exposure At same time as HBIG, then at 1 & 6 mo
Sexual Exposure	Globulin & HB Vaccine X 3	0.6 ml/kg 1 ml 1M	Within 14 days of last sexual contact; At same time as HBIG, then at 1 & 6 mo

Contact Center for Disease Control Hotline for most current and more specific information (404) 332-4555

Acute Gastroenteritis

- Definition: Acute inflammation of the gastrointestinal mucosa

- Etiology/Incidence

    1. Commonly due to infectious agents—viruses, bacteria, and parasites (Giardia, amoebae)

        a. Exotoxins produced by some organisms, (e.g., staphylococcus) induce hypersecretion or increased peristalsis resulting in diarrhea or vomiting

        b. Bacteria such as *E. coli*, and salmonella penetrate and invade the gastric mucosa and lead to diarrhea accompanied by fever and fecal leukocytes

    c. See Table 4 for characteristics of some etiologic agents in gastroenteritis

2. Second leading cause of morbidity in the U.S.

    a. Occurs universally in all age groups

    b. Epidemic outbreaks of bacterial enteritis occur in groups of persons who have ingested contaminated food

    c. Viral gastroenteritis occurs more frequently in the winter months

    d. Primarily a self-limiting disease

    e. The very young, elderly, and those with concomitant chronic debilitating disease are at higher risk for mortality

Table 4
Characteristics of Select Etiologic Agents in Gastroenteritis

	Incubation or Onset	Fever	Fecal leukocytes	Other
E. coli	24-72 hr	+	+	Common cause of travelers' diarrhea; Doxycycline used preventively
Campylobacter	2-5 days	+	+	Erythromycin & Tetracycline used in treatment
Staphylcoccus	1-6 hr	−	−	Grows in meats; dairy foods
Shigella/ Salmonella	8-24 hr	+	+	Highly Infectious
Botulism	12-36 hr	−	−	Neuro. signs—diplopia, vertigo, dysphagia; respiratory support may be needed
Giardia lamblia	7-21 days	−	−	Metronidazole, quinacrine used in treatment; cause of travelers' diarrhea

- Signs and Symptoms

1. Abrupt onset of nausea, vomiting

2. Explosive flatulence

3. Crampy abdominal pain

4. Frequent, watery diarrhea

5. Myalgia

6. Headache

7. Fever

8. Generalized weakness/malaise

■ Differential Diagnosis

1. Acute appendicitis

2. Cholecystitis

3. Inflammatory bowel disease, e.g., colitis

4. Fecal impaction with overflow

5. Pelvic Inflammatory Disease

■ Physical Findings

1. General appearance—ill

2. Vital Signs—fever moderate to high 101-102 °F in bacterial; up to 103 °F in viral

3. Abdomen—diffuse tenderness; no spasm or rebound tenderness except with salmonella infection; hyperactive bowel sounds; slight distention; absent or hypoactive bowel sounds common with botulism

4. Neurological—dizziness, difficulty in swallowing and other neurological deficits are indication of botulism and require emergency intervention; with other etiologies findings are expected to be normal

■ Diagnostic Tests/Findings

1. CBC—normal indices

2. Stool guaiac—usually negative in viral infections; positive with invasive bacterial infections

3. Stool examination—if etiologic agent is an invasive bacteria, leukocytes will be present

4. Stool culture—diagnostic for bacteria

   a. Done in suspected cases of bacterial infection, food poisoning, and if symptoms do not begin to abate in 48 hours

   b. Special cultures needed for suspected campylobacter, cholera

■ Management/Treatment

1. Immediately refer to a physician those with

   a. Dehydration

      b. Rebound tenderness

      c. Severe abdominal pain

      d. Neurological symptoms

      e. Concomitant debilitating ilness

  2. Most can be treated for 24 to 48 hours without laboratory testing with

      a. Bedrest as needed progressing to regular activity

      b. NPO except for cracked ice while nausea and vomiting are present, then restriction to clear liquids for 24 hours; follow with addition of toast and crackers proceeding to a bland then regular diet

      c. Antiemetics and antidiarrheals are usually not indicated and may prolong the problem; treatment of salmonella has been noted to prolong the carrier state

      d. If necessary provide for parenteral administration of prescription medications

- General Considerations

  1. Consult with physician if major symptoms do not abate in 48 hours; approach may include stool for ova and parasites, specialized stool cultures and proctosigmoidoscopy

  2. Report bacterial infections and food poisoning to the health department

  3. Patient Education

      a. Disease course and expected outcome; symptoms usually resolve in 24 to 48 hours but mild diarrhea may persist for a week or two

      b. Explain proper food preparation and storage

      c. Appropriate dosage and side effects of medications

      d. Proper methods of hygiene including hand washing and disposal of stool and emesis

      e. Signs of dehydration; neurological involvement that require contacting health care professional

  4. Follow up

      a. Usually self-limiting; return visit warranted if symptoms (other than mild diarrhea) do not abate in 48 to 72 hours or worsen

b. Diarrhea may continue for 1 to 2 weeks with salmonella infection

Irritable Bowel Syndrome (IBS) (Functional Bowel Syndrome)

- Definition: Functional disturbance of intestinal motility marked by a common symptom complex which includes abdominal pain and alternating bouts of constipation and diarrhea

- Etiology/Incidence
  1. Disturbance in bowel motor activity thought to include a normal response to severe stress and learned visceral response to stress leading to
     a. Nonpropulsive colonic contractions which lead to constipation
     b. Increased contraction in the small bowel and proximal colon with diminished activity in the distal colon leading to diarrhea
  2. Influenced by emotional factors
  3. Common GI disorder
     a. Accounts for about 50% of most GI complaints seen by health care professionals and a major cause of morbidity in the U.S.
     b. Onset usually occurs before age 40
     c. Women affected more often than men

- Signs and Symptoms
  1. Aching or cramping periumbilical or lower abdominal pain often precipitated by meals and relieved by defecation; does not awaken patient at night.
  2. Pain may radiate to left chest or arm (gas in splenic flexure)
  3. Changes in bowel function
     a. Diarrhea
        (1) 4 to 6 movements/day
        (2) Small watery stools with clear mucus
        (3) No nocturnal diarrhea
     b. Constipation with irregular passage of small hard stools

    c. Alternating episodes of diarrhea and constipation

  4. Flatulence

  5. Exaggerated response to and preoccupation with bowel symptoms

  6. Bleeding, weight loss, and nocturnal diarrhea are not characteristic of IBS

- Differential Diagnosis
  1. Inflammatory bowel disorder, e.g., ulcerative colitis
  2. Viral or bacterial gastroenteritis
  3. GI neoplasms
  4. Parasitic infections
  5. Lactose deficiency
  6. Laxative abuse
  7. Side effects of drugs affecting bowel motility

- Physical Findings
  1. General Appearance—"worried well," anxious, depressed
  2. Vital Signs—normal
  3. Abdomen—mild abdominal tenderness, normal or mildly hyperactive bowel sounds
  4. Rectal examination—normal

- Diagnostic Tests/Findings
  1. Stool examination—negative for blood, ova, parasite, and pathogenic bacteria
  2. CBC—normal
  3. Barium enema—decreased motility otherwise normal
  4. Proctosigmoidoscopy—normal

- Management/Treatment
  1. Confer with physician before ordering Barium enema or proctosigmoidoscopy
  2. Provide emotional support, reassurance, information on stress reduction
  3. High fiber diet

4. Pharmacologic agents

   a. Bulk laxatives—psyllium hydrophilic mucilloid (Metamucil)

   b. Narcotics, depressants, and long term pharmaceutical use to be avoided

   c. Consult with physician regarding

      (1) Anticolinergics

         (a) Dicyclomine hydrochloride (Bentyl) 20-40 mg orally q.i.d. or propantheline (Pro-banthine) 15 mg orally q.i.d.

         (b) Usually given only after nonpharmacologic measures have failed

         (c) Side effects—dry mouth, tachycardia, orthostatic hypotension

      (2) Immodium (loperamide) or other opiate derived antidiarrheals are reserved for only very severe cases; potential for abuse in these patients is great

      (3) Mild tranquilizers

5. Patient Education

   a. Disease course and expected outcomes

   b. Rationale for treatment

   c. High fiber diet

6. Planned exercise (may help in stress reduction)

7. Need for annual rectal examination and sigmoidoscopy after age 40

8. Some patients may benefit from psychological counseling

Colorectal Cancer

- Definition: Malignancy of gastrointestinal tract primarily colon or rectum

- Etiology/Incidence

  1. Causes remain unclear

  2. Risk factors include history of colonic polyps, breast or female genital tract cancer, chronic inflammatory bowel disorders,

positive family history; high fat, low fiber, high-caloric diet

3. Second most common cancer in western world, more common over the age of 50; peaks in the eighth decade

- Signs and Symptoms: Vary by location

    1. Right sided colon cancer

        a. Usually asymptomatic

        b. Vague or crampy, colicky abdominal pain

        c. Unexplained weight loss

        d. Occult blood in stool

        e. Anemia

    2. Left sided colon cancer

        a. Alternating constipation with diarrhea

        b. Change in stool caliber (narrow, ribbon-like)

        c. Lower abdominal pain

        d. Red blood mixed in stool

        e. Sensation of incomplete evacuation

    3. Rectal cancer

        a. Tenesmus

        b. Rectal bleeding (bright red)

        c. Mucous discharge

- Differential Diagnosis

    1. Diverticular disease

    2. Lymphoma

- Physical Findings

    1. Palpable mass primarily in right colon

    2. Lymphadenopathy

    3. Rectal mass found on rectal examination

    4. Stools positive for occult blood

- Diagnostic Tests/Findings

    1. Barium enema radiograph—air contrast preferable to single

contrast, may see an apple core lesion or mass

2. Colonoscopy—may allow for biopsy of lesion found by barium enema

3. Fiberoptic sigmoidoscope—may find distal tumors

4. Testing of stools for occult blood—cancers detected with this technique are usually early stage and have a high cure rate

5. Carcinoembryonic antigen (CEA) test—often performed, although not specific for colon cancer; normal level of CEA does not exclude possibility of malignancy

6. CBC can demonstrate an anemia

- Management/Treatment

1. Referral for surgical excision or resection depending upon the depth of invasion of tumors

2. Patients with metastatic lesions, noted at the time of diagnosis, have a poor prognosis; palliative treatment is then indicated

3. Patients with a resection often require a temporary colostomy

- General Considerations

1. Screening for colon cancer

a. Test stools for occult blood annually

b. Digital rectal examination annually

c. Sigmoidoscopy every 3 to 5 years after age 50

2. Monitor for signs of dehydration during colon preps

3. Instruct patient on possibility of a colostomy after procedure and begin patient teaching on care of colostomy preoperatively

4. Encourage patient and family to ventilate feelings regarding the diagnosis

5. Make referrals to pastoral care or mental health liaison as indicated

6. Refer to community agencies for assistance after discharge, i.e., American Cancer Society, Ostomy Association (Cacchione, 1993)

Questions

Select the best answer

1. Mr. P., 55 year old of Irish decent, complains of pain in his chest and stomach for the past two weeks. He has been taking Alka Seltzer which seems to give him temporary relief. The pain is intermittent but has awakened him at night. The pain has a burning quality, and radiates up into his chest. He has hypertension which is controlled with diuretics.

   Which of the following would least likely be the cause of his pain?

   a. Coronary artery insufficiency.
   b. Diverticulitis
   c. Duodenal ulcer
   d. Esophageal reflux

2. Your next step would be to

   a. Start Mr. P. on antacids
   b. Discontinue his diuretic and switch to another class of antihypertensive
   c. Order an endoscopy
   d. Obtain additional medical history data

3. The fact that Mr. P.'s pain is not increased with activity and is unrelieved by rest makes it less likely that his problem is

   a. Coronary artery insufficiency
   b. Gastric ulcer
   c. Duodenal ulcer
   d. Esophageal reflux

4. Which fact favors a diagnosis of gastric ulcer in this case?

   a. The patient's gender
   b. The patient's age
   c. The pain quality and pattern
   d. The use of diuretics

5. Which of the following would be most beneficial in distinguishing a duodenal from a gastric ulcer in this patient?

   a. A history of a confirmed healed duodenal ulcer in the past year
   b. Reported unexplained weight loss in the past 6 months
   c. Pain aggravated by food intake
   d. An endoscopy or upper GI barium radiograph

6. Predisposing factors for duodenal ulcer include all of the following except:

   a. Genetic factors
   b. Stress
   c. Frequent laxative use
   d. Use of anti-inflammatory drugs

7. Bleeding from a duodenal ulcer

   a. Usually causes increased pain
   b. In large amounts can cause diarrhea
   c. Is associated with constipation
   d. Indicates perforation

8. If Mr.P. has a peptic ulcer and his physical exam is unremarkable except for mild epigastric tenderness, it

   a. Would not be unusual
   b. Indicates further diagnostic testing is unnecessary
   c. Is evidence that neoplastic disease is not present
   d. Rules out bleeding

9. If further testing revealed mild anemia and a negative stool guaiac, the next step would be to

   a. Start iron supplementation and antacid therapy
   b. Start H_2 receptor antagonists and reschedule return visit for 4 to 6 weeks
   c. Repeat the stool guaiac
   d. Order an endoscopy and barium study

10. If further testing revealed Mr. P. has a small, non-bleeding duodenal ulcer and after 4 weeks of therapy with an H_2 antagonist and antacids his symptoms abated, you

    a. Need to confirm healing with and upper GI barium radiograph or endoscopy
    b. Instruct him to continue treatment for at least 4 more weeks
    c. Instruct him to stop medications and start a bland diet
    d. Stop medications and place him on anticholinergics

11. Further testing revealed Mr. P's problem was a small, nonbleeding duodenal ulcer. He is placed on antacids and H_2 antagonists. After three days he calls complaining of diarrhea. You tell him

    a. This is a transient and not unusual side effect
    b. To discontinue the H_2 immediately
    c. To take the antacids with the H_2 antagonists
    d. Take an antidiarrheal medication, e.g., Imodium

12. Mr. J. is an overweight 38 year old who has had intermittent heartburn for several months. He has been taking Tums which do provide temporary relief. During the past week he has been awakening during the night with a burning sensation in his chest. He is on no medication and has had no other major health problems.

    Which additional information would lead you to believe that gastroesophageal reflux is the cause of his pain?

    a. The pain seems better when he smokes to relieve his nerves
    b. Constipation has been a chronic problem and he uses over the counter laxatives at least weekly
    c. He often awakens at night with coughing and a bad taste in his mouth
    d. Coffee and fried foods never bother him

13. Mr. J. had no weight loss or dysphagia and his physical examination is unremarkable. Your next step would be to

    a. Order an endoscopic exam
    b. Refer him to a gastroenterologist
    c. Start him on liquid antacids
    d. Tell him to eat a snack before bedtime

14. If you had decided his problem was esophageal reflux, you should tell him

    a. He probably has a hiatal hernia causing the reflux
    b. He will probably require surgery
    c. He should avoid all fruit juices
    d. Smoking, alcohol, and caffeine can aggravate his problem

15. The most definitive test for LES incompetence and gastroesophageal reflux is

    a. Stool guaiac
    b. Upper GI barium radiograph
    c. Cardiac and abdominal examination
    d. Bernstein test

16. Mary L. is 26 years old, slightly overweight, and 2 months post partum. She is complaining of heartburn, flatulence, and anorexia. During her pregnancy she had experienced similar symptoms but they have become more severe in the last week and she vomited twice. She has an intermittent pain in her right hypochondrium. She also thinks she pulled a shoulder muscle as she has an almost constant dull ache there. Your first step is to

    a. Order liver function tests
    b. Obtain a more detailed history
    c. Refer her back to her obstetrician

    d. Refer her to a gastroenterologist

17. Mary's physical examination is unremarkable except for RUQ tenderness and a positive Murphy's sign. Which of the following could be excluded from your diagnosis at this point?

    a. Appendicitis
    b. Salpingitis
    c. Diverticulitis
    d. Cholecystitis

18. Which would be the most helpful diagnostic test at this point?

    a. CBC and liver function studies
    b. Ultrasound
    c. Liver scan
    d. Chest radiograph and ECG

19. On further testing Mary is diagnosed with cholecystitis and in consultation with a physician is put on a conservative treatment plan. Which of the following would be included in this plan?

    a. Encourage her to undertake a rapid weight reduction plan
    b. Put her on oral contraceptives if she isn't already on them
    c. Decrease fiber in her diet and eliminate all fats
    d. Direct her to contact a health provider if her pain increases or fever or chills develop

20. A 22 year old male student comes to the student health service complaining of generalized abdominal pain and nausea. He had been out with a group of friends the night before and had been eating pizza and drinking beer. He awoke with generalized abdominal pain this morning and took some Alka Seltzer without much effect. The pain has gotten steadily worse throughout the day and he now feels nauseated. He wonders if he might have food poisoning. Examination reveals hypoactive bowel sounds, and some tenderness in the RLQ. There is no guarding or rebound tenderness. His temperature is 100 °F.

The absence of guarding and rebound tenderness

    a. Suggests a psychogenic cause of his pain
    b. Rules out appendicitis
    c. Makes peritonitis unlikely
    d. Indicates irritable bowel syndrome

21. The next step you would take is

    a. Refer to the physician
    b. Obtain a WBC and differential

    c. Obtain a stool culture

    d. Continue careful observation

22. Since he does not appear severely ill at this point, absence of vomiting and decreased bowel sounds and mild fever 15 hours after his last pizza and beer makes it highly unlikely that

    a. Food poisoning is the problem

    b. He has appendicitis

    c. Perforation of the appendix can occur

    d. Surgery will be needed

23. In the meantime you

    a. Encourage him to walk around to stimulate bowel activity

    b. Have him sip fluids to avoid dehydration

    c. Tell him you suspect appendicitis

    d. Give him an analgesic for pain relief

24. In elderly patients which of the following would not be an expected indication of appendicitis?

    a. Mild fever

    b. Abdominal distention with little pain

    c. Flatulence and hyperactive bowel sounds

    d. Shift to the left without leukocytosis

25. Ms. J is a 29 year old accountant who comes in complaining of frequent crampy abdominal pain after meals. She is often constipated and takes over the counter laxatives which are followed by a couple of days of diarrhea. She does feel better after having a bowel movement but only temporarily. She has also been embarrassed by flatulence and has noticed some abdominal distention. She has had no weight loss and has not noticed any blood in her stool. This problem has gone on for at least 6 months

Your next step would be to

    a. Obtain a complete history

    b. Order a barium enema

    c. Order a Bernstein test

    d. Suggest a trial of antispasmodics

26. Which of the following makes diverticulitis an unlikely diagnosis in this patient?

    a. Her age

    b. Frequent constipation

    c. Flatulence

d. Crampy, intermittent pain

27. Which of the following might be expected to occur with irritable bowel syndrome?

a. Rectal bleeding
b. Nocturnal diarrhea
c. Pain radiating to the left chest and arm
d. Leukocytosis

28. Which of the following would be the reason for hospitalizing a patient with acute diverticulitis?

a. LLQ tenderness
b. Advanced age
c. Leukocytosis
d. Increased pain with defecation

29. Conservative treatment of acute diverticulitis includes all of the following except

a. Bedrest
b. Liquid diet
c. Antibiotics
d. Colonic irrigations

30. A positive stool guaiac in a person suspected of having diverticulitis is

a. Not an uncommon finding
b. An ominous sign indicating need for hospitalization
c. Requires immediate barium enema
d. An indication of pending perforation

31. Bacturia in persons with acute diverticulosis may indicate

a. Abscess formation
b. Bowel-bladder fistula
c. Free perforation into the abdomen
d. Reason for leukocytosis

32. Ms. S., a 19 year old college freshman has just completed exam week. She comes in complaining of fatigue, headache, anorexia, and a runny nose. Symptoms began about 2 weeks ago. She has been taking vitamins and over the counter cold preparations but feels worse. "Just the smell" of food makes her nauseated. Her boy friend had mono about a month ago and she wonders if she might have it. Physical examination reveals cervical lymphadenopathy, a slightly enlarged tender liver and enlarged spleen.

Which laboratory tests in addition to a CBC, throat culture, and mono spot test would be most helpful in the differential diagnosis at this point?

a. HAV IgG antibody test
b. Anti $HB_s Ag$
c. Liver enzymes
d. Stool culture

33. There is no indication in Ms. S's history to indicate IV drug abuse or exposure to blood products. Given the duration of her symptoms and a confirmed increase in her liver enzymes which test would be most helpful in confirming your diagnosis.

a. IgM antibody to HAV
b. IgG antibody to HAV
c. $HB_s Ag$
d. Anti-HB_s

34. Highly elevated AST and ALT in this patient may indicate

a. She will soon exhibit jaundice
b. She is more severely ill than she appears
c. She is more infectious than if these values were lower
d. Severity of disease process

35. A normally healthy young adult diagnosed as having salmonella food poisoning should be told

a. To take Doxycycline 100 mg t.i.d.
b. That Imodium may decrease his diarrhea temporarily but may also prolong the problem
c. That he should try to force fluids despite his nausea and vomiting to prevent dehydration
d. The diarrhea should abate in about 24 hours

36. Which is the next laboratory test to obtain if diarrhea and vomiting persist for more than 48 hours?

a. Stool guaiac
b. Sigmoidoscopy
c. Flat plate of the abdomen
d. Stool culture and microscopic examination

37. Blurred vision and dizziness in a patient with suspected food poisoning requires

a. Gastroenterologic consult
b. Antibiotic therapy
c. Immediate hospitalization

d. Follow up in 24 hours

38. An 18 year old previously healthy female presents with a case of a sudden onset of nausea, vomiting, generalized crampy abdominal pain followed by explosive diarrhea. The stools are uniformly thin and watery, without blood or pus. Physical exam reveals hyperactive bowel sounds and bilateral lower quadrant tenderness but no guarding or rebound. Rectal exam is negative and she is afebrile.

The hypothesis that best explains these findings is

a. Acute appendicitis
b. Acute salpingitis
c. Acute gastroenteritis
d. Ruptured ovarian cyst

Answers

1. b	22. a
2. d	23. c
3. a	24. c
4. b	25. a
5. d	26. a
6. c	27. c
7. b	28. b
8. a	29. d
9. c	30. a
10. b	31. b
11. a	32. c
12. c	33. a
13. c	34. a
14. d	35. b
15. d	36. d
16. b	37. c
17. c	38. c
18. b	
19. d	
20. c	
21. a	

Bibliography

Bartlett, J. G. (1993). *1993 Pocketbook of infectious disease therapy*. Baltimore, MD: Williams & Wilkins.

Bass, N., Smith, L. H., & Van Dyke, R. (1990). Gastrointestinal disease. In T. E. Andreoli, C. C. Charles, F. Plum, & L. H. Smith (Eds.), *Cecil essentials of medicine* (2nd ed.). (pp. 253-309). Philadelphia: W. B. Saunders.

Berg, D. (1993). *Handbook of primary care medicine*. Philadelphia: J. B. Lippincott Co.

Brannon, D. P., & Drossmann, D. A. (1990). Irritable bowel syndrome: Recognition and management. *Hospital Medicine, 26*(6), 95, 99-99.

Buekhart, C. (1992). Guidelines for rapid assessment of abdominal pain indicative of acute surgical abdomen. *Nurse Practitioner, 17*(6), 39-49.

Cave, D. (1992). Therapeutic approaches to recurrent peptic ulcer disease. *Hospital Practice, 27*(9A), 36-49.

Cacchione, P. (1993). Gastrointestinal disorders. In C. Kopac & V. Millonig (Eds.), *Gerontological nursing certification review guide for the generalist, clinical specialist, nurse practitioner* (pp. 177-207). Potomac, MD: Health Leadership Associates.

Dudley, S. L., & Borstelmann Satrin, R. (1991). Cholelithiasis: Diagnosis and current therapeutic options. *Nurse Practitioner, 16*(3), 12-18, 23,24.

Friedman, L., & Knauer, M. (1994). Liver, biliary tract, and pancreas. In L. Tierney, S. McPhee, and M. Papadakis, *Current medical diagnosis and treatment*. (pp. 528-562). Norwalk, CT: Appleton & Lange.

Hauptman, W., Hitscherich, R., & Miskovitz, P. (1993). Update on acute and chronic viral hepatitis. *Hospital Medicine, 29*(1), 83-85, 88.

Huether, S., McCance, K., & Tarmina, M. (1990). Alterations in digestive function. In K. McCance & S. Huether, *Pathophysiology: The biologic basis for disease in adults and children* (pp. 1212-1266). St. Louis: C. V. Mosby.

Richter, J. E. (1992). Gastroesophageal reflux: Diagnosis and management. *Hospital Practice, 27*(1), 59-66.

Steinhart, M. J. (1992). Irritable bowel syndrome. *Postgraduate Medicine, 91*(6), 315-322.

Endocrine Disorders

Sister Maria Salerno

Diabetes Mellitus

- Definition: Genetically influenced metabolic disorder of carbohydrate, fat, and protein metabolism characterized by abnormally high blood glucose levels due to inadequate or absent insulin production and/or impaired insulin action.

- Etiology/Incidence
  1. Type I (Insulin-dependent (IDDM), formerly called juvenile onset, ketosis prone)
     a. Genetic susceptibility (HLA-DR3 gene) with environmental exposure to virus or other infectious processes leading to abnormal immune response and destruction of insulin producing pancreatic beta cells is suspected
        (1) Family history of autoimmune disorders
        (2) Islet cell antibodies
        (3) Insulin autoantibodies
        (4) Absence of C-peptide
     b. Occurs more often in those < 20 years of age; those with European Ancestry; 10 to 15% of diabetics are of this type
  2. Type II (Non-insulin-dependent (NIDDM), formerly called adult or maturity onset, ketosis resistant)
     a. Strong genetic link—familial pattern
        (1) Impaired insulin production response of beta cells to increased demands of obese state
        (2) Insulin resistance mediated by decreased insulin receptors in target cells
        (3) Post cell receptor defect impairing glucose transport into the cells
        (4) No specific HLA antigens or islet cell antibodies
     b. More frequent in those > 40 years of age, overweight (80 to 90%), sedentary, with a family history of Type II; 80 to 90% of diabetics are of this type.
  3. Other-Secondary
     a. Pancreatic disease

    b. Hormonal

    c. Drug/chemical induced

        (1)   Diuretics

        (2)   Steroids

        (3)   Tricyclics

        (4)   Phenylthiazines

    d. Genetic syndromes

4. About 6 million diagnosed cases and estimated 5 million undiagnosed; after thyroid disease and obesity most common metabolic disorder encountered in primary care settings. Third leading cause of death in U.S.

- Signs and Symptoms

   1. Type I

    a. Usually sudden and severe in onset

    b. Early

        (1)   Polyuria

        (2)   Polydipsia

        (3)   Polyphagia

        (4)   Weight loss with normal or increased appetite

        (5)   Blurred vision

        (6)   Fatigue/weakness

        (7)   Nausea/vomiting

        (8)   Vaginal itching/infections

        (9)   Ketones in blood and urine

        (10) Skin rashes

    c. With advanced disease and long-term complications

        (1)   Loss of appetite

        (2)   Bloating

        (3)   Dehydration

        (4)   Decreased level of consciousness

        (5)   Ketosis

        (6)   Neurogenic and microvascular changes

            (a) Paresthesias

            (b) Progressive visual impairment

            (c) Cold extremities

            (d) Decreased or absent pedal pulses

            (e) Constipation, nocturnal diarrhea

            (f) Nocturia, neurogenic bladder, uremia, impotence

  2.   Type II

     a. Onset more insidious

     b. Early may not be noticed

        (1)   Polyuria

        (2)   Polyphagia

        (3)   Polydipsia

        (4)   Blurred vision

        (5)   Fatigue

        (6)   Sores that heal slowly

        (7)   Recurrent infections (vaginitis, especially Candida; urinary tract, furuncules)

        (8)   Spontaneous abortion

     c. With advanced disease and long term complications

        (1)   Similar to Type I, but macrovascular changes more prominent than microvascular

            (a) Atherosclerosis

            (b) Vascular insufficiency

            (c) Coronary heart disease

        (2)   Hyperosmolar, hyperglycemic, nonketotic coma

■ Differential Diagnosis

  1.   Pancreatitis

  2.   Cushing's syndrome

3. Pheochromocytoma

4. Acromegaly

5. Cirrhosis

6. Secondary effects of drug therapy

    a. Oral contraceptives

    b. Corticosteroids

    c. Thiazides

    d. Phenytoins

- Physical Findings

    1. Type I

        a. Early

            (1) Thin, decreased weight

            (2) Ill appearance

            (3) Orthostatic hypotension

            (4) Skin infections

        b. With more advanced disease

            (1) Skin—ulcerations of feet and legs, "shin spots" over tibial bones; loss of hair over lower legs and toes

            (2) Eyes—retinopathy, including microaneurysms; yellow hard or fluffy "cotton wool" exudates; neovascularization, cataracts, glaucoma

            (3) Cardiovascular—diminished or absent pedal pulses; decreased capillary filling, pretibial edema, cool extremities

            (4) Neurologic—sensory loss, absent knee and ankle jerks, deficits in extraocular movements

    2. Type II

        a. Early

            (1) Usually obese

            (2) Hypertension

        b. With advanced disease similar to Type I

- Diagnostic Tests/Findings

  1. Plasma blood sugar—criteria for confirmation

     a. Repeated documentation of increased fasting glucose level > 140 mg/dl on two occasions

     b. Overt clinical symptoms (polydipsia, polyphagia, polyuria, nocturia, and weight loss) with a random plasma glucose > 200 mg/dl

     c. Abnormal oral glucose tolerance test— fasting plasma glucose < 140 mg/dl, plus plasma glucose > 200 mg/dl at 2 hour and one other time during a two hour oral GTT with a 75 g load

        (1) Carbohydrate loading essential to test accuracy. High carbohydrate meal of 200 to 300 g each day for three consecutive days preceding test, test in the morning, after an overnight fast of 10 to 14 hours

        (2) Serum potassium should be greater than 3.6 mEq/L

        (3) Contraindicated in presence of intercurrent illness, recent trauma, surgery, or known fasting blood glucose > 140 mg/dl

        (4) Rarely needed for diagnosis

  2. Urinalysis—presence of glucose, acetone, and in advanced stages protein

  3. Blood urea nitrogen and urine creatinine—elevated in acute dehydration and with renal involvement

  4. Serum cholesterol and triglyceride levels—often elevated especially in Type II

  5. Electrocardiogram and chest radiography—for coronary and pulmonary pathology

  6. Hemoglobin A_{1c}— predominately used as a measure of glycemic control; indicates average plasma glucose level for previous 60 to 90 days; tested every 3 to 6 months—5.5 to 8.5% considered good control

- Management/Treatment

  1. Goals of therapy are to attain best possible metabolic control while avoiding potential side effects

  2. Unless acutely ill treatment can be instituted on an outpatient basis

3. Consult physician for

   a. Newly diagnosed

   b. Anyone refractory to treatment

   c. Anyone with a blood sugar > 400 mg/dl

4. Give consideration to work schedule, life style, economic, social, and cultural aspects in management approach, e.g., persons who are homeless, persons working a night shift

5. Diet

   a. Consistent dietary schedule; ideally 3 meals and 3 snacks; especially important for Type I Diabetics and Type II on insulin; teach use of exchange lists to those on insulin; for Type II, space meals 5 hours apart with few or no snacks

   b. Avoid refined carbohydrates and simple sugars

   c. Total carbohydrate intake should be 50 to 60% of total caloric intake

   d. Limit fats to 25 to 30% of total calories

   e. Increase fiber to 25 g/1,000 calories

   f. Moderate protein intake, < 0.8 g/kg/day or < 20% of total caloric intake

   g. Total caloric intake to maintain or achieve ideal body weight (IBW)

      (1) Calculation of IBW

         (a) Females—allow 100 lb for first 5 feet of height plus 5 lb for each additional inch of height

         (b) Males—allow 106 lb for first 5 feet of height and add 6 lb for each additional inch of height

         (c) Small frame subtract 10%

         (d) Large frame add 10%

      (2) Caloric requirement

         (a) Multiply IBW by 10 = baseline calories

         (b) Add 3 X IBW if activity level is sedentary (most fall in this category); 5 X IBW if moderate; and 10 X IBW if strenuous

         (c) IBW = 125 lb

$125 \times 10 = 1250$ (baseline calories)
$125 \times 3 = 375$ (activity calories)
$1250 + 375 = 1625$ (total calories needed per day)

   (d) In Type II—obese where weight reduction is primary treatment subtract 500 calories from the total number needed per day

6. Exercise

  a. Planned daily exercise is an essential component for all diabetics

  b. Older diabetics may be limited in types of exercise due to other concurrent problems such as arthritis

  c. Diminishes need for insulin by enhancing oxidation of sugar and facilitating absorption of insulin from injection sites

  d. Those on insulin should be instructed to inject insulin furthest from site of intensive exercise, e.g., abdomen rather than arms or thighs

  e. Additional carbohydrate should be ingested prior to exercise

  f. Contributes to weight and lipid control

7. Oral hypoglycemic agents

  a. Oral hypoglycemic agents (See Table 1) indicated in symptomatic NIDDM—Type II when diet management (weight reduction) is not feasible or adequate to control plasma glucose

  b. First generation drugs—potent with long duration of action, increased risk of hypoglycemia, especially in the elderly

  c. Contraindicated in those with allergy to sulfa

Table 1
ORAL HYPOGLYCEMICS

Agent	Daily Dose mg	Doses/day hours	Half-life hours	Onset hours	Duration	Metabolism
First Generation Sulfonylureas						
Tolbutamide (a) (Orinase)	500-3000	2-3	4-5	1	6-12	Hepatic
Acetohexamide (b) (Dymelor)	250-1500	1 or 2	6-8	1	10-14	Hepatic
Tolazamide (c) (Tolinase)	100-250	1 or more	4-6	4-6	10-14	Hepatic
Chlorpropamide (d) (Diabinese)	100-500	1	24-48	1	72	Renal
Second Generation Sulfonylureas						
Glyburide (e) (Diabeta) Micronase	2.5-20	1 or 2	biphasic 8-10	1.5	24	Hepatic
Glipizide (f) (Glucotrol)	2-40	1 or 2	3.5-6	1	12-18	Hepatic

(a) Most benign, least potent, especially useful in renal disease.
(b) Little advantage over Tolbutamide; uricosuric effects.
(c) Equipotent to tolbutamide with less severe side effects.
(d) Potent; contraindicated for use in elderly and renal disease; disulfiram-like reaction with alcohol; may cause hyponatremia.
(e) Take on empty stomach; low toxicity, NO disulfiram reaction; caution in elderly.
(f) 50-200 times more potent than other hypoglycemics; no disulfiram-like reaction; low toxicity; caution in the elderly.

Table 2
INSULINS

Type	Action	Onset (Hours) (a)	Peak (Hours)	Duration (Hours) (b)
Regular	Rapid	.25-1	1-2	5-6
Semilente	Rapid	.5-2	1-2	12-16
NPH	Intermediate	1-2	2-8	24-48
Lente (isophane)	Intermediate	1-2	2-8	24-48
NPH (70%) with Regular (30%) (Mixtard, Novalin 70/30)	Intermediate	.5	4-8	24
PZI (protamine zinc)	Long	2-4	8-12	38
Ultralente	Long	2-4	8-12	36

NOTE: Beef, pork, beef-pork, and human synthetic insulin available in rapid and intermediate acting. Long acting are not currently available in human insulin.

(a) Onset depends on site of injection and dose size
(b) Duration is proportional to dose size and is increased in renal failure

8.   Insulin (See Table 2)

   a. Indicated for

       (1)   Type I-IDDM

       (2)   Type II-NIDDM when hyperglycemia persists after attempts of diet management and/or diet management and use of oral hypoglycemics

       (3)   In mild diabetics during periods of intercurrent stress

       (4)   In gestational diabetes

   b. Purity

       (1)   Standard Beef or Pork - > 10 but < 25 parts per million (ppm) proinsulin (immunogenic agent)

       (2)   Purified Beef or Pork - < 10 ppm proinsulin

       (3)   Human synthetic < 10 ppm proinsulin

       (4)   Beef more antigenic than pork species; human insulin least antigenic of all

   c. Initiation and adjustment of dosage

       (1)   Exogenous insulin replacement begins with 10 to 30 units of intermediate acting insulin before breakfast each morning

           (a) Lower doses for thin patients and higher for obese (tend to have more insulin resistance)

           (b) Change dose no more than every 2 to 3 days

       (2)   As long as plasma glucose is > 150 mg/dl before the evening meal, dose is increased by 2 to 5 units every 2 to 3 days

       (3)   Once all urine glucose tests approach negative and afternoon postprandial plasma glucose is consistently < 150 mg/dl fasting plasma glucose is checked for sustained effect of single insulin dose. If glucose is elevated dose will be split with about 2/3 given before breakfast and 1/3 before the evening meal. Doses are adjusted until fasting plasma glucose is 120 to 150 mg/dl

       (4)   Once afternoon and before breakfast regulation is achieved, late morning levels are assessed; if needed, Regular insulin can be combined with morning injection to keep late morning plasma glucose levels < 150 mg/dl

(a) THE AMOUNT OF REGULAR INSULIN NORMALLY SHOULD NOT EXCEED 50% OF THE INSULIN GIVEN AT ANY TIME

(b) Do not mix Lente or Ultra lente with Regular; zinc in Lente precipitates Regular, decreasing effective proportion of regular and increasing that of the Lente

(c) Do not mix Lente with Velosulin short acting (Nordisk)—phosphate buffer increases concentration of unmodified soluble insulin and diminishes effect of intermediate acting preparation

(d) Regular insulin should be drawn up first if mixing regular and NPH in the same syringe

(5) Once daily regimen is established, urine and self-monitored plasma glucose levels are tested 3 to 4 times a day as indicated by the insulin schedule and severity of the disease

(a) Daily dose requirement decreases with progressive renal failure

(b) Control is assessed at 3 to 6 month intervals; glycosylated Hgb which reflects average glucose levels of the preceding 8 to 12 weeks may be helpful

9. Combined insulin-sulfonylurea

a. Morning sulfonylurea and NPH-Lente insulin in the evening for select Type II diabetics

(1) No proof of superiority to traditional approach

(2) Helps control morning hyperglycemia without concomitant hypoglycemia seen with insulin alone

(3) May help patient avoid need for multiple insulin injections

b. Seems to work best in those who are less than 150% of Ideal Body Weight and have had the disease for less than 15 years

■ General Considerations

1. Patient Education—should begin at time of diagnosis and will extend over several weeks

a. Cause and general management of diabetes

b. Importance of diet and weight control

    c. Self-monitoring of blood and urine glucose

    d. Administration of insulin or dosing, action, and side effects

    e. Administration of oral hypoglycemic agents, dosing, action and side effects

    f. Potential alteration in glucose metabolism with acute illness, exercise, and emotional stress

    g. Test for and significance of ketonuria

    h. Recognition and treatment of hypoglycemia

    i. Proper leg and foot care

    j. Sick-day guidelines

    k. Guidelines for economizing with repeated use of needles and splitting glucose test strips

  2. Complications

    a. Hypoglycemia

      (1) Causes

        (a) Insulin overdosage

        (b) Omission or delay of meals

        (c) Heavy exercise

        (d) Errors in injection technique

        (e) Renal failure

        (f) Weight loss

        (g) Development of hepatitis, pituitary or adrenal insufficiency, or other conditions that cause hypoglycemia

        (h) Drugs that affect insulin metabolism/action see Table 3

Table 3
MEDICTION EFFECT ON INSULIN METABOLISM/ACTION

Medication	Action
Alcohol	Decreased half-life of sulfonylureas in alcoholics, can cause severe hypoglycemia in those on hypoglycemics
Beta-adrenergic	Inhibit insulin secretion; block most hypoglycemia symptoms; prolong effect of insulin
Calcium channel blockers	Inhibit insulin secretion
Diazoxide	Inhibits insulin secretion
Glucocorticoids	Insulin antagonism
Nicotinic acid	Insulin resistance
Oral contraceptives	Insulin resistance
Phenytoin	Inhibits insulin secretion
Sympathomimetics	Insulin antagonism Inhibit insulin secretion
Thiazide diuretics	Inhibit insulin secretion
MAO inhibitors	Increase effects of antidiabetic agents
Salicylates	Increase effects of antidiabetic agents
Coumarin	Increase effects of sulfonylureas
Phenylbutazone	Increase effects of sulfonylureas

(2) Symptoms

    (a) Weakness

    (b) Sweating

    (c) Shakiness

    (d) Tremors

    (e) Nervousness

    (f) Headache

    (g) Dizziness

    (h) Hunger

    (i) Irritability

    (j) Convulsions, confusion, coma

  b. Somogyi phenomenon

(1) Cause—morning rebound hyperglycemia and ketonuria; occurs in response to nocturnal hypoglycemia with excessive insulin administration

(2) Clues—erratic plasma glucose and urine ketone values; symptoms of nocturnal hypoglycemia (night sweats, nightmares, low serum glucose 2 to 3 a.m.), weight gain in presence of heavy glycosuria

(3) Treatment—reduce insulin dose 10 to 20%

(4) Distinguish from *Dawn Phenomenon* which is early morning fasting hyperglycemia without nocturnal hypoglycemia; thought to be related to circadian rhythm secretion of growth hormone and treated by evening or bedtime dose of insulin

c. Lipodystrophy

   (1) Atrophy—subcutaneous fat atrophy at insulin injection sites

   (a) Cause—impurities in the insulin, possible autoimmune mechanism

   (b) Treatment—switch to purified insulin, inject directly into atrophic areas

   (2) Hypertrophy—over-growth of subcutaneous tissue

   (a) Cause—growth promoting effects of insulin; improper rotation of injection sites

   (b) Treatment—prevent by proper rotation of injection sites

d. Insulin Allergy

   (1) Rare and usually localized

   (2) Treatment—change to human synthetic insulin

   (3) Localized allergies may be treated with antihistamines or corticosteroid; consultation required

e. Insulin resistance requiring more than 200 units per day

   (1) Rare and even less common with increased use of human insulins

   (2) Cause—over-production of insulin-binding immunoglobulins

   (3) Treatment—change to less immunogenic pork or human synthetic insulins

(4) May require glucocorticoid treatment; consultation required

f. Diabetic ketoacidosis (DKA) — hyperglycemia with ketonuria and disruption of the fluid, electrolyte, and pH balance leading to coma and even death; marked by hyperglycemia, metabolic acidosis, and ketonemia; sometimes PRESENTING SIGN in undiagnosed Type I

(1) Cause — infection, trauma, myocardial infarction, other severe stress, and noncompliance with therapeutic regimen

(2) Treatment — emergency fluid replacement, insulin therapy, sodium bicarbonate therapy, and close monitoring of blood chemistries

g. Hyperosmolar nonketotic syndrome — severe hyperglycemia, hyperosmolarity, and dehydration in the absence of ketoacidosis which may lead to coma; most often occurs in elderly on oral hypoglycemics and those with undiagnosed Type II

(1) Precipitating Factors — calcium channel blockers, corticosteroids, thiazide diuretics, propanolol, phenytoin

(2) Treatment — similar to ketoacidosis, but need less insulin and more fluid replacement

(3) Prognosis is poor in elderly, particularly those with concurrent renal disease, hypertension, or congestive heart failure

3. Follow Up

a. Well controlled patients — minimum every 3 to 4 months

b. Yearly ECG, chest radiograph, creatinine, urinalysis, lipid profile, physical examination including fundoscopic, full neurologic examination

c. Annual ophthalmologic examination by ophthalmologist

d. Skin inspection, fundoscopic, and evaluation of glycemic control by fasting or postprandial plasma glucose measurements at each visit

e. Hemoglobin A_{1c} every 3 to 6 months

4. Referrals to local support groups and identification of local chapters of the American Diabetes Association for information, support, and publications

Hyperthyroidism (Thyrotoxicosis)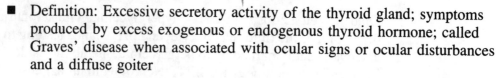

- **Definition**: Excessive secretory activity of the thyroid gland; symptoms produced by excess exogenous or endogenous thyroid hormone; called Graves' disease when associated with ocular signs or ocular disturbances and a diffuse goiter

- Etiology/Incidence
  1. Causes
     a. Autoimmune response (Graves' disease accounts for more than 85% of cases)
     b. Subacute thyroiditis
     c. Toxic multinodular goiter; toxic uninodular goiter (autonomous thyroid adenoma)
     d. Metastatic follicular thyroid carcinoma
     e. Thyrotoxicosis factitia
     f. TSH-secreting pituitary tumor (secondary hyperthyroidism)
     g. hCG secreting tumors (choriocarcinoma, hydatiform mole)
     h. Testicular embryonal carcinoma
  2. One of the most common endocrine disorders
  3. Highest incidence in women between 20 and 40 years of age

- Signs and Symptoms
  1. Most frequent
     a. Anxiety
     b. Diaphoresis
     c. Fatigue
     d. Hypersensitivity to heat
     e. Nervousness
     f. Palpitations
     g. Weight loss
     h. Insomnia
  2. Frequent
     a. Dyspnea

b. Weakness

c. Increased appetite

d. Eye complaints, e.g., difficulty focusing

e. Swelling of legs

f. Hyperdefecation without diarrhea, hyperactive bowel sounds

g. Diarrhea

h. Oligomenorrhea or amenorrhea

3. Infrequent

a. Anorexia

b. Constipation

c. Weight gain

d. Signs of pseudobulbar palsy

4. Elderly patients may present with few signs or symptoms noted in younger patients (apathetic hyperthyroidism). May present with cardiovascular problems unresponsive to digitalis, quinidine, or diuretics

a. Atrial fibrillation

b. Angina

c. Congestive heart failure

■ Differential Diagnosis

1. Diagnosis is indicated by presence of elevated T_4 (or index) and/or elevated free T_3 (or index) and a clinical pattern consistent with the diagnosis

a. In primary hyperthyroidism a depressed TSH (thyroid stimulating hormone) is also detectable

b. In secondary states TSH levels are inappropriately elevated in the presence of elevated levels of thyroid hormone

2. Distinguish from

a. Anxiety neurosis, especially in menopause

b. Other diseases associated with hypermetabolism, e.g., pheochromocytoma and acromegaly

c. Myasthenia gravis (causes the same ophthalmoplegic signs)

d. Orbital tumors can cause exophthalmos

- Physical Findings

    1. General—thin, muscle wasting may be evident; nervous; quick motions

    2. Vital Signs—tachycardia, irregular pulse, widened pulse pressure

    3. Integumentary—skin moist, velvety, may show increased pigmentation or vertiligo; hair thin, fine; spider angiomas and gynecomastia may be evident

    4. Eyes—prominent; appear to "stare"; lid lag; lack of accommodation; exophthalmos

    5. Neck—enlarged thyroid gland (goiter) smooth or nodular, symmetric or asymmetric; thyroid bruit or thrill; absence of these signs does not rule out hyperthyroidism

    6. Cardiovascular—paroxysmal atrial fibrillation, harsh pulmonary systolic murmur, congestive failure, possible enlargement

    7. Neurologic—hyperactive reflexes; fine tremors of fingers, tongue; mental changes ranging from mild exhilaration to delirium. In the elderly, apathy, lethargy and severe depression may be manifested

    8. Lymphatic—lymphadenopathy and splenomegaly may be present

- Diagnostic Tests/Findings
  See Table 4 for list of thyroid function tests

Table 4
THYROID ASSESSMENT TESTS

Thyroxine (T_4)	Major hormone secreted by the thyroid gland and effective indicator of thyroid function
T_4 (RIA-serum)	By radioimmunoassay (RIA); normal adult is 5 to 12 μg/dl
Free T_4 (FTI)	Unaffected by TBG and is a better reflection of the true Index hormonal status; serum T_4 and T_3 resin uptake (T_3, RU) used to calculate this index; normal adults 0.9-2.2ng/dl
T_3 Resin Uptake (T_3RU)	Indirect measure of T_4 levels by assessing T_4 binding sites; may be thought of as the reciprocal of the T_4 RIA; in hyperthyroidism there is a high T_3 Resin Uptake; in hypothyroidism the T_3 is low; normal adult is 25 to 35%
T_3 RIA (Serum)	Direct measure of triiodothyronine (T_3) thyroid hormone; helpful in diagnosing thyrotoxicosis when T_4 is normal; in hypothyroidism T_3 often normal; T_4 more helpful; normal adult is 80 to 200ng/dl(RIA)
Thyroid Antibodies, Thyroglobulin	High titers indicate autoimmune disease, e.g., Hashimoto's thyroiditis; also elevated in carcinoma of the thyroid; normal adult is 1:20, 0-50 ng/ml (RIA)
Thyroid stimulating Hormone (TSH)	Direct measure of TSH secreted from the anterior pituitary in response to thyroid-releasing hormone (TRH); normal adult is 2 to 5.4 μU/ml. < 10 μU/ml (RIA)
TSH immunoradiometric assay (IRMA)	Newer assay replacing TSH (RIA); normal adult is 0.5 to 5.0 μU/ml; more clearly detects suppressed TSH in hypothyroidism
Radioactive iodine Uptake (RAIU)	Used primarily to detect hyperthyroidism; radioactive iodine given orally or intravenously; the thyroid is scanned at 3 different intervals to determine iodine uptake of the thyroid gland; an elevated RAIU indicates hyperthyroidism; normal adult is 2 hr., 1 to 13%; 6 hr., 2 to 25%; 24 hr., 15 to 45%

1. Free Thyroxine Index (FTI) usually elevated; if normal and clinical impression is strong for hyperthyroidism then do

2. T_3, radioimmunoassay (T_3, RIA)—elevated with a normal T_4 in early hyperthyroidism and T_3 toxicosis

3. T_4 level elevated in later stages

4. If diagnosis of primary hyperthyroidism is equivocal TSH immunoradiometric assay (IRMA) to detect suppressed TSH levels

5. TRH suppression test can be done if TSH (IRMA) is not available. Patients who have primary hyperthyroidism will have a suppressed TSH response to TRH stimulation. Some drugs, e.g., thyroid replacement hormones and glucocorticoids, fasting, and severe illness can produce a similar effect

■ Management/Treatment

1. Refer for hospitalization for suspected "thyroid storm"

a. High fever

b. Severe agitation

c. Confusion

d. Cardiovascular collapse

e. Malignant exophthalmus

f. Difficulty in breathing due to enlarged or tender thyroid gland

2. Obtain physician consult for clients suspected of/or newly diagnosed with hyperthyroidism for treatment which may include

a. Propranolol 10 to 60mg orally every 6 hours to control symptoms while other treatment is in progress

b. Radioactive Iodine (^{131}I)

   (1) Therapeutic dose is 80 to 120 mCi administered in doses of 5 to 15mCi based on estimated weight of the thyroid gland

   (2) Most become euthyroid after 3 to 6 months

   (3) Hypothyroidism is frequent and can occur anytime after radioactive iodine therapy

c. Antithyroid drugs are indicated for initial control of thyrotoxicosis especially in pregnant women, those not wanting to take ^{131}I, or in preparation for surgical removal. Especially effective in patients with small goiters

   (1) Propylthiouracil (PTU) 150 mg orally t.i.d.; preferred for use in pregnant women

   (2) Methimazole (MMI, Tapazole 5 to 10 mg tablets) 20 mg orally b.i.d.

   (3) Side effects

      (a) Dermatitis

      (b) Nausea

      (c) Agranulocytosis (most serious)

      (d) Hypothyroidism which can cause a TSH stimulated increase in goiter size

   (4) Patient education:

      (a) Medication is to be taken for about two years and not

abruptly discontinued

    (b) However, at first sign of infection or fever drug should be stopped and healthcare professional contacted

    (c) Therapeutic effect of medication is not usually evident for about three weeks

  d. Surgery

    (1) Not used as frequently now

    (2) Indicated for children, adolescents, pregnant women unable to tolerate PTU, adults nonresponsive to thiourea treatment who refuse RAI

- General Considerations
  1. Client education
     a. Rationale for treatment; dosage and side effects of medications; takes at least three weeks before antithyroid medications become effective
     b. Instructions regarding nutritional needs: high carbohydrate, high caloric diet until medication takes effect; avoidance of stimulants such as caffeine
     c. Symptoms of "thyroid storm"
  2. Follow up
     a. Periodic examinations until euthyroid
     b. All patients who have been treated for hyperthyroidism should be periodically checked for hypothyroidism which may occur anytime during treatment

Adult Hypothyroidism (Myxedema)

- Definition: Decreased or deficient thyroid hormone—primary (glandular dysfunction) or secondary (pituitary insufficiency); occurs in all age groups
- Etiology/Incidence
  1. Major classifications
     a. Primary—caused by damage to the hormone producing capabilities of the thyroid gland itself
        (1) Most common cause in adults is autoimmune thyroiditis (Hashimoto's, chronic lymphocytic)

(2) Can also be caused by ablation of the gland by surgery, medication, radiation, and goitrogens (thiocynates, rutabagas, lithium carbonate)

(3) More common than secondary

b. Secondary—often related to destructive lesions of the pituitary gland as with chromophobe adenoma or postpartum necrosis (Sheehan's syndrome). Frequently associated with signs of adrenal and gonadal disorders

c. Tertiary—TRH deficiency arising in the hypothalmus; sometimes grouped with secondary

2. Occurs in all age groups; more prevalent in women and those

a. With a history of thyroiditis

b. With previously treated hyperthyroidism (all modalities)

c. Being treated with lithium or paraaminoslicylic acid

d. With coexistent autoimmune disorders (e.g., rheumatoid arthritis, lupus, pernicious anemia)

■ Signs and Symptoms

1. Most Frequent

a. Cold intolerance

b. Coarse skin

c. Decreased sweating

d. Dry skin

e. Lethargy

f. Swelling of eye lids

2. Frequent

a. Anemia (normocytic, normochromic, microcytic, or macrocytic)

b. Anorexia

c. Coarse hair

d. Cold skin

e. Constipation

f. Hair loss

g. Hoarseness or aphonia, thick tongue

      h. Hyperlipidemia including hypercholesterolemia

      i. Leg edema

      j. Menorrhagia

      k. Memory impairment

      l. Swelling of face

      m. Paresthesias

- Differential Diagnosis

  1. Rule out coexisting autoimmune disease or secondary hypothyroidism
  2. Nephrotic syndrome
  3. Chronic renal disease

- Physical Findings

  1. Vital signs—bradycardia, mild hypotension, hypertension
  2. Edema of hands, face, eyelids
  3. Integumentary—dry, scaly skin with carotenemic tone; brittle nails; alopecia; puffy eyelids; temporal thinning of the eye brows
  4. ENT—enlarged tongue, possible hearing decrease, thyroid often enlarged
  5. Cardiovascular—bradycardia, decreased intensity of heart tones, cardiac enlargement (myxedemic heart may be related to pericardial effusion)
  6. Respiratory—pleural effusion
  7. Abdominal—ascites, possible decreased bowel sounds
  8. Neuromuscular—slow or delayed deep tendon reflexes, cerebellar ataxia, dementia (myxedema madness, manifested with hallucinations, paranoid ideation, and hyperactive delirium), pseudomyotonia, carpal tunnel syndrome

- Diagnostic Tests/Findings

  1. Free Thyroxine Index (FTI) or T_4; if low a TSH is helpful in determining etiology
  2. TSH elevated in primary hypothyroidism
  3. If T_4 is normal and TSH is elevated, may be mild hypothyroidism
  4. Thyrotropin-releasing hormone (TRH) stimulation done if low TSH

with low T_4 or low FTI; may indicate secondary hypothyroidism

5. CBC—may demonstrate anemia

■ Management/Treatment

1. Refer for immediate hospitalization any client suspected of developing myxedemic coma—severe hypothyroidism associated with hypothermia, decreased mentation, hypoventilation, respiratory acidosis, relative hypotension, hyponatremia, hypoglycemia

2. Obtain physician consultation for clients with suspected or newly diagnosed hypothyroidism for further testing and/or initiation of treatment which would include

   a. Administration of synthetic T_4 (Levothyroxine); desiccated thyroid is no longer used due to variability in composition

      (1) Average replacement dose of T_4 is thyroxine 0.125 mg/day in healthy, nonelderly adults and may range from 0.025 to 0.3 mg/day

      (2) Dosage starts with 0.1 mg/day for those < 50 years of age, and 0.025 to 0.05 mg/day in those > 50 years of age or with known ischemic heart disease without angina

      (3) Dosage is increased by 0.025 mg/day every two weeks until the patient is clinically euthyroid

      (4) Patients with coexisting adrenal insufficiency, coronary insufficiency, or angina require particular care

      (5) Initial effects of replacement not usually perceptible for at least two weeks after initiation of therapy and are initially demonstrated by decreased facial edema and increased urination

3. On follow-up visits, after replacement therapy has been instituted

   a. Check cardiopulmonary status; if pulse is > 100/minute consult with physician

   b. Monitor for symptoms or signs of too vigorous therapy, side effects, and toxic effects of replacement therapy; ask about dyspnea, orthopnea, angina, palpitations, nervousness, insomnia

   c. Be alert to concomitant use of opiates, barbiturates, other central nervous system depressants, digitalis, and insulin; persons with hypothyroidism are particularly sensitive to these agents; as they become euthyroid dosages may have to be increased

4. Monitor control of clinical symptoms and periodically monitor serum

FTI and TSH. Persistently high TSH or low FTI may indicate underreplacement. A high T_4 and low TSH with symptoms of hyperthyroidism usually indicates over replacement

5. Patient Education

   a. Nature and chronicity of the disease and the need for life long treatment

   b. Rationale for treatment—dosage, side effects, and toxic effects of treatment

   c. Teach signs of hyperthyroidism

   d. Management of symptoms of hypothyroidism until abatement with replacement therapy

     (1) Fatigue

     (2) Dry skin

     (3) Constipation (increased fiber, fluids)

Thyroid Nodule

- Definition: Discrete enlargements within the thyroid gland
- Etiology unknown but nodules are common

   1. Palpable in 5 to 10% of U.S. population

   2. Majority are benign

   3. Risk of nodule malignancy less than 10% in most adults

   a. Men have a higher incidence than women

   b. Papillary and follicular carcinoma are most common types of malignancy

     (1) Papillary tends to spread intrathyroidally or to cervical lymphatics

       (a) Twice as common in women as men

       (b) Accounts for 80% of thyroid malignancies in adults < 40

     (2) Follicular carcinoma accounts for approximately 20% of all thyroid cancers

       (a) Incidence somewhat higher in older individuals

       (b) Usually slow growing but more aggressive than

papillary; can spread rapidly to lymph nodes and to distant sites via the blood stream, often to lung, bone, brain, or liver

   c. Medullary and anaplastic carcinoma are rarer but tend to metastisize very early. Anaplastic carcinoma, because of high invasiveness and early metastasis, results in death in weeks or months regardless of treatment modality

   d. Risk of carcinoma is increased with a history of radiation exposure, particularly during childhood, to the head or neck for acne, tonsils, adenoids; the risk is also increased in those with a family history of thyroid cancer. This is especially true for medullary carcinoma

- Signs and Symptoms
  1. Thyroid mass
  2. Expanding goiter or nodule which is hard and/or tender
  3. Hoarseness or dysphagia

- Differential Diagnosis: Distinguish between nonneoplastic enlargements, e.g., cystic nodules, multinodular goiters; malignancy confirmed by biopsy

- Physical Findings
  1. Single hard thyroid nodule (or multiple nodules) fixed to overlying tissue
  2. Regional lymphadenopathy

- Diagnostic Tests/Findings
  1. Free Thyroxine Index (FTI)—usually normal; if elevalted chances of malignancy are decreased
  2. RAI scan—nonfunctioning (cold) nodule
  3. Ultrasonsgraphy—if cystic rarely malignant
  4. Thyrocalcitonin—increased in medullary carcinoma
  5. Biopsy (open or needle)—positive cytology if malignant

- Management/Treatment
  1. Any individual with the signs and symptoms or physical findings previously described should be referred
  2. Treatment may include
     a. Excision of the nodule (complete thyroidectomy in the case of

medullary carcinoma) and regional lymph nodes

    b. Ablation of metastasis with large doses of radioactive iodine

    c. Suppression of thyroid function with L-thyroxine

    d. Chemotherapy for anaplastic carcinoma; (thyroid suppression and radioactive ablation of metastasis are not effective in medullary thyroid carcinoma)

3. Client education related to diagnostic tests

4. Follow up for detection of metastasis, recurrence, and subsequent treatment is usually on an annual basis

Cushing's Syndrome

- Definition: A constellation of clinical abnormalities due to an excess of glucocorticoids

- Etiology/Incidence

    1. Excessive or prolonged administration of glucocorticoids (most common)

    2. Excessive pituitary ACTH secretion (Cushing's disease)

    3. Secretion of ACTH by a non-pituitary tumor (ectopic tumor), e.g., carcinoma of the lung or other malignant growths

    4. Tumors within the adrenal cortex-adenomas or carcinoma

    5. Cushing's disease and primary adrenal tumors are more common in females

    6. Ectopic corticotropin production is more common in males

- Sign and Symptoms

    1. Central obesity with slender extremities

    2. Full face

    3. Muscular weakness

    4. Back pain

    5. Mental changes

    6. Thin fragile skin

    7. Poor wound healing

    8. Acne

9. Menstrual Disorders

- Differential Diagnosis: Differentiation between the etiological causes of Cushing's syndrome
- Physical Findings
  1. Moon face with facial plethora
  2. Hirsutism
  3. Skin—thin and atrophic
  4. Purplish-red striae on abdomen, breast or buttocks
  5. Truncal obesity with wasting of limbs
  6. Prominent supraclavicular and dorsal cervical fat pads ("buffalo hump")
  7. Hypertension
- Diagnostic Tests/Findings
  1. Plasma cortisol—evening cortisol levels and 24 hour total levels are elevated
  2. Urinary cortisol—elevated
  3. Dexamethasone test (most reliable for distinguishing among causes of Cushing's syndrome)
  4. MRI, CT and ultrasonographic imaging for identification of pituitary tumor, non-pituitary ACTH-producing neoplasms
- Management/Treatment
  1. Treatment of choice for Cushing's Disease—surgery
  2. Adrenal tumors or hyperplasia-removal
  3. If surgery is contraindicated radiation and drug therapy (used to control cortisol excess) may be used which includes Ketoconazole 400 to 500 mg b.i.d.; Metyrapone 2 g per day; Aminoglutethimide 1 g per day
  4. For Cushing's syndrome due to prolonged administration of steroids
     a. Discontinuation of therapy gradually
     b. Reduction of steroid dose
     c. Changing to an alternate-day schedule

Addison's Disease (Primary adrenocortical insufficiency)

- Definition: An insidious, usually progressive disease due to destruction of the adrenal cortex

1. Primary-due to destruction of adrenal cortex

2. Secondary-lack of corticotropin stimulation

- Etiology/Incidence

    1. Idiopathic autoimmune destruction of adrenal tissue (over 80%); two to three times more common in females; usually diagnosed between ages 30 to 50 years

    2. Tuberculosis—second most frequent cause (common cause in underdeveloped countries)

    3. Acquired immunodeficiency syndrome (AIDS)—becoming a more frequent cause

    4. Less common—hemorrhage, fungal infections, antineoplastic chemotherapy, abrupt withdrawal of exogenous steroids

    5. Primarily a rare disease

- Signs and Symptoms

    1. Chronic primary adrenocortical insufficiency—develops gradually

        a. Weakness and fatigue, orthostatic hypotension may be early symptoms

        b. Anorexia, weight loss

        c. Tan appearance to the skin

        d. Gastrointestinal symptoms

    2. Acute adrenocortical insufficiency—seen more often in patients without previous diagnosis or those with a diagnosis who are exposed to stress with related increased requirement for glucocorticoids; symptoms of chronic are exaggerated especially profound hypotension

    3. Most dangerous feature of Addison's disease is hypotension which may cause shock, especially during stress AND is nonresponsive to usual treatment; requires glucocorticoid replacement

- Differential Diagnosis

    1. ADH syndrome

    2. Salt-losing nephritis

    3. Diabetes mellitus

- Physical Findings

    1. Hyperpigmentation of skin

2. Hypotension

3. Black freckles over forehead, face, neck, and shoulders

4. Areas of vitiligo

5. Bluish-black discolorations of the areolae and of the mucous membranes of the lips, mouth, rectum, vagina

- Diagnostic Tests/Findings

    1. Sodium levels—low (< 130 mEq/L)

    2. Potassium levels—high (> 5 mEq/L)

    3. BUN—elevated

    4. Plasma renin level—increased

    5. ACTH plasma levels—increased

    6. Ratio of serum sodium to potassium (< 30:1)

    7. Low fasting blood glucose (< 50 mg/dl)

    8. Hematocrit—elevated

    9. WBC—low

    10. Eosinophils—increased

- Management/Treatment

    1. In acute crisis referral with hospitalization

    2. Chronic

        a. Lifetime of treatment

        b. Cortisol 15 to 20 mg orally every a.m.; 5 to 10 mg 4 to 6 p.m.

        c. 9χ—Fluorocortisol 0.05 to 0.1 mg every a.m.

        d. Monitor weight, blood pressure, and electrolytes

- General Considerations

    1. Education regarding increasing cortisol during times of stress

    2. Education regarding carrying an identification bracelet or card

    3. Salt additives for excess heat or humidity

    4. Prognosis is excellent with continued substitution therapy

Questions

Select the best answer

Mrs. O. is a 46 year whose hypertension has been controlled with hydrochlorothiazide 50 mg every day for the past three years. She is 5'8" and weighs 220 lb. Although no other abnormal physical findings were noted, blood work done as part of her routine annual physical examine reveals a fasting blood glucose of 300 mg/dl. Other abnormal laboratory tests included elevated serum cholesterol (250) and triglyceride level (170), a K+ of 3.4, and 4+ glycosuria.

1. You should then

   a. Discontinue her hydrochlorothiazide
   b. Order a glucose tolerance test
   c. Repeat a fasting glucose
   d. Start insulin therapy

2. Mrs. O is about how many pounds over her ideal body weight?

   a. 80
   b. 105
   c. 140
   d. 154

3. Type II diabetics (NIDDM)

   a. Are apt to develop ketosis
   b. Account for less than 10% of diabetes
   c. Macrovascular changes are more prominent than microvascular
   d. Often present with severe polydipsia and polyphagia

4. Mrs. O has led a fairly sedentary life style and asks if enrolling in an exercise club would help get her sugar down. You would tell her that

   a. Exercise is an important part of control of her blood sugar
   b. She should start a virgorous exercise program as soon as possible
   c. Exercise at this point won't affect her blood sugar
   d. Exercise will probably increase her appetite

5. Given her sedentary life syle and need to lose weight, how many calories/day should Mrs. O be consuming? Wt. 220 lb, Hgt. 5'8".

   a. 1,000
   b. 1,300
   c. 1,400
   d. 1,800

6. Mrs. O's second fasting blood sugar is 296 and she has been diagnosed as a Type II diabetic. Mrs. O does not want to take insulin. You tell her

    a. Most Type II diabetics never have to take insulin

    b. Before considering the use of insulin it is usual to try a modified dietary plan and exercise

    c. It would be a lot easier if she started insulin as soon possible

    d. The value of using insulin to control Type II Diabetes is not clear

7. Dietary recommendations for diabetics do not include

    a. Strict carbohydrate restriction

    b. Limiting fats and cholesterol

    c. Limiting protein intake

    d. Eating meals at regular intervals

8. Indications for starting a diabetic on oral hypoglycemics include

    a. Allergy to sulfa drugs

    b. Pregnancy in a Type II diabetic controlled by diet

    c. Diagnosis of Type I diabetes

    d. Failure to control hyperglycemia with diet in a Type II diabetic

9. A Type II diabetic has had good control of his blood glucose with oral hypoglycemics. He is in for a routine three month check. He had a complete work up 6 months ago. Which of the following is LEAST likely to be done at this visit?

    a. Urinalysis.

    b. Blood glucose.

    c. Fundoscopic examination

    d. ECG

10. Mr. P. is on 30 units of NPH and 5 units of regular insulin each morning and 15 units of NPH each evening to control his Type I diabetes. His blood glucose levels for the past three days have been

Fasting	Before Lunch	Before Supper	At hs
200-250	95-110	110-120	95-130

He should be instructed to

    a. Add 2 units of NPH to his pm dose

    b. Add 2 units NPH before breakfast

    c. Add 2 units of regular insulin to his pm dose

    d. Do nothing

11. Hemoglobin A_{1c} gives an indication of glucose control over the past

    a. Week
    b. Four to six weeks
    c. Month
    d. 60 to 90 days

12. Synthetic human insulin

    a. Causes more antibody formation
    b. Contains more impurities than purified pork insulin
    c. Is least antigenic of all insulins
    d. None of the above

13. Mr. J. is a 50 year old type II diabetic who has been on insulin for the past six months. He reports that his fasting blood glucose levels have been running above two hundred but they have been great during the rest of the day. His evening dose of NPH insulin has been increased three times in the last two weeks with no improvement in the fasting values. Currently he is on 30 units NPH/4 units Regular in the morning and 18 Units NPH/4 units Regular before supper. This is his most recent glucose pattern

B	L	S	hs
250-280	130-144	120-132	100-120

    If he has fairly good dietary compliance, you should instruct him to

    a. Increase the evening NPH by 2 more units
    b. Check his blood glucose between 2 and 3 a.m. for the next 2 days
    c. Increase the morning dose of regular insulin by 2 units
    d. Increase the morning dose of NPH insulin by 2 units

14. High fasting glucose after a nocturnal hypoglycemia in a diabetic otherwise in good control with insulin would indicate

    a. Dawn phenomenon
    b. Somogyi effect
    c. Insulin allergy
    d. Lipodystrophy

15. Which action would counteract this problem?

    a. Increase his morning dose of NPH
    b. Have him use human insulin instead of pork insulin
    c. Decrease his evening NPH insulin dose
    d. Increase his morning dose of Regular insulin

16. Mrs. J. is a Type II diabetic who has been on pork insulin for the past two years

and she has begun to develop hard lumpy raised areas in her right thigh where she has been placing injections. The only action that will prevent further development of such areas would be to

   a. Switch to human synthetic insulin
   b. Inject insulin directly into the lumpy areas
   c. Rotate the injection sites
   d. Switch to oral hypoglycemics

17. Ms. W. is a 34 year old who is seeking care because of increased irritability, weight loss "despite a great appetite" and diarrhea (not watery but 2 to 3 stools a day). She feels exhausted but can't seem to sleep and states she "feels like I could jump out of my skin."

    If excess thyroid hormone is the problem which of the following might be noted?

   a. Yellowing skin
   b. Fine tremor
   c. Delayed tendon reflex
   d. Sinus bradycardia

18. Graves disease is caused by

   a. Viral infection
   b. Use of Lithium
   c. An autoimmune response
   d. Excessive ingestion of thyroid hormone

19. In Graves disease you would expect

   a. TSH to be decreased
   b. T_3 to be decreased
   c. T_3 resin uptake to be decreased
   d. T_4 to be decreased

20. If Ms. W. is diagnosed with Graves disease and placed on antithyroid medication you will include which of the following in your initial patient teaching?

   a. The need of life long use of antithyroid medications
   b. Initial signs of the effectiveness of treatment will be increased urination
   c. The possibility of developing myxedemic coma
   d. Signs of hypothyroidism

21. The most serious side effect of both PTU and methimazole is

   a. Skin rash
   b. Diarrhea
   c. Agranulocytosis
   d. Hepatitis

22. The best guide to adequacy of the dosage of antithyroid medication in thyrotoxicosis is

    a. Thyroid antibodies
    b. T_3 (RIA)
    c. TSH
    d. T_4

23. Sally G. is a 44 year old who thinks she is begining menopause because her menstrual periods have become irregular. Her major complaint is a lack of energy and weight gain. Physical examination reveals dry skin, thinning hair, a puffy facial appearance, and an enlarged, nontender thyroid. Her B.P. is 130/92 with a heart rate of 60.

    These findings are consistent with

    a. Graves disease
    b. Hypothyroidism
    c. Plummer's disease
    d. Thyrotoxicosis

24. Which of the following findings would be consistent with a hypothyroid state?

    a. Hyperactive bowel sounds
    b. Lid lag
    c. Insomnia
    d. Parethesias

25. Ms. H. is diagnosed with hypothyroidism and placed on levothyroxine 0.1 mg per day. After a week she calls to tell you she hasn't seen any improvement and wants to discontinue her medication. Your best response would be to

    a. Add propranolol to her regimen
    b. Change to desiccated thyroid
    c. Increase her dosage .125 mg/day
    d. Encourage her to take this dose for at least another week

26. Ms. L. is a 50 year old female who has been diagnosed as having primary myxedema. An initial dose of 0.15 mg/day of levothyroxine has been prescribed. Patient education would include which of the following?

    a. Discussion of the chronicity of the disease and the life-long medication use
    b. That it will take six months to a year for her fatigue to disappear
    c. Avoidance of foods causing increased peristalsis
    d. Explanation that after two years of therapy this medication may not be needed

27. Your 57 year old patient has been on prednisone for her rheumatoid arthritis. She has the typical "moon face," excess weight in her torso area, and is complaining

that she bruises easily when she bumps herself. As her primary care provider the best action would be to

a. Discontinue her prednisone immediately
b. Add a NSAID to her treatment regimen
c. Convert to an alternate-day schedule
d. Discontinue prednisone immediately and start on naproxen 250 mg b.i.d.

28. Skin changes in Addison's disease include

a. Circumoral pallor
b. Maculopapular eruptions associated with stress
c. Hyperpigmentation
d. Facial plethora and hirsutism

Answers:

1. c
2. a
3. c
4. a
5. b
6. b
7. a
8. d
9. d
10. a
11. d
12. c
13. b
14. b
15. c
16. c
17. b
18. c
19. a
20. d
21. c
22. b
23. b
24. d
25. d
26. a
27. c
28. c

Bibliography

Albisser, A. M., & Sperlich, M. (1992). Adjusting insulins. *Diabetic Educator, 18*(3), 211-219.

Armstrong, J. (1991). A brief overview of diabetes mellitus and exercise. *Diabetic Educator, 17*(3), 175-178.

Bartuska, D. (1991). Thyroid disease in the elderly. *Hospital Practice, 26*(12), 85-89, 92, 95-98, 102, 107.

Bell, D. (1992). Exercise for patients with diabetes. *Postgraduate Medicine, 91*(1), 83.

Beaser, R. (1992). Fine tuning insulin therapy. *Postgraduate Medicine, 91*(3), 323-330.

Federman, D. D. (1991). Hyperthyroidism in the geriatric population. *Hospital Practice, 26*(1), 61-76.

Griffin, J. E. (1990). Review. Hypothyroidism in the elderly. *American Journal of the Medical Sciences, 295*(2), 125-128.

Johnson, J. L., & Felicetta, J. V. (1992). Hyperthyroidism: A comprehensive review. *Journal of the American Academy of Nurse Practitioners, 4*(1), 8-14.

Johnson, J. L., & Felicetta, J. V. (1992). Hypothyroidism: A comprehensive review. *Journal of the American Academy of Nurse Practitioners. 4*(4), 131-138.

Vitale, B. P., & Littler, J. E. (1990). Gastroenterology. In J. E. Littler & T. Mammany (Eds.), *The Family Practice Handbook* (pp. 133-158). Chicago: Yearbook Medical Publishers.

Yates, A. J., & DeFronzo, R. H. (1993). Metabolic disorders. In I. H. Stein *Internal medicine: Diagnosis and therapy* (3rd ed.) (pp 497-535). Norwalk CT: Appleton & Lange.

Yeomans, A. C. (1990). Assessment and management of hypothyroidism. *Nurse Practitioner, 15*(11), 8,11-12,14,16.

Genitourinary and Gynecologic Disorders

Pamela A. Shuler

Acquired Immunodeficiency Syndrome (AIDS)

- Definition: Secondary immunodeficiency syndrome resulting from HIV infection and characterized by opportunistic infections, neurologic dysfunction, malignancies and a variety of other disorders

- Etiology/Incidence

    1. HIV invades and multiplies within one or more types of susceptible cells; circulating CD4 lymphocytes and macrophages are most commonly affected, destroying the host's immune system

    2. Median time from HIV infection to AIDS is 10 years

    3. Over 1 million Americans are infected with HIV

    4. Most diagnoses are made in persons 20 to 49 years old; women aged 15 to 44 constitute one of the fastest growing segments of the U.S. epidemic

    5. HIV is transmitted through direct contact with bodily fluids (blood, semen, vaginal secretions)

    6. Major routes of HIV transmission

        a. Sexual intercourse (homosexual and heterosexual)

        b. Needle sharing (IV drug users)

        c. Transfusions of blood and blood products

        d. Needle stick, open wound and mucous membrane exposure to health care workers (0.4% incidence according to the Center for Disease Control [CDC])

        e. Injection with previously used unsterilized needle (acupuncture, tattooing, medical injection)

        f. Pregnancy (mother to unborn fetus)

        g. Breastfeeding (mother to infant)

    7. Trends

        a. Decreasing number of newly infected homosexual males

        b. African American and Hispanic women are disproportionately represented in AIDS cases

        c. Younger U.S. groups of infected people have higher proportion of females than do older groups

- Signs and Symptoms—CDC Classification

    1. Asymptomatic HIV infection (may last > 10 years)

        a. Inoculation to seroconversion 90% by three months and 98% by six months

    2. Acute HIV infection

        a. Two to eight weeks after infection may have

            (1) High fever, lymphadenopathy, rash, sometimes aseptic meningitis

            (2) Usually mistaken for flu or mononucleosis

        b. Months to years before AIDS—may have chronic fatigue, weight loss, nightsweats, persistent dermatitis, shingles, persistent diarrhea, oral candidiasis, hairy leukoplakia, chronic vaginal candidiasis, tuberculosis, cognitive changes

    3. Persistent generalized lymphadenopathy (PGL)

        a. Palpable lymph node enlargement (2 sites other than inguinal)

        b. No concurrent illness to explain lymphadenopathy

    4. HIV diseases that contribute to progression of AIDS

        a. *Pneumocystis carinii* pneumonia, Kaposi's sarcoma, Cytomegalovirus and/or other opportunistic infections/cancers

        b. Encephalopathy

        c. Wasting syndrome (involuntary weight loss greater than 10% of baseline body weight, plus either chronic diarrhea or chronic weakness and documented fever)

- Differential Diagnosis: Other diseases that lead to immune suppression or are related to patient's symptoms, e.g., cancer, tuberculosis, enterocolitis and endocrine diseases

- Physical Findings: Variable, depending upon infection stage

- Diagnostic Tests/Findings

    1. Initial blood test for antibody detection, e.g., Enzyme-linked immunosorbent assay (ELISA)

    2. Confirmatory blood tests for HIV specific antibody profile

        a. Western blot assay

      b. Indirect immunofluorescence assay (IFA)

- Management/Treatment
(All STD treatment regimens throughout this chapter based on *1993 Sexually transmitted treatment guidelines*, published by CDC)

  1. Currently, no cure or vaccination for HIV infection

  2. Experimental treatment regimens are constantly evolving

  3. Treatment of HIV and opportunistic infections, malignancies and prophylaxis against opportunistic infections continue to evolve rapidly; basic guidelines include

    a. Therapy for opportunistic infections and malignancies

      (1) Conditions include *P. carinii* pneumonia, toxoplasmosis, cryptcoccis, lymphoma, cytomegalovirus, esophageal candidiasis, Herpes simplex and zoster, Kaposi's sarcoma

      (2) Medications include antibiotics, antifungals and corticosteroids

    b. Antiviral treatment

      (1) Zidovudine (ZDV)

        (a) Indication—symptomatic persons with 500 CD4 + T cells/μL or less and asymptomatic persons with 300 CD4 + T cells/μL or less

        (b) Dose—500 mg orally daily in three divided doses

        (c) Common side effects—anemia, neutropenia, nausea, malaise, headache, insomnia

        (d) Monitoring—complete blood count (CBC) with differential every three months once stable

      (2) Didanosine (ddI)

        (a) Indication—CD4 cell count of 500/mm^3 or less and intolerance to ZDV or with progression of disease on ZDV

        (b) Dose—125 to 300 mg orally b.i.d.

        (c) Common side effects—peripheral neuropathy, pancreatitis, dry mouth, hepatitis

        (d) Monitoring—CBC with differential, potassium, amylase, triglycerides, monthly neurological examination

c. Prophylaxis of opportunistic infections

    (1)   *P. carinii* pneumonia

        (a) Trimethoprim—sulfamethoxazole (TMP-SMX) one double-strength tablet daily

        (b) Aerosolized pentamidine—300 mg monthly if unable to tolerate TMP-SMX

    (2)   *M. tuberculosis*

        (a) Isoniazid—10 mg/kg/day up to 300 mg daily for 1 year

        (b) All patients with positive PPD reaction (5 mm of induration or greater) should receive prophylactic treatment

    (3)   The use of prophylaxis for other infections including toxoplasmosis, *M. avium*-intracellulare infection, cytomegalovirus infection, cryptococcal infection and histoplasmosis is under study.

d. Recommended immunizations for HIV infected persons

    (1)   Pneumococcal vaccination

    (2)   Annual influenza vaccination

    (3)   Three-dose schedule of hepatitis B vaccine for those who lack immunity

4. Discuss therapeutic and diagnostic plans

5. Educate regarding prevention, transmission and treatment of the disease

6. Emphasize importance of behavioral measures to protect and enhance the immune system

    a. No tobacco, street drug, alcohol use

    b. Nutritious diet

    c. Stress management, imagery

    d. Exercise as tolerated

    e. Decrease exposure to infectious agents since the HIV virus is spread when the immune system is activated

7. Encourage continued "safer sex" practices, and/or abstinence

8. Assist patient, as appropriate, in meeting physical, psychological, social, cultural, environmental and spiritual needs

9. Report AIDS cases to local health department

Gonorrhea (Uncomplicated Gonococcal Infections)

■ Definition: A sexually transmitted bacterial infection that produces urethritis in men and cervicitis in women

■ Etiology/Incidence

1. Causative organism is *Neisseria gonorrhoeae*, a gram-negative diplococcus

2. Approximately 1.0 million infectious new cases annually

3. Has greatest incidence in the 15 to 29 year old age group

4. Incubation period usually 2 to 8 days

5. Spectrum of infection—cervicitis, urethritis, salpingitis, proctitis

6. A leading cause of infertility among U.S. females

■ Signs and Symptoms

1. Female

    a. Often asymptomatic

    b. Dysuria, urinary frequency, urgency with a purulent urethral discharge

    c. Vaginal discharge

    d. Pelvic pain

    e. Intermenstrual bleeding

2. Male

    a. One quarter are asymptomatic

    b. Dysuria (urethra most common site in male), frequency

    c. Penile discharge (serous/milky to yellow with blood-tinge)

    d. Testicular pain

■ Differential Diagnosis

1. Nongonococcal cervicitis, vaginitis or urethritis

2. Reiter's syndrome (chlamydia)

3. Pelvic inflammatory disease (PID)

4. Proctitis (other origin)

- Physical Findings

  1. Female

     a. Purulent discharge from cervix (primary site in reproductive age women)

     b. Inflammation of Bartholin's glands

     c. Evidence of PID (untreated infection)

  2. Male

     a. Evidence of urethritis, prostatitis

     b. Evidence of epididymitis (with untreated infection)

- Diagnostic Tests/Findings

  1. Female tests

     a. Gram stain of endocervical canal discharge shows WBCs with gram negative intracellular diplococci; sensitivity only 40 to 70% in women; greater than 90% in men

     b. Wet prep of purulent cervical discharge may show polymorphonuclear leukocytes (WBCs) > 10 (high-power)

     c. Culture material from endocervix and other suspect sites on to Thayer-Martin or Transgrow media to confirm diagnosis

  2. Male tests

     a. Gram stain of urethral discharge smear shows gram-negative diplococci and WBCs

     b. Culture of urethra and other suspect sites

  3. Test for concomitant infection from other STDs including HIV, syphilis, and chlamydia

  4. Test partners

- Management/Treatment

  1. Treat all contacts

  2. First choice—Ceftriaxone 125 mg IM once, or Ciprofloxacin 500 mg orally once, or Cefixime 400 mg orally once, or Ofloxacin 400 mg

orally once, *plus* Doxycycline 100 mg orally b.i.d. for 7 days, or Erythromycin base or stearate 500 mg orally q.i.d. for seven days if the patient is pregnant; high incidence of co-existing chlamydia

3. Alternative regimens—Spectinomycin 2 g IM once or Ceftizoxime 500 mg IM once, or Cefotaxime 500 mg IM once, or Cefotetan 1g IM once, or Cefoxitin 2g IM once, Cefuroxim axetil 1 g orally once, or Cefpodoxime proxetil 200 mg orally once, or Enoxacin 400 mg orally once, or Lomefloxacin 400 mg orally once, or Norfloxacin 800 mg orally once, *plus* Doxycycline as above

4. Test of cure not essential; rescreening one to two months after treatment recommended, or sooner for repeat culture if symptoms persist or recur

5. Discuss therapeutic and diagnostic plans

6. Emphasize importance of complete treatment

7. Avoid sexual intercourse until patient and partner(s) cured

8. Educate regarding prevention, transmission and treatment of the disease; encourage continued use of condoms

9. Report cases to health department

Genital Chlamydial Infection

- Definition: A sexually transmitted disease that produces urethritis in men and cervicitis in women

- Etiology/Incidence

  1. *Chlamydia trachomatis*

  2. Approximately 4 million new cases occur annually

  3. The most common bacterial sexually transmitted disease in the U.S.

  4. A leading cause of female infertility and ectopic pregnancy in U.S.

- Signs and Symptoms

  1. Female

     a. Often asymptomatic

     b. Dysuria

     c. Vaginal discharge/spotting

     d. Lower abdominal/pelvic pain

     e. Dyspareunia

    f. Dysmenorrhea, menstrual irregularity

    g. Infertility

    h. Enlarged, tender inguinal lymph nodes

  2. Male

    a. Often asymptomatic

    b. Urethral discharge (any color)

    c. Dysuria

    d. Testicular pain/swelling

    e. Enlarged, tender inguinal lymph nodes

- Differential Diagnosis
  1. Gonococcal cervicitis
  2. Urethritis
  3. Proctitis
  4. PID
  5. Urinary tract infection
  6. Epididymitis
  7. Prostatitis from other infective agent
  8. Vaginitis
- Physical Findings
  1. Female
     - a. Mucopurulent urethral and/or cervical discharge
     - b. Hypertropic, eroded and friable cervix (maybe)
     - c. Evidence of PID (advanced infection)
  2. Male
     - a. Mucopurulent urethral discharge
     - b. Evidence of prostatitis
     - c. Evidence of epididymitis (untreated infection)
- Diagnostic Tests/Findings
  1. Female
     - a. Wet prep or gram stain shows WBCs > 10 (high-power)

b. Direct immunofluorescent assay and the enzyme-linked immunosorbent assay (ELISA) are positive

(1) Reliability of tests in population with low prevalence of infection is questionable

(2) Indirect antigen-detection tests usually used since cultures expensive and cumbersome

2. Male

a. Gram stain or wet prep shows WBCs > 10 (high-power)

b. Same indirect antigen-detection tests

3. Test for concomitant infection from other STDs in patient (HIV, Gonorrhea, Syphilis)

4. Test partners

- Management/Treatment

1. Treat all contacts

2. First choice—Doxycycline, 100 mg orally b.i.d. for 7 days or Azithromycin one g orally once

3. Ofloxacin 300 mg orally b.i.d. for 7 days, or Erythromycin base 500 mg orally q.i.d. for 7 days, or Erythromycin ethylsuccinate 800 mg orally q.i.d. for 7 days, or Sulfisoxazole 500 mg orally q.i.d. for 10 days

4. During pregnancy—Erythromycin base or stearate, 500 mg orally q.i.d. for 7 days or Erythromycin base 250 mg orally q.i.d. for 14 days, Erythromycin ethylsuccinate 800 mg orally q.i.d. for 7 days or Erythromycin ethylsuccinate 400 mg orally q.i.d. for 14 days, or Amoxicillin, 500 mg orally t.i.d. for 7 days

5. No test-of-cure 3 to 4 weeks after treatment unless symptoms persist or re-infection suspected

6. Discuss therapeutic and diagnostic plans

7. Emphasize importance of complete treatment

8. Avoid sexual intercourse until patient and partner(s) complete treatment

9. Educate regarding prevention, transmission and treatment of the disease; encourage continued use of condoms

Syphilis

- Definition: A complex infectious disease that can affect almost any organ or tissue in the body and mimics many diseases

- Etiology/Incidence

  1. Causative organism is *Treponema pallidum*, a spirochete

  2. Transmission primarily occurs through minor skin or mucosal lesions during sexual encounters; genital and extragenital areas may be inoculated

  3. Can be transmitted via placenta (after 10th week) from mother to fetus (congenital rate—1 in 10,000 pregnancies)

  4. Incidence has steadily increased since 1985; approximately 40,000 cases (primary and secondary types) reported in U.S. annually

  5. Risk of contraction—30 to 50% (partner-primary syphilis)

- Signs and Symptoms

  1. Primary

     a. Painless chancre

  2. Secondary

     a. Skin rash—especially palmar and plantar

     b. Malaise, anorexia

     c. Alopecia

     d. Arthralgias/myalgias/flu-like symptoms

     e. Other symptoms depending on affected organs

  3. Latent

     a. May be asymptomatic

     b. Integumentary, ocular, cardiovascular, gastrointestinal, respiratory or neurological manifestations may be present

  4. Neurosyphilis

     a. May occur during any stage of syphilis

     b. Optic, auditory, cranial nerve and/or meningeal symptoms are most common

■ Differential Diagnosis

   1. Primary

      a. Herpes genitalis

      b. Chancroid

      c. Neoplasm

      d. Lymphogranuloma venereum (LGV)

      e. Superficial fungal infections

   2. Secondary

      a. Conditions associated with rash or other presenting symptoms, e.g., flu, mononucleosis, pityriasis rosea, drug eruptions

      b. Infectious hepatitis

   3. Latent

      a. Neoplasms of skin, liver, lung, stomach or brain

      b. Other forms

         (1) Meningitis

         (2) Cardiovascular disorders

         (3) CNS disorders

         (4) Arthritis

         (5) Primary neurologic lesions

■ Physical Findings

   1. Neurological signs may be present at any stage

   2. Primary

      a. Indurated ulcer (chancre) on

         (1) Genitals

         (2) Mouth

         (3) Rectum

         (4) Nipple

      b. Regional lymphadenopathy

   3. Secondary

    a. Low-grade fever

    b. Highly variable skin rash (including palms and soles)

    c. Mucous patches

    d. Evidence or manifestations of condyloma latum

    e. Generalized lymphadenopathy

    f. Evidence of meningitis, iritis, hepatitis, glomerulonephritis

4. Latent

    a. May have no clinical signs of infection

    b. Granulomatous lesions (gummas)—skin, mucous membranes, bone

    c. Leukoplakia

    d. Evidence of periostitis, osteitis or arthritis

    f. Gummatous infiltrates in larynx, trachea, pulmonary parenchyma, stomach and/or liver

    g. Diminished coronary circulation

    h. Acute myocardial infarction

    i. Cardiac insufficiency

    j. Aortic aneurysm

    k. Meningitis

    l. Hemiparesis

    m. Hemiplegia

    n. Tabes dorsalis

    o. General paresis

■ Diagnostic Tests/Findings

1. Early syphilis—primary, secondary or latent syphilis of less than one year's duration

    a. Definitive methods

        (1) Darkfield microscopy

        (2) Direct fluorescent antibody tests of lesion exudate or tissue

    b. Presumptive methods (neither test alone is sufficient for diagnosis)

          (1)   Treponemal serologic tests—once positive, always positive regardless of treatment or disease activity

               (a)   Fluorescent treponemal antibody absorption (FTA-ABS) test

               (b)   Microhemagglutination assay for antibody to *T. pallidum* (MHA-TP)

               (c)   Tests/titers should be reported as positive or negative and used to confirm nontreponemal tests

               (d)   FTA-ABS or MHA-TP confirmation tests positive in 85 to 95% of primary and in 100% of secondary cases

2. Nontreponemal serologic tests

   a. Veneral Disease Research Laboratory (VDRL)

   b. Rapid Plasma Reagin (RPR)

   c. VDRL and RPR titers correlate with disease activity and reported quantitatively

3. Latent syphilis of more than one year's duration and cardiovascular syphilis

   a. VDRL or RPR test (+ in 75% of cases)

   b. FTA-ABS or MHA-TP confirmation test (+ in 98% cases)

   c. Lumbar puncture with tests on cerebrospinal fluid (CSF)

4. Neurosyphilis (occurs at any stage)

   a. Treponemal and nontreponemal serologic tests results dependent upon stage of disease

   b. CSF examinations as above

5. Test for concomitant infection from other STDs in patient and contacts

   a. HIV

   b. Gonorrhea

   c. Chlamydia

6. Test partners

■ Management/Treatment

1. Pregnant patients allergic to penicillin should be treated with penicillin after desensitization for all stages

2. Early syphilis and persons exposed within last 90 days

   a. Treat all partners

   b. First choice—Benzathine penicillin G, 2.4 million units IM once

   c. Penicillin allergy—Doxycycline 100 mg orally b.i.d. for 2 weeks or Tetracycline 500 mg orally q.i.d. for 2 weeks

3. Late latent cases and cardiovascular syphilis (normal CSF examination)

   a. First choice—Benzathine, penicillin G, 2.4 million units IM weekly for 3 weeks

   b. Penicillin allergy—Doxycycline 100 mg orally b.i.d. for 4 weeks or Tetracycline 500 mg orally q.i.d. for 4 weeks

4. Neurosyphilis

   a. First choice—12 to 24 million units aqueous crystalline penicillin G daily, administered as 2 to 4 million units IV every 4 hours for 10 to 14 days

   b. Alternate regimen if compliance assured—2.4 million units procaine penicillin IM daily, plus probenecid 500 mg orally q.i.d., both for 10 to 14 days

5. Post-Treatment Follow-Up

   a. Primary and secondary baseline RPR or VDRL at time of treatment and repeated every 3 months; titer should fall fourfold in 3 months, eightfold in 6 months and become negative within 2 years (MHA-TP and FTA-ABS will be positive for lifetime)

   b. Latent—RPR or VDRL repeated at 6 month and 12 month intervals; titer should fall fourfold in 12 to 24 months

   c. Neurosyphilis—CSF examination every 6 months until normal

6. Discuss therapeutic and diagnostic plans

7. Emphasize importance of complete treatment

8. Avoid sexual intercourse until patient and partner(s) cured

9. Educate regarding prevention, transmission and treatment of the disease; encourage continued use of condoms

10. Report cases to health department

Herpes Genitalis

- Definition: A viral STD that recurrently produces painful genital lesions and has no cure
- Etiology/Incidence
  1. Caused by herpes simplex virus (HSV) types 1 (5-10%) and 2 (90-95%)
  2. Initial (primary) and recurrent infections affect approximately 200,000 and 30 million persons respectively annually
  3. Duration of initial infection—10 to 14 days; recurrent 7 to 10 days; viral shedding (without clinical symptoms) occurs during latency (interval between outbreaks)
  4. Virus resides in presacral ganglia during latency
  5. Can lead to neuralgia, meningitis, ascending myelitis, urethral strictures, and lymphatic suppuration
  6. Infection during pregnancy can lead to spontaneous abortion or fetal morbidity/mortality; risk for transmission to neonate appears highest among women with first episode near time of delivery
- Signs and Symptoms
  1. First clinical episode
     a. Fever/chills
     b. Malaise
     c. Headache
     d. Dysuria
     e. Vaginal discharge, abnormal bleeding
     f. Dyspareunia
     g. Pruritic/burning genital vesicles that rupture and become painful ulcers—mean duration 12 days
  2. Recurrent episodes
     a. Pruritic/burning vesicles that rupture into less painful ulcers—mean duration 4.5 days
- Differential Diagnosis
  1. Syphilis
  2. Lymphogranuloma venereum

3. Gonorrhea

4. Chlamydia

5. Chancroid

6. Vaginitis

7. Herpes zoster

8. Condyloma latum

9. Erythema multiforme

10. Neoplasm (especially cervical)

- Physical Findings

  1. Fever—first episode

  2. Single or multiple vesicles surrounded by inflammation/edema on external genitalia, penis, scrotum, anus, vagina or cervix (75%); vesicles spontaneously rupture and form painful, erythematous ulcers, scab over and heal

  3. Cervix may appear diffusely inflamed, edematous with large punched-out ulcers or a granulomatous-appearing tumor-like mass covered with gray exudate may be present

  4. Profuse, watery vaginal discharge often present and may be only sign

- Diagnostic Tests/Findings

  1. Papanicolaou or other histochemical stain—identification of multinucleated giant cells with intranuclear inclusions in a cytologic smear

  2. Identification of HSV virus(es) from tissue (vulvar, vaginal, cervical) cultures or antigen test

  3. Serologic tests for HSV types 1 and 2 antibodies are also available

  4. Test for concomitant infection of other STDs in patient and contacts

     a. HIV

     b. Syphilis

     c. Condyloma acuminata

     d. Gonorrhea

     e. Chlamydia

     f. Chancroid

- Management/Treatment

  1. Symptomatic treatment—drying and antipruritic agents and topical anesthetic agents

  2. Chemotherapeutic agents—Acyclovir (Zovirax), available in topical, oral and intravenous formulations

     a. Topical therapy—minimal benefit except may be useful for immunocompromised patients

     b. Oral therapy

        (1) Recurrent herpes simplex infections—200 mg 5 times a day or 500 mg 3 times a day or 800 mg 2 times a day for 10 days

        (2) Uncomplicated primary herpes simplex infections—200 mg 5 times per day for 7-10 days

        (3) Prophylactic or suppressive therapy (if 6 or more outbreaks per year)—200 mg 5 times a day or 400 mg twice daily for 1 year

     c. Intravenous therapy

        (1) Used in severe disease and when complications necessitate hospitalization

        (2) Acyclovir 5 to 10 mg/kg IV every 8 hours for 5 to 7 days

     d. Acyclovir is eliminated by the kidneys; hydration is particularly important

     e. Safety of systemic treatment has not been established during pregnancy

  3. Discuss therapeutic and diagnostic plans

  4. Avoid sexual intercourse when lesions present; encourage continued use of condoms

  5. Educate regarding prevention, transmission and treatment of the disease and dangers during pregnancy

Genital Warts (Condylomata acuminata)

- Definition: Sexually transmitted warty growths appearing on any part of the genitalia.

- Etiology/Incidence

  1. More than 60 types of human papillomavirus (HPV) cause the warts;

types 16, 18, 31, 33, 35, 45 and 56 are predominately detected in high-grade neoplastic lesions

2. HPV increases risk of penile, vulvar and cervical cancers

3. Has its greatest incidence in the 15 to 25 year old age group; is correlated with multiple sex partners, early coitus and lack of contraceptive barrier methods

4. Approximately 3 million cases diagnosed annually

5. The most common symptomatic viral STD in the U.S.; highly contagious

- Signs and Symptoms

    1. Painless, pruritic or burning warts on external genitalia (male and female)

    2. Possibly—dyspareunia, dysuria, bleeding

- Differential Diagnosis

    1. Condyloma latum

    2. Neoplasm

    3. Granuloma inguinale

    4. Moles

- Physical Findings

    1. Single or multiple soft, fleshy, papillary or sessile, painless keratinized growths (may be multilobulated papules and quite large) around anus, vulvovaginal area, penis, urethra, perineum or oral cavity

    2. In women, similar lesions may appear in vagina/on cervix; vaginal discharge from co-existing infection(s) may be present; men may have lesions in urethra

    3. May have no signs since flat warts often difficult to visualize

- Diagnostic Tests/Findings

    1. Tissue sample (biopsy) for detection of viral DNA is widely available, but clinical utility is questionable

    2. Application of 5% acetic acid and colposcopy aids in diagnosis—turns lesions white; biopsies may be taken to rule out displasia and carcinoma

    3. Pap smear may indicate koilocytosis (indicative of HPV infection) on

cervix

4. Test for concomitant infection of other STDs

    a. HIV

    b. Gonorrhea

    c. Syphilis—RPR or VDRL to rule out Condyloma latum

    d. Chlamydia

- Management/Treatment

1. New treatment regimens are evolving to ameliorate symptoms; no current methods are curative

    a. Small vulvar and perianal warts

       (1) Self-treatment with Podafilox 0.5% solution—apply with cotton tip applicator b.i.d. for 3 days followed by no treatment for 4 days; cycle can be repeated 4 times

       (2) 80 to 90% solution of trichloroacetic acid (TCA) or tincture of podophyllin weekly for 6 weeks (patient must wash off podophyllin in 4 hrs); protect surrounding skin with petroleum jelly

       (3) TCA is preferred since it is more effective, not absorbed and can be used during pregnancy and on penis; treatment may be slightly more painful than podophyllin; immediate application of sodium bicarbonate paste following treatment will decrease pain

    b. Large warts (> 2 cm), vulvar/vaginal warts

       (1) CO_2 laser

       (2) Electrodesiccation, electrocautery, cryocautery

2. NO MORE THAN 1/3 OF LESION ENCIRCLING AN ORIFICE SHOULD BE TREATED AT SINGLE VISIT

3. Cervical warts—see section on dysplasia

4. Discuss therapeutic and diagnostic plans

5. Educate regarding prevention, transmission and treatment of the disease; encourage continued use of condoms

6. Emphasize importance of follow-up particularly if Pap abnormal

7. Discuss possible chronicity

a. Treatment may not be successful

b. High recurrence rate due to dormant and asymptomatic viral shedding

c. Individuals who smoke have more difficulty with recurrence

d. Smoking is a HPV co-factor for cervical cancer

Pelvic Inflammatory Disease (PID)

- Definition: Infection of the upper genital tract, including the endometrium, oviducts, ovaries, uterine wall/serosa, broad ligaments and pelvic peritoneum

- Etiology/Incidence

  1. A disease of polymicrobial infection caused by a variety of aerobic and anaerobic bacteria including *N. gonorrhoeae*, Chlamydia, group b streptococcus, *Escherichia coli*, bacteroides and bacterial vaginosis organisms

  2. Clinical PID is usually a polymicrobial infection

  3. More than 1 million episodes occur annually

  4. Most prevalent serious infection for women 16 to 25 years

  5. After initial infection, women more susceptible to reinfection, ectopic pregnancy and infertility

  6. Oral contraceptives and barrier methods with spermicide provide significant protection

  7. Annual costs of PID and its sequelae is—$4.2 billion

- Signs and Symptoms

  1. Often symptoms are mild, atypical, subtle or absent

  2. Fever/chills

  3. Nausea/vomiting

  4. Dysuria

  5. Vaginal discharge

  6. Dysmenorrhea

  7. Menstrual irregularity

  8. Lower abdominal/pelvic pain (usually < 1 week duration)

9. Dyspareunia

10. Infertility

■ Differential Diagnosis

1. Appendicitis

2. Ectopic pregnancy

3. Septic abortion

4. Hemorrhagic or ruptured ovarian cysts or tumors

5. Twisted ovarian cyst

6. Degeneration of a myoma

7. Enteritis

■ Physical Findings and Diagnostic Tests/Findings
Clinical criteria for diagnosing PID

1. Minimum criteria—empiric treatment required if all three present

    a. Direct abdominal tenderness, with or without rebound tenderness

    b. Tenderness with motion of cervix and uterus

    c. Adnexal tenderness

2. Additional criteria to increase specificity of diagnosis

    a. Laboratory documentation of cervical infection with *C. trachomatis* or *N. gonorrhoeae*

    b. Fever > 38.3 °C

    c. Abnormal cervical or vaginal discharge

    d. Elevated erythrocyte sedimentation rate and/or C-reactive protein

3. Elaborate criteria for diagnosis

    a. Histopathologic evidence of endometritis on endometrial biopsy

    b. Tubo-ovarian abscess on sonography or other radiologic tests

    c. Laparoscopic abnormalities consistent with PID

■ Management/Treatment

1. Resolution of symptoms and preservation of tubal function are the primary goals in management of PID; ideally all patients are hospitalized; however, for economic and practical reasons many are treated as outpatients

2. Hospitalization is highly recommended if

   a. Diagnosis is uncertain and surgical emergencies cannot be excluded

   b. Pelvic abscess is suspected

   c. Patient is pregnant, an adolescent or HIV infected

   d. Severe illness, e.g., nausea and vomiting precludes outpatient treatment

   e. Patient unable to follow or tolerate outpatient regimen

   f. Patient has failed to clinically respond to outpatient treatment

   g. Clinical follow-up within 72 hours of starting antibiotic therapy cannot be arranged

3. Outpatient Treatment

   a. First choice—cetoxitin 2g IM plus probenecid, 1 g orally once or ceftriaxone 250 mg IM or other parenteral third-generation cephalosporins plus Doxycycline 100 mg orally twice daily for 14 days

   b. Ofloxacin 400 mg orally b.i.d. plus clindamycin 450 mg orally q.i.d. or metronidazole 500 mg orally b.i.d. for 14 days

4. Follow-up appointment in 72 hours, then tests-of-cure conducted 7 to 10 days and 4 to 6 weeks post-treatment

5. Test and treat partners

6. Discuss therapeutic and diagnostic plans

7. Emphasize importance of complete treatment

8. Avoid sexual intercourse until patient and partner(s) cured

9. Education regarding prevention, transmission and treatment of the disease; encourage continued use of condoms

10. Discuss fertility issues as appropriate

Vulvovaginitis

- Definition: Inflammation and infection of the vulva/vagina
- Etiology/Incidence

  1. Commonly caused by *Trichomonas vaginalis* (a motile protozoan), Bacterial vaginosis (a polymicrobial bacterial vaginal infection) or *Candida albicans* (a fungi or yeast)

2. Trichomonas—transmitted through intercourse and also infects the lower urinary tract in men as well as women

3. Bacterial vaginosis (BV)—the most frequently diagnosed symptomatic vaginitis in the U.S.; not necessarily sexually acquired

4. Candida vaginitis—occurs in close to 30% of women; is not considered to be a STD; is predisposed by pregnancy, diabetes, use of broad-spectrum antibiotics or corticosteroids; heat, moisture and occlusive clothing also increase risk

5. Several types of vaginitis may co-exist

- Signs and Symptoms
  1. Trichomonas
     a. Malodorous yellow-green discharge with pruritus
     b. Dyspareunia
     c. Dysuria (male partners may also have dysuria)
  2. Bacterial vaginosis
     a. Malodorous ("fishy") discharge
     b. Spotting
  3. Candida vaginitis
     a. Thick discharge with pruritus
     b. Erythema of vagina and vulva

- Differential Diagnosis
  1. Chlamydia
  2. Gonorrhea
  3. Herpes genitalis
  4. Condyloma acuminata
  5. Allergy, contact dermatitis
  6. HPV discharge
  7. Atrophic vaginitis

- Physical Findings
  1. Trichomonas
     a. Diffuse vaginal erythema

b. Intensely inflamed lesions on cervix and vaginal mucosa— "strawberry patches"

c. Discharge

   (1)   Ranges from white/watery to green, thick and frothy

   (2)   Vaginal pH—higher than 4.5

2. Bacterial vaginosis

   a. Watery, grayish discharge

   b. Amine-like odor present when discharge alkalinized with 10-20% potassium hydroxide (KOH)—"whiff test"

   c. Vaginal pH of 5 or more

3. Candida vaginitis

   a. White, "cottage-cheese" discharge

   b. Marked vulvovaginal erythema/edema with intense pruritis

■ Diagnostic Tests/Findings

1. Wet prep microscopic examination of vaginal secretions viewed on low or high power

   a. Trichomonas—discharge mixed with saline will show motile trichomonads on microscopic examination

   b. Bacterial vaginosis—discharge mixed with saline will show clue cells on microscopic examination

   c. Candida vaginitis—discharge mixed with 10% KOH will show branched and budding pseudohyphae on microscopic examination

2. Test for concomitant infection from other STDs

   a. HIV

   b. Syphilis

   c. Condyloma acuminata

   d. Gonorrhea

   e. Chlamydia

■ Management/Treatment

1. Trichomonas—metronidazole (Flagyl), 2 g orally as a single dose or 500 mg b.i.d. for 7 days

2. Bacterial vaginosis

    a. Drug of choice—metronidazole (Flagyl), 500 mg orally b.i.d. for 7 days

    b. Alternative regimens

        (1) Clindamycin, 300 mg orally b.i.d. for 7 to 10 days (safe during pregnancy)

        (2) Metronidazole 2 g orally in a single dose *or*

        (3) Clindamycin cream, 2%, one full applicator (5g) intravaginally at hs for 7 days *or*

        (4) Metronidazole gel, 0.75%, one full applicator (5 g) intravaginally b.i.d. for 5 days

3. Candida vaginitis—many different preparations and treatment regimens exist; the following are commonly prescribed

    a. Miconazole or clotrimazole 1% cream, 5 g intravaginally at bedtime for 7 days

    b. Terconazole 80 mg suppository, 1 suppository intravaginally at bedtime for 3 days

    c. Resistant cases may need partner treatment

4. Discuss therapeutic and diagnostic plans

5. Avoid sexual intercourse until patient and partner(s) cured

6. Education regarding prevention, transmission and treatment of the disease; encourage continued use of condoms

7. Education regarding dangers of douching and incidence of infection

8. Education regarding P.I.D. association with bacterial vaginosis

Urinary Tract Infection (UTI, Cystitis: Acute, Uncomplicated)

- Definition: Inflammation and infection of the urinary bladder; urethra may be involved

- Etiology/Incidence

1. Most common causative organisms—*Escherichia coli*, (women) and Proteus species (men)

2. More common in women than men; urological evaluation required for men with UTI

3. 30 to 40% of women will experience at least 1 UTI

4. Contributing factors in women
   a. Sexual intercourse; diaphragm use
   b. Pregnancy
   c. Diabetes
   d. Catherization
   e. Instrumentation
5. Contributing factors in men
   a. Residual urine (prostatic enlargement)
   b. Neuropathic bladder
   c. Calculi
   d. Prostatitis
   e. Catherization
   f. Instrumentation

- Signs and Symptoms
  1. Dysuria, frequency, urgency
  2. Suprapubic discomfort
- Differential Diagnosis
  1. Vaginitis (females)
  2. Prostatitis (males)
  3. Gonorrhea
  4. Chlamydia infection
  5. Renal calculi
  6. Pyelonephritis
- Physical Findings
  1. Urinary meatus may be erythematous/edematous
  2. Negative costovertebral angle tenderness
  3. Negative pelvic or prostate examination
- Diagnostic Tests/Findings
  1. Pyuria—> 5 WBC/HPF (may not be present)
  2. Complete urinalysis (clean catch) with culture and sensitivity testing

      a. Bacteria count over 100,000 organisms per mililiter in fresh "clean catch" midstream specimen is reliable indicator of active urinary tract infection; women with acute cystitis may have more than 10^3 but less than 10^5 per milliliter in midstream urine cultures

      b. Leukocyte esterase dipstick test—positive

      c. Urine dipstick positive for protein, blood, nitrites suggestive of UTI

■ Management/Treatment

1. Single-dose regimens—due to higher than expected relapse rates, 3-day course is recommended

2. Three-day regimens (uncomplicated lower tract infection)—bactrim DS orally b.i.d. for 3 days, or ciprofloxacin 500 mg orally b.i.d. for 3 days, or augmentin 500 mg orally t.i.d. for 3 days

3. Standard oral regimens—sulfisoxazole 2 g orally then 1 to 2 g orally q.i.d. for 10 days or nitrofurantoin 50 mg orally q.i.d. for 7 to 10 days or cephalexin 500 mg orally q.i.d. for 7 to 10 days or bactrim DS orally b.i.d. for 7 to 10 days or ciprofloxacin 250 mg orally b.i.d. for 7 to 10 days

4. Treatment during pregnancy—ampicillin 500 mg orally q.i.d. for 7 to 14 days or amoxicillin 500 mg orally t.i.d. for 7 to 14 days; cephalosporin 500 mg q.i.d. for 7 to 14 days

5. Consider adding phenazopyridine hydrochloride 200 mg orally t.i.d. for 2 days for discomfort associated with urinary tract irritation (caution patient of orange/red tinge to urine)

6. Increase water and decrease carbonated drink intake

7. Repeat urinalysis with culture and sensitivity after medication regimen completed

8. Discuss therapeutic and diagnostic plans

9. Advise return appointment if symptoms increase or no improvement

10. Emphasize importance of complete treatment and follow-up appointment for repeat urinalysis

Acute Pyelonephritis (Upper UTI)

- Definition: An acute bacterial infection of the upper urinary tract (kidney and renal pelvis); usually results from an ascending infection.

- Etiology/Incidence

  1. *Escherichia coli* (gram negative) accounts for 80% of infections; *Staphylococcus saprophyticus* and *Streptococcus faecalis* (gram positive) account for 5 to 10%

  2. If urologic abnormalities or calculi present, the following organisms may cause infection Enterobacter, Proteus, Klebsiella, Serratia and Pseudomonas

  3. Majority of infections occur in young women; rare occurrence in men under age 50 years

  4. Most commonly occurs in patients who are pregnant or have disruptive urinary flow, neurogenic bladder dysfunction or vesicoureteral reflux

- Signs and Symptoms— usually develop rapidly over a few hours

  1. Shaking chills

  2. Malaise, generalized muscle tenderness

  3. Nausea, vomiting and diarrhea

  4. Flank/back pain (unilateral or bilateral)

  5. Abdominal pain

  6. Dysuria, frequency or urgency (may be absent)

- Differential Diagnosis

  1. Cystitis

  2. Prostatitis

  3. Musculoskeletal back pain

  4. Appendicitis

  5. Diverticulitis

  6. Pelvic inflammatory disease

  7. Ectopic pregnancy

- Physical Findings

  1. Fever, tachycardia

  2. Costovertebral angle pain (unilateral or bilateral) upon percussion

     3.   Peritoneal signs are usually absent

     4.   Patient appears very ill

■ Diagnostic Tests/Findings

     1.   Microscopic urinalysis

        a. 5 to 10 WBCs per high-power field present

        b. Occasional erythrocytes present

        c. White cell casts may be present

        d. Mild proteinuria

     2.   Urine culture— > 100,000 bacteria per ml of urine present; sensitivity testing should be done

     3.   Gram stain of uncentrifuged urine—one bacterium per oil-immersion correlates with 100,000 bacteria per ml of urine or more

     4.   Complete blood count (CBC)—leukocytosis with left shift

     5.   Elevated ESR

     6.   BUN and creatinine are usually normal

     7.   Electrolytes may be abnormal if dehydrated

■ Management/Treatment

     1.   M.D. referral or consult required

     2.   Inpatient therapy

        a. Patients who are pregnant, have underlying illness, have decreased renal reserve, very toxic (high fever, hypotensive, etc) or unable to tolerate oral therapy should be hospitalized for parenteral antibiotics

        b. IV antimicrobial therapy is based upon culture and sensitivity report

        c. IV hydration is also required

     3.   Outpatient therapy—if compliant/reliable and have immediate access to health care services if condition worsens

        a. Antibiotics may include Trimethoprim-sulfamethoxazole (if gram stain indicates gram negative organism), norfloxacin or ciprofloxacin

        b. Resistance to ampicillin is 30%, therefore it should not be used as

> sole therapy

   c. Follow-up by phone or in office in 24 hours

   d. Hydration measures

4. Repeat urine culture 1 week after completed course of antibiotics

5. Second repeat of urine culture in 6 months is optimal

6. Discuss therapeutic and diagnostic plans

7. Emphasize importance of complete treatment and follow-up appointments

8. Instructions regarding no sexual intercourse until treatment completed

9. Education regarding emergency signs and symptoms if managed as outpatient

Acute Bacterial Prostatitis

- Definition: Inflammation/infection of the prostate gland

- Etiology/Incidence

  1. *Escherichia coli* or other gram-negative bacteria are common causative agents

  2. Occasionally acute urinary retention develops, requiring urgent hospitalization, suprapubic drainage may be necessary; URINARY CATHETERIZATION SHOULD BE AVOIDED

  3. Absence of zinc in prostatic fluid can predispose patient to infection

  4. Young adult men may be more prone to nonbacterial prostatitis or prostatosis

     a. WBCs are present in expressed prostatic secretions, but no organisms are cultured

     b. Causative agents include mycoplasma, gardernella and chlamydia

- Signs and Symptoms

  1. Fever/chills, malaise

  2. Low back pain

  3. Dysuria, urgency, nocturia, frequency

  4. Perineal pain increased with defecation

- Differential Diagnosis

1. Acute/chronic bacterial cystitis (urinary retention)
2. Chronic prostatitis
3. Nonbacterial prostatosis
4. Prostatodynia
5. Prostatic or seminal vesicle abscesses
6. Benign prostatic hypertrophy
7. Prostatic cancer
8. Epididymitis

- Physical Findings
  1. Fever
  2. Prostate—edematous, firm or "boggy," warm and tender; AVOID VIGOROUS MASSAGE—CAN LEAD TO BACTEREMIA

- Diagnostic Tests/Findings
  1. Urine cultures—positive
  2. Prostatic secretions—expressed prostatic secretions (EPS), WBCs > 20 cells/high powered field is abnormal
  3. Diagnosis is best made by performing simultaneous quantitative bacterial cultures of urethral urine, bladder urine, and EPS
  4. Patient often treated based only on physical findings and urine culture

- Management/Treatment
  1. Patients who appear septic and/or have urinary retention should be hospitalized
  2. Outpatient treatment
     a. First choice if age > 35 years is bactrim DS orally b.i.d. for 2 to 4 weeks; if age < 35 years Doxycycline 100 mg orally b.i.d. for 10 days
     b. Alternative choices are carbenicillin 2 tablets orally q.i.d. for 2 to 4 weeks or ciprofloxacin 250 to 500 mg orally b.i.d. for 2 to 4 weeks
  3. Bed rest
  4. Sitz bath t.i.d. for 30 minutes
  5. Follow-up appointment 48 to 72 hours
  6. Discuss therapeutic and diagnostic plans

7. Avoid sexual intercourse until acute phase resolved; encourage continued use of condoms if multiple partners

8. Education regarding signs/symptoms of urinary retention and epididymitis

9. Emphasize importance of follow-up appointments

Chronic Bacterial Prostatitis

- Definition: Chronic inflammation/infection of prostate gland
- Etiology/Incidence
  1. Causative organisms are *Escherichia coli*; Enterobacter organisms, Proteus species, *Chlamydia trachomatis*
  2. Often associated with urethritis or infection of lower urinary tract
  3. One of the most common causes of recurrent urinary tract infection in men
- Signs and Symptoms
  1. Symptoms similar to, but milder than acute bacterial prostatitis
  2. Hallmark of disease is relapsing UTI due to same pathogen found in prostatic secretions
  3. Urinary frequency, dysuria
  4. Vague lower abdominal pain
  5. Lumbar and perineal pain
  6. Fever and urethral discharge uncommon
  7. May experience swelling and severe tenderness of scrotum
- Differential Diagnosis: Same as acute bacterial prostatitis
- Physical Findings
  1. May involve scrotal contents, producing intense local discomfort, swelling, erythema, and severe tenderness to palpation
  2. Prostate may be tender, irregularly indurated or boggy
- Diagnostic Tests/Findings
  1. Diagnosis made by examination of EPS and quantitative bacterial cultures
     a. EPS—abnormal if greater than 10 WBC/hPF

        b. More than 1 or 2 lipid-laden macrophages/hPF—abnormal

- Management/Treatment
    1. Often difficult to treat
    2. Usual antibiotics—trimethroprim/sulfamethoxazole, carbenicillin, ciprofloxacin, norfloxacin for 4 to 12 weeks
    3. Sitz baths, prostatic massage, intercourse, masturbation

Epididymitis

- Definition: An acute intrascrotal infection
- Etiology/Incidence
    1. Caused by infection from bladder urine, the prostate, or an ascending urethral infection
    2. Common affliction of men 35 years and younger; chlamydia usual causative organism for this population (*Neisseria gonorrhoeae* far less common)
    3. Infection in men > 35 years usually arises from bladder bacteriuria secondary to coliform organisms or following instrumentation, catheterization or surgery (prostatectomy)
    4. "Sterile" epididymitis associated with vigorous physical activity is caused by vasal reflux of sterile urine which leads to a chemical inflammation of the epididymis
    5. Epididymitis in boys may indicate underlying congenital anatomic abnormalities (i.e., ectopic ureter, posterior urethral valve)
    6. Condition is usually unilateral
    7. Epididymitis may be complicated by development of testicular necrosis, testicular atrophy or infertility
- Signs and Symptoms
    1. Painful, scrotal swelling (pain may radiate up the spermatic cord into the lower abdomen)
    2. Sensation of scrotal heaviness
    3. Symptoms of prostatitis or UTI may be present
    4. Systemic symptoms may develop—fever, chills and malaise
- Differential Diagnosis

1. Acute orchitis (mumps)
2. Testicular torsion
3. Testicular abscess
4. Tumor of testicle with or without hemorrhage
5. Hydrocele
6. Trauma

- Physical Findings
  1. Enlarged, tender indurated epididymis
  2. Urethral discharge may be present
- Diagnostic Tests/Findings
  1. Men
     a. STD testing (chlamydia, gonorrhea and syphilis)
     b. Culture and gram-stained smear of uncentrifuged urine
     c. Scrotal ultrasonography if condition initially severe or if fever continues while on antibiotics (rule out abscess)
  2. Boys—require more extensive work-up
     a. Intravenous urography
     b. Cystourethroscopy
     c. Voiding cystourethrography
     d. Scrotal ultrasonography (with or without Doppler imaging)
     e. Radionuclide scanning
     f. Surgical exploration may be required
- Management/Treatment
  1. M.D. referral or consult required if
     a. Patient is a child
     b. Systemic symptoms of infection (leukocytosis, fever) present in adults; patient should be hospitalized for parenteral antibiotics
  2. Outpatient therapy
     a. Antibiotic therapy based on patient's age and symptoms
        (1) Adult < 35 years of age—first choice is ceftriaxone 250 mg

IM in a single dose plus Doxycycline 100 mg orally b.i.d.; alternative choice for men 17 years of age or older is ofloxacin 300 mg orally b.i.d. for 10 days

   (2)   Adult > 35 years of age—Trimethoprim-sulfamethoxazole one double-strength tablet b.i.d. or ciprofloxacin 250 mg b.i.d. for 10 days; treat for 4 weeks if underlying prostatitis present

   b.   Scrotal elevation, support and bed rest

   c.   Analgesics—nonsteroidal anti-inflammatory agents

   d.   Ice (early), heat (late)

   e.   Spermatic cord block with lidocaine may be used

3.   Follow-up appointment 48 hours if symptoms persist or worsen

4.   Discuss therapeutic and diagnostic plans

5.   Emphasize importance of complete treatment

6.   Avoid sexual intercourse until course of antibiotics completed

7.   Inform patient that swelling and discomfort may persist for weeks or months after eradication of infecting organism; epididymis may remain enlarged or indurated indefinitely

8.   Educate regarding prevention, transmission and treatment of sexually transmitted disease (if causative agent); encourage continued use of condoms

9.   Encourage patient to discuss concerns and/or fears

Benign Prostatic Hypertrophy (BPH)

- Definition: Progressive, benign hyperplasia of prostate gland tissue

- Etiology/Incidence

1.   Cause is uncertain

2.   Approximately 50% of men have BPH by age 50; incidence increases to 80% by age 80

3.   The most common cause of bladder outlet obstruction in males > 50 years

4.   Symptoms are attributed to mechanical obstruction of the urethra by the hyperplastic prostate gland

- Signs and Symptoms
  1. Frequency, urgency
  2. Nocturia
  3. Weak urinary stream, dribbling
  4. Sensation of full bladder immediately after voiding
  5. Retention
- Differential Diagnosis
  1. Urethral stricture
  2. Prostate or bladder cancer
  3. Neurogenic bladder
  4. Bladder calculus
  5. Acute or chronic prostatitis
  6. Bladder neck contracture
  7. Medications that affect micturition
- Physical Findings
  1. Abdomen—may indicate distended bladder from retention
  2. Prostate (patient should void prior to examination)
     a. Nontender with asymmetrical or symmetrical enlargement; gross enlargement not typical
     b. Consistency is smooth and rubbery (consistency of a pencil eraser)
     c. Distinct nodules (spheroids) may be present
        (1) M.D. referral/consultation required
        (2) Differentiation between BPH nodules and cancerous ones is based on induration or hardness of gland
        (3) Urology referral and biopsy may be required
- Diagnostic Tests/Findings
  1. Urinalysis—NO hematuria, urinary tract infection
  2. Urinary flow rate—voided volume and peak urinary flow rate (uroflowmetry) tests prostatic obstruction
  3. Abdominal ultrasound—rules out associated upper tract pathology

4. Serum creatinine and BUN—normal

5. Prostate-specific antigen (PSA) levels may be elevated between 4 to 10 ng/ml; levels > 10 ng/ml may be indicative of carcinoma

- Management/Treatment

1. Observation

2. Urology consult required for pharmacologic, mechanical, or surgical treatments

3. Pharmacologic—drugs selected that reduce bulk and/or tone of gland

4. Mechanical—balloon dilation of prostatic urethra

5. Surgery—indications

   a. Acute urinary retention (urgent urology referral)

   b. Gross hematuria

   c. Epididymitis (especially if recurrent)

   d. Recurrent urinary tract infections

   e. Renal failure from obstruction

   f. Intolerable chronic symptoms

6. Discuss therapeutic and diagnostic plans

7. Educate regarding signs/symptoms of urinary retention, renal failure and epididymitis

8. Emphasize importance of follow-up appointments

9. Avoid caffeine and alcohol to decrease bladder irritation

Prostate Cancer

- Definition: A malignant neoplasm of the prostate gland

- Etiology/Incidence

1. Etiology is unknown; environmental factors may be involved; adenocarcinoma is most common type

2. Second most common malignancy in American men and third most common cause of cancer deaths in men over 55

3. The relative survival rates have improved over the past 30 years (due to increased awareness and early detection, rather than improved

therapy)

    4.   May be associated with high-fat diet

■ Signs and Symptoms

    1.   Many patients are asymptomatic

    2.   Symptoms may mimic BPH with frequency, dribbling, nocturia

    3.   Occasionally bone pain from metastases (advanced stage)

    4.   Occasionally symptoms of uremia due to urethral obstructions (advanced stage)

■ Differential Diagnosis

    1.   BPH, urethral stricture

    2.   Bladder cancer

    3.   Neurogenic bladder

    4.   Bladder calculus

    5.   Acute/chronic prostatitis

    6.   Bladder neck contracture

    7.   Medications that affect micturition

■ Physical Findings

    1.   May present with lymphadenopathy, signs of uremia or urinary retention with distended bladder

    2.   More common physical findings are confined to prostate—on rectal examination prostate feels harder than normal and normal boundaries of gland may be obscured; nodules may be present

■ Diagnostic Tests/Findings (performed by consultant M.D.)

    1.   Transperineal or transrectal needle biopsy of prostate—diagnostic accuracy rate > 90%

    2.   PSA levels between 4 to 10 ng/ml may indicate BPH, levels > 10 ng/ml are suggestive of carcinoma; false negatives occur

    3.   Transrectal ultrasound can aid in identification of solid nodules and is used to guide biopsy

    4.   Other tests such as bone scans may be conducted

■ Management/Treatment

    1.   Consult/referral required

2. Treatment predicated largely on stage of tumor; accurate staging is therefore essential

3. Methods of treatment include surgery, radiation, hormonal therapy

4. Assistance as appropriate in meeting physical, psychological, social, cultural, environmental and spiritual needs

5. Emphasize importance of follow-up appointments

Fibrocystic Breast Changes

- Definition: Benign breast condition characterized by increased growth of fibrous tissue, proliferation of the ductal epithelial lining and/or formation of cysts

- Etiology/Incidence

1. Cause is unknown, estrogen dependency is suspected; condition occurs clinically in 50% and histologically in 90% of women

2. Three types of fibrocystic changes have been identified

   a. Nonproliferative lesions

   b. Proliferative lesions without atypia

   c. Atypical hyperplasia

3. Presence of atypical hyperplasia is associated with an increased risk of breast cancer

- Signs and Symptoms (more pronounced premenstrually)

1. Cyclic breast tenderness, engorgement, increased density, increased nodularity, enlargement of cystic lump(s)

2. Nipple discharge may be present

3. Symptoms of discomfort decrease after menopause

- Differential Diagnosis

1. Fibroadenosis

2. Fat necrosis

3. Fibroadenoma

4. Carcinoma (especially in women > 40 years)

- Physical Findings

1. Breasts

    a. Skin and contour usually normal

    b. Mass or thickened area present

        (1)   Location—UOQ or any area

        (2)   Size—varies

        (3)   Shape—round, oval or nodular

        (4)   Mobility—mobile

        (5)   Consistency—soft to firm (depends on tension of fluid within cysts)

        (6)   Number—solitary or multiple (may give impression of "beads on a string")

        (7)   Nipple—clear/serous discharge may be present (rare)

- Diagnostic Tests/Findings

    1. Fine Needle Aspiration (FNA) fluid should return

    2. FNA biopsy or excisional biopsy—no cancer cells

    3. Mammography—negative (For women > 35 years)

    4. Ultrasound—distinguishes cyst vs solid mass

- Management/Treatment

    1. Warm compresses applied t.i.d.; supportive brassiere

    2. Low-salt diet; diuretics may also be given premenstrually

    3. Elimination of dietary methylxanthines (coffee, tea, colas, chocolate)

    4. Vitamin E—400 to 600 international units orally daily

    5. Vitamin B_6—50 to 100 mg daily

    6. Hormonal and anti-hormonal therapy are controversial; the following agents may be used in severe cases

        a. Oral contraceptives

        b. Danazol

        c. Bromocriptine

        d. Tamoxifen

    7. Surgical excision is controversial

    8. Discussion of diagnostic and therapeutic plans

9. Reassurrance of low-risk for malignancy

10. Instruction and demonstration of breast self-examination

11. Encouragement to report new mass that does not resolve following menstruation

12. At follow-up appointments, assess for progression of condition and/or concurrent malignancy

Breast Cancer

- Definition: A malignant neoplasm of the breast
- Etiology/Incidence
  1. The most common site of cancer in women
  2. Second leading cause of death from cancer
  3. Frequency increases steadily after age 35
  4. One in 10 women may develop breast cancer in the U.S.
  5. Family history increases a woman's risk twofold to threefold
  6. Approximately 150,000 new cases occur annually
  7. Risk factors include
     a. Positive family history (premenopausal more significant)
     b. Nulliparity
     c. Late first pregnancy (over age 34)
     d. Early menarche and late menopause
     e. Fibrocystic changes associated with atypical hyperplasia
     f. Previous unilateral breast or endometrial cancer
     g. Alcohol intake
     h. High fat diet
  8. Whites have a higher incidence than non-whites
- Signs and Symptoms
  1. Often asymptomatic
  2. Nontender, painless mass is usual presenting sign
  3. Later manifestations
     a. Skin erythema, dimpling, ulceration

    b. Breast pain

    c. Nipple retraction, eczema, or ulceration

■ Differential Diagnosis

  1. Fibrocystic breast changes

  2. Fibroadenoma

  3. Intraductal papilloma

  4. Lipoma

  5. Fat necrosis

  6. Mastitis (inflammatory breast cancer)

  7. Dermatitis (Paget's disease)

■ Physical Findings

  1. Most common manifestation is single, firm, nontender, ill-defined breast lump

    a. Associated findings may include

      (1) Diffuse nodularity

      (2) Skin dimpling

      (3) Nipple retraction, discharge (usually bloody)

      (4) Lymphadenopathy

      (5) Ulcerated/fungating mass (rare)

      (6) Palpable supra-clavicular and/or axillary lymph nodes

  2. Inflammatory cancer—skin erythema/edema, pain

  3. Paget's disease

    a. Associated with about 5% of mammary carcinomas

    b. Nipple erosion, crusting, bloody discharge

    c. Eczema-like change in skin

■ Diagnostic Tests/Findings

  1. Mammography—mass or calcifications indicated; may be negative since 10% of palpable masses are missed on mammogram

  2. Ultrasound—distinguishes cyst vs solid mass

  3. FNA cytology—fluid vs solid mass, 10% false-negative

4. Large-needle (core needle) biopsy—histological examination reveals cancer cells (problems with sampling occur)

5. Excisional biopsy—most reliable diagnostic test where staging of the tumor is done

6. Determination of hormone receptor tumor cells

7. Various tests may be conducted if metastasis is suspected including bone and organ scans

- Management/Treatment

1. Referral to an oncology team is required

2. Dependent upon tumor stage, presence of hormone receptors and patient's symptoms/preferences

3. May include surgery, chemotherapy, radiation therapy and/or hormonal therapy

4. Discussion of diagnostic and therapeutic plans

5. Encouragement to express concerns and fears

6. Education and demonstration of breast self-examination to patient and family members, especially daughters

7. Encouragement to report new mass or changes

8. Assistance, as appropriate, in meeting physical, psychological, social, cultural, environmental and spiritual needs

9. Emphasis on importance of keeping follow-up appointments with specialists and primary care providers

Dysfunctional Uterine Bleeding— Premenopausal (DUB)

- Definition: Excessive, abnormal uterine bleeding with no demonstrable organic cause that occurs at irregular intervals

- Etiology/Incidence

1. DUB usually results from the irregular sloughing of endometrium during anovulatory cycles (90% of cases); but occasionally occurs with poor quality ovulatory cycles

2. Is most frequently due to abnormalities of endocrine function

3. Usually represents estrogen withdrawal or estrogen breakthrough bleeding

4. Heaviest bleeding due to high sustained levels of estrogen and seen

with

    a. Polycystic ovarian disease

    b. Obesity

    c. Immaturity of the hypothalamic-pituitary-ovarian axis (postmenarchal teenagers)

    d. Late ovulations (perimenopausal women)

  5. Not related to oral contraceptive use

- Signs and Symptoms

  1. A carefully obtained history is critical to assist in ruling-out other conditions, as well as characterizing bleeding pattern

  2. Bleeding is usually characterized by one or more of the following

    a. Persistent or intermittent uterine bleeding

    b. Episodes of extremely heavy bleeding

    c. Oligomenorrhea

  3. DUB bleeding patterns

    a. Intermenstrual bleeding—variable amounts of bleeding that occur between regular menstrual periods

    b. Menometrorrhagia—prolonged, frequent, excessive uterine bleeding that occurs at irregular intervals

    c. Menorrhagia (hypermenorrhea)—prolonged (> 7 days) and excessive (> 80 ml) uterine bleeding occurring at regular intervals

    d. Metrorrhagia—uterine bleeding between normal cycle

    e. Polymenorrhea—frequent, irregular bleeding < 18 day intervals

    f. Oligomenorrhea—infrequent, irregular uterine bleeding that occurs at intervals > 40 days

- Differential Diagnosis

  1. It is *inappropriate* to assume that abnormal uterine bleeding is endocrine in origin. Other conditions must be ruled-out, often according to reproductive age.

  2. Adolescents

    a. Vaginal trauma secondary to athletics or early sexual exposure

    b. Hypothalamic-pituitary dysfunction secondary to exercise

    c. Pregnancy

    d. Genital infection

    e. Oral contraceptive use/misuse

    f. Blood dyscrasias

3. Women in reproductive years

    a. Above noted causes

    b. Endocrine-related anovulatory abnormal uterine bleeding, common with exercise

    c. Organic pathology

        (1) Uterine fibroids

        (2) Endometrial polyps

        (3) Chronic systemic illness, e.g., liver cirrhosis, renal failure

    d. Neoplasia

4. Perimenopausal women

    a. Above listed causes

    b. Follicular dysfunction (predominant cause)

■ Physical Findings

1. A thorough general and pelvic examination should be performed to assist in ruling out conditions included in the differential diagnosis; the source of bleeding must be determined

2. For DUB, the examination may be essentially negative, or an adnexal mass may indicate polycystic ovaries

■ Diagnostic Tests/Findings

1. Of secondary importance and usually only substantiates a diagnosis already determined by history and physical examination findings

2. Three most important initial tests

    a. Pregnancy test (quantitative Beta hCG)

    b. Prolactin determination (hyperprolactinemia may initially present as ovulatory dysfunction or anovulation and abnormal uterine bleeding)—may be elevated after breast examination

    c. Thyroid stimulating hormone (TSH)

3. Additional initial tests should include

    a. Follicle stimulating hormone (FSH) and luteinizing hormone (LH)

    b. Complete blood count, blood smear, platelet count, prothrombin time, bleeding time

    c. Cervical Pap smear

    d. STD screening tests

    e. Urinalysis

4. Additional tests may be done to rule out other conditions as indicated by the history and physical examination, such as

    a. Coagulation profile

    b. Serum iron studies

    c. Pelvic ultrasound

5. Tests more important in older women

    a. Endometrial biopsy

    b. Endometrial aspiration

    c. D & C

- Management/Treatment

1. Should be considered according to amount of blood loss and in an age-related manner

2. Medical consult is usually required

3. Arrest of heavy acute or prolonged bleeding may require intravenous conjugated estrogens followed by combined oral contraceptives or medroxyprogesterone acetate to prevent recurrence

4. Induction of ovulation is reserved for those desiring pregnancy (use of Clomiphene citrate)

5. Iron supplementation if indicated

6. Patient should maintain a basal body temperature chart and record symptoms during cycles

7. Discussion of therapeutic and diagnostic plans

8. Review of emergency instructions for acute, heavy bleeding

9. Review of nutritional requirements and encourage intake of iron-rich foods

10. Instruction regarding basal body temperature monitoring

11. Encouragement of expression of concerns and fears

12. Emphasis on importance of keeping follow-up appointments

Dysplasia—Abnormal Papanicolaou (Pap) Smear Management

- Definition: Squamous intraepithelial lesions (SIL) refers to precancerous cellular development of the cervix (includes mild, moderate and severe dysplasia) and carcinoma in situ of the cervix

- Etiology/Incidence

   1. Etiology is most likely related to a sexually transmitted factor; the human papillomavirus (HPV) is suspected to be an initiator of malignant transformation

   2. Suspected HPV co-factors include cigarette smoking and folate deficiency

   3. Major risk factors for cervical cancer

      a. Sexual intercourse prior to age 20

      b. More than three sexual partners in a lifetime

      c. Intercourse with a male who has had multiple sexual partners

      d. Smoking or history of smoking

      e. Presence or history of HPV (types 16, 18, 31, 33, 35, 45 and 56) more commonly associated with high-grade lesions—see section on Genital Warts or Condylomata acuminata

      f. Intercourse with man who has HPV

   4. Approximately 90% of cases are squamous cell carcinomas

   5. Globally, carcinoma of the cervix is the most common female malignancy; in the U.S. it ranks as the third most common gynecologic malignancy (behind endometrial and ovarian cancer)

- Cervical Cancer Screening

   1. The Papanicolaou (Pap) smear has reduced disease-related mortality in the U.S. by 50% in the past 40 years

   2. Screening has also increased detection of preinvasive cervical neoplasms including dysplasia and carcinoma in situ (CIS)

   3. 30% of Pap smears may have false-negative results

   4. Risk of invasive cervical cancer significantly increases when screening

exceeds 3 year intervals

5. Recommended screening criteria (U.S. Preventive Task Force)

   a. Initiate at age 18 or at the age of first intercourse

   b. Between the ages of 18 and 65, Pap smears should be repeated every one to three years depending upon patient's risk factors for cervical cancer

   c. After age 65

      (1) Routine screening may be discontinued if findings are normal on two consecutive Pap smears

      (2) If abnormal Pap smear, annual screening should occur until two consecutive Pap smears are normal

- Pap smear interpretation: The Bethesda Classification System is most commonly used

   1. Statement on specimen adequacy

      a. Satisfactory for interpretation

      b. Less than optimal

      c. Unsatisfactory

   2. General categorization

      a. Within normal limits

      b. Other

         (1) Infection

         (2) Reactive or reparative changes

         (3) Squamous cell abnormalities

            (a) Atypical—undetermined significance

            (b) Low grade squamous intraepithelial lesion (SIL)—associated with HPV and/or mild dysplasia (cervical intraepithelial lesion 1 (CIN 1)

            (c) High grade squamous intraepithelial lesion (SIL)—moderate dysplasia (CIN 2), severe dysplasia (CIN 3) or carcinoma in situ (CIS)

            (d) Squamous cell carcinoma

         (4) Glandular cell abnormalities

(a) Presence of endometrial cells—menstruating or postmenopausal women

(b) Atypical—undetermined significance (endometrial or endocervical)

(c) Adenocarcinoma

(d) Other epithelial malignant neoplasm

(5) Nonepithelial malignant neoplasm

(6) Hormonal evaluation (vaginal smears only, i.e., hysterectomy)

- Management of Pap smear results

1. Within normal limits—repeat annually or as indicated according to cervical cancer risk factors and age

2. Infection

    a. Treat based on agent causing inflammation

    b. Repeat Pap smear 3 months after treatment

3. Reactive or reparative changes

    a. Treat if infectious agent present

    b. May be related to contraceptive mechanical devices (IUD), atrophic changes, chemotherapy and/or radiotherapy etc.

    c. Repeat Pap smear 3 months after treatment

4. Atypical squamous or glandular cells of undetermined significance

    a. Indicates abnormality, cause unclear but often an infection

    b. Repeat Pap smear 3 months after appropriate treatment

    c. Colposcopy and cervical biopsies with endocervical curettage (ECC) if atypia persists

5. Low and high grade SIL

    a. Colposcopy and cervical biopsies with endocervical curettage (ECC) if atypia persists

    b. Low-grade lesions may be monitored with Pap smears and colposcopy every 6 months if ECC is negative

    c. Common treatments include Cryotherapy, large loop excision of transformation zone (LLETZ), laser vaporization

    d. Referral to M.D. specialist if carcinoma in situ present

6. Squamous cell carcinoma, adenocarcinoma and other epithelial or nonepithelial malignant neoplasm—refer to M.D. specialist

7. Hormonal evaluation—treat atropic changes if present (see section on Menopause)

8. Discuss therapeutic and diagnostic plans

9. Emphasize importance of regular screening

10. Review patient's individual risk factors as appropriate

11. Educate regarding recommended management and treatment as appropriate

12. Encourage patient to discuss concerns and/or fears

Amenorrhea

- Definition

  1. Primary amenorrhea—absence of normal spontaneous menstrual period by age 16

  2. Secondary amenorrhea—cessation of menses after a variable period of normal function, usually 3 to 6 consecutive cycles

- Etiology—potential underlying conditions

  1. Primary amenorrhea

     a. Hypergonadotropic hypogonadism

     b. Turner's Syndrome (gonadal dysgenesis)

     c. Severe malnutrition

     d. Pituitary tumors

     e. Head trauma

     f. Encephalitis

     g. Uterine malformations, congenital absence of uterus

     h. Imperforate hymen

     i. Androgen insensitivity

     j. Polycystic ovaries

  2. Secondary amenorrhea

     a. Pregnancy (most common cause)

    b. Oral contraceptives

    c. Menopause

    d. Emotional stress

    e. Malnutrition

    f. Excessive exercise

    g. Lactation

    h. Hyperprolactinemia (pituitary tumor)

    i. Anorexia/obesity

    j. Drug use

    k. Polycystic ovaries

    l. Hypothalamic suppression

    m. Hyper and hypothyroidism

    n. Addison's disease

    o. Anovulation

- Signs and Symptoms

  1. Primary amenorrhea

    a. Absence of menarche

    b. Failure to develop pubic hair and other secondary sex characteristics

    c. Abnormal growth and development may be present

    d. Normal breast development may or may not occur

    e. Patient symptoms are dependent upon the etiology of the amenorrheic condition

  2. Secondary amenorrhea

    a. Absence of menses at expected time intervals

    b. Previous regular menses

- Differential Diagnosis

  1. First, rule out pregnancy

  2. All the potential underlying conditions listed under ETIOLOGY should be considered in the differential diagnosis

3. A thorough and complete history/physical examination, with supplemental diagnostic/laboratory testing will assist in ruling out unrelated etiologies

- Physical Findings
    1. A thorough general and pelvic examination should be performed, partially directed by the history
    2. Findings will be related to the underlying etiology
    3. The examination may be essentially negative if the amenorrhea is secondary to such conditions as oral contraceptive use or unreported emotional stress

- Diagnostic Tests/Findings
    1. Primary amenorrhea—refer to endocrinologist if suspected
    2. Secondary amenorrhea
        a. Pregnancy test (quantitative Beta hCG)—first test done
        b. Prolactin (if negative pregnancy test), FSH, LH
        c. Progestin challenge test
        d. TSH
            (1) Elevated TSH—hypothyroid
            (2) Normal TSH—rule out pituitary adenoma
        e. Cervical Pap smear
        f. STD screening tests
        g. Urinalysis
    3. Additional tests may be done to rule out other conditions as indicated by the history and physical examination

- Management/Treatment
    1. Dependent upon underlying etiology
    2. Medical consult is often required
    3. Discuss therapeutic and diagnostic plans
    4. Encourage expression of concerns and fears
    5. Emphasize importance of keeping follow-up appointments

Dysmenorrhea

- Definition: Crampy pain that accompanies menstruation, often with a constellation of other symptoms
    1. Primary—usually begins in women under 20 years; no other pelvic disease identified
    2. Secondary—usually occurs after age 20 in women with pelvic pathology
- Etiology/Incidence
    1. Primary—probably the result of excessive uterine prostaglandin production; usually appears shortly after onset of ovulatory cycles; affects approximately 50% or more of all menstruating females
    2. Secondary—usually occurs in the presence of organic disease, e.g., endometriosis, pelvic adhesions, adenomyosis, cervical stenosis, uterine fibroids, chronic pelvic infection
- Signs and Symptoms
    1. Primary
        a. Pain usually crampy in nature, may radiate to back, thighs and lower abdomen
        b. May also have other symptoms, e.g., nausea, vomiting, diarrhea, headache, fatigue
        c. Usually begins at onset of menstruation or several hours before; duration is usually 48 to 72 hours
    2. Secondary
        a. Signs and symptoms associated with organic disease listed under Etiology/Incidence
        b. Pain occurs at any point in cycle
- Differential Diagnosis
    1. Differentiation between primary and secondary dysmenorrhea
    2. Rule out secondary pathologic conditions as noted under Etiology/Incidence
- Physical Findings
    1. Primary—usually no significant physical findings; uterine corpus may be tender during menstruation; no pelvic masses or uterine fixation
    2. Secondary—findings associated with organic disease

- Diagnostic Tests/Findings
    1. Primary—prostaglandin F_{2x} elevated
    2. Secondary—tests related to suspected organic pathology
- Management/Treatment
    1. Primary
        a. Prostaglandin synthetase inhibitors (PGSI), e.g., naproxen, indomethacin, mefenamic acid, ibuprofen
        b. Oral contraceptives for sexually active individuals
        c. Moderate exercise on a regular basis
        d. Diet high in whole grains, beans, vegetables, fruit
        e. Elimination of or decreased salt, sugar, caffeine
    2. Secondary—treatment related to organic pathology

Premenstrual Syndrome (PMS)

- Definition: A group of somatic and affective symptoms occurring during the luteal phase of the menstrual cycle and decreasing shortly after the onset of menstruation
- Etiology/Incidence
    1. Exact cause unknown
    2. Postulated etiologic factors include insufficient progesterone, fluid retention, nutritional problems, glucose metabolism disorders, vitamin deficiencies, ovarian infections, altered serotonin, endorphin levels; elevated prolactin levels
    3. Peak prevalence is in the thirties with a decline noted in the forties
    4. Incidence ranges from 5% to 95%; generally agreed about 40% of women are significantly affected at one time or another; only 2% to 3% of women of childbearing age suffer severe symptoms
    5. Most women experience some physical and emotional changes before onset of menstrual flow (molimina)
- Signs and Symptoms
    1. Bloated feeling, feeling of weight increase
    2. Breast pain or tenderness
    3. Skin disorders

4. Hot flushes

5. Headache

6. Pelvic pain

7. Change in bowel habits

8. Irritability, aggression, tension, anxiety, depression, crying, lethargy

9. Insomnia

10. Change in appetite, thirst

11. Change in libido

12. Loss of concentration

13. Poor coordination, clumsiness, accidents

- Differential Diagnosis

    1. Depression

    2. Anxiety Disorders

    3. Marital Discord

    4. Substance abuse

- Physical Findings

    1. Because etiology is still unknown, diagnosis is made by history

    2. Complete history and physical examination should be conducted to rule out any medical problems that could be influencing symptomatology

- Diagnostic Tests/Findings: No laboratory tests are available to make diagnosis

- Management/Treatment

    1. Exercise 3 to 4 times per week, especially during luteal phase

    2. Appropriate diet, low in carbohydrates with reasonable amounts of protein (from fish and poultry rather than red meats), vegetables, and fruit

    3. Elimination of tobacco, alcohol, caffeine

    4. Pyridoxine

    5. Diuretics

    6. Progesterone

7. Prostaglandin—inhibitors, e.g., mefenamic acid, naproxen sodium
8. Oral contraceptives
9. Danazol
10. Bromocriptine
11. PMS support group referral

Questions

Select the best answer

1. The following statements regarding AIDS are correct except
   a. Most diagnoses are made in persons 20 to 49 years old
   b. Over 1 million Americans are infected with HIV
   c. HIV is transmitted through casual kissing
   d. The ELISA blood test detects HIV-specific antibodies

2. During the acute phase of HIV infection (first 2 to 8 weeks) the following symptoms may be present
   a. Rash
   b. Shingles
   c. Persistant dermatitis
   d. Pulmonary symptoms

3. The following are HIV treatment measures except
   a. Zidovudine (AZT)
   b. Didanosine (ddI)
   c. Nutritious diet and stress management
   d. Isolation from the general public

4. The following may develop with AIDS
   a. Kaposi's sarcoma
   b. Cytomegalovirus
   c. Wasting syndrome
   d. All the above

5. Which of the following is a diagnostic test for gonorrhea?
   a. Western blot assay
   b. VDRL
   c. Wet prep with WBCs
   d. Culture of endocervix on Thayer-Martin media

6. Correct statements about *Neisseria gonorrhoeae* include all of the following except
   a. One of the leading causes of infertility among U.S. females
   b. The majority of male patients are asymptomatic
   c. PID is a possible complication
   d. Fever may indicate systemic complications

7. The following treatment regimens are recommended for the treatment of gonorrhea except

a. Ceftriaxone
b. Ciprofloxacin
c. Acyclovir
d. Ofloxacin

8. The most serious gonococcal complication that can occur in women is
    a. PID
    b. Cervicitis
    c. Arthritis
    d. Conjunctivitis

9. The most common sexually transmitted disease in the U.S is
    a. Gonorrhea
    b. Syphilis
    c. Chlamydia
    d. Herpes

10. The causative organism of Chlamydia is
    a. *Chlamydia coli*
    b. *Chlamydia megalovirus*
    c. *Chlamydia trachomotis*
    d. *Chlamydia hominos*

11. A 20 year female presents to your clinic with dysuria, dyspareunia, mucopurulent discharge. She reports that her boyfriend was recently treated for nongonococcal urethritis, what STD has she most probably been exposed to?
    a. Gonorrhea
    b. HPV
    c. Chlamydia
    d. Trichomonas

12. Which of the following is a diagnostic test for chlamydia?
    a. Culture of endocervical smear streaked on Thayer-Martin
    b. Indirect antigen-detection test
    c. RPR
    d. VDRL

13. The following statements regarding syphilis are correct except
    a. It cannot be transmitted via the placenta
    b. Incidence has steadily increased since the mid-1980's
    c. Risk of contraction through sexual intercourse approaches 50%
    d. It can affect any organ or tissue in the body

14. All of the following are characteristics of secondary syphilis except

    a. Skin rash
    b. Arthralgias
    c. Chancre
    d. Malaise

15. The treatment of choice for a 32 year old male with early syphilis who is allergic to penicillin is
    a. Ciprofloxacin
    b. Doxycycline
    c. Erythromycin
    d. Augmentin

16. A 38 year old female presents to your clinic with meningeal symptoms; what stage of syphilis must you rule-out?
    a. Primary
    b. Secondàry
    c. Latent
    d. Any stage

17. One of the definitive methods of diagnosis of early syphilis is
    a. FTA-ABS
    b. Darkfield microscopy
    c. VDRL
    d. MHA-TP

18. A 24 year old female seen in your clinic has been diagnosed with urethral strictures. What STD is probably included in her past history?
    a. Chlamydia
    b. Herpes genitalis
    c. Syphilis
    d. HPV

19. The following statements regarding herpes genitalis are correct except
    a. Causative agent is a virus
    b. Genital lesions are painless
    c. Infection during pregnancy can lead to spontaneous abortion
    d. Treatment focuses on relieving symptoms

20. The most common symptomatic STD in the U.S. is
    a. Gonorrhea
    b. Chlamydia
    c. Genital warts (HPV)
    d. Herpes genitalis

21. The following statements regarding genital warts are correct except
    a. More than 60 types of HPV cause warts
    b. Increased risk of developing cervical, penile and vulvar cancer
    c. Lesions on the vulva, cervix and penis are treated with Cryotherapy
    d. RPR aids in diagnosing cervical lesions

22. All of the following conditions are included in the differential diagnosis for PID except
    a. Enteritis
    b. Appendicitis
    c. Degeneration of a myoma
    d. Cholecystitis

23. After an initial case of PID, a woman is more susceptible to experience
    a. Ectopic pregnancy
    b. Reinfection
    c. Infertility
    d. All the above

24. In order to clinically diagnose PID all the following criteria must be met except
    a. Direct abdominal tenderness
    b. Cervical motion tenderness
    c. Fever
    d. Adnexal tenderness

25. A 22 year old female seen in your clinic has the following signs and symptoms— malodorous, greenish discharge, perineal itching, red macular cervical lesions, and a vaginal pH of 5.0 to 7.0. What type of vulvovaginitis does she probably have?
    a. Candida
    b. Gardnerella
    c. Bacterial vaginosis
    d. Trichomonas

26. All of the following statements regarding bacterial vaginosis are correct except
    a. Multiple bacterial causative agents
    b. "Curdy" white discharge
    c. Positive "whiff test"
    d. Flagyl is the treatment of choice

27. A classic description of the discharge associated with candida vaginitis is
    a. "Cottage-cheese"
    b. "Fishy" odor
    c. "Strawberry patches"

    d. None of the above

28. One of the most common causative organisms of UTIs is
    a. Klebsiella
    b. Beta-hemolytic streptococci
    c. Chlamydia
    d. *E. coli*

29. The following statements regarding UTI are correct except
    a. 30 to 40% of women will experience at least 1 UTI in life-time
    b. Men with UTIs should be referred to a urologist
    c. Condom use by sex partner is a contributing factor in women
    d. Prostatitis is a contributing factor in men

30. Which of the following is not a characteristic sign or symptom associated with a UTI
    a. Fever
    b. Pyuria
    c. Urgency
    d. Negative CVA tenderness

31. Which of the following activities is contraindicated in a patient with suspected acute bacterial prostatitis?
    a. Ejaculation
    b. Urinary catherization
    c. Prostate exam
    d. All of the above

32. The drug of choice for a 40 year old, monogamous male with prostatitis is
    a. Ciprofloxacin
    b. Doxycycline
    c. Bactrim DS
    d. Carbenicillin

33. The cause of benign prostatic hypertrophy (BPH) is
    a. Chronic prostatitis
    b. Pre-cancerous changes in prostate gland tissue
    c. Uncertain
    d. Long-term use of hypertensive medications

34. Which of the following statements regarding BPH is incorrect?
    a. 80% of men by 80 years of age have BPH
    b. BPH often leads to bladder outlet obstruction
    c. Drugs to reduce bulk of gland may be prescribed

d. Upon palpation, the prostate is firm/hard to touch

35. The most common type of prostate cancer is
    a. Adenocarcinoma
    b. Squamous cell
    c. Lymphoma
    d. Sarcoma

36. What is the most common physical finding associated with prostate cancer?
    a. Boggy prostate
    b. Tender prostate
    c. Enlarged, smooth prostate
    d. Hard, nodular prostate

37. Which of the following statements regarding prostate cancer is incorrect?
    a. The largest cancer mortality rate in men 55 to 74 years of age
    b. Relative survival rates have improved over the past 30 years
    c. Prostate-specific antigen is used as a laboratory marker
    d. Bladder calculus is considered in the differential diagnosis

38. The type of fibrocystic breast change that has been associated with malignancy is
    a. Proliferative changes without atypia
    b. Nonproliferative changes
    c. Atypical hyperplasia
    d. Dysplasia

39. What diagnostic test is most definitive in diagnosing fibrocystic changes?
    a. Mammography
    b. Fine needle aspiration
    c. Excisional biopsy
    d. Ultrasound

40. A 30-year-old woman is diagnosed with fibrocystic breast changes in your office. All of the following components may be included in the treatment plan except
    a. Yearly mammograms starting now
    b. Low-salt diet
    c. Limited consumption of caffeine
    d. Oral contraceptives

41. The most common site of gynecological cancer in women is
    a. Cervical
    b. Breast
    c. Ovarian
    d. Endometrial

42. All of the following are breast cancer risk factors except
    a. Nulliparity
    b. Alcohol intake
    c. Positive family history
    d. Late menarche and early menopause

43. Which description is most characteristic of breast cancer?
    a. Single, firm, non-tender, ill-defined breast lump
    b. Multiple, firm, non-tender, ill-defined breast lumps
    c. Single, firm, tender, circumscribed breast lump
    d. Single, rubbery, non-tender, circumscribed breast lump

44. Which of the following statements regarding breast cancer is incorrect?
    a. 10% of palpable masses are missed on mammography
    b. Core needle biopsy is the most reliable diagnostic test
    c. Paget's disease affects the nipple
    d. Inflammatory breast cancer may be painful

45. Dysfunctional uterine bleeding is most often (90%) associated with
    a. Polycystic ovaries
    b. Ovulatory cycles
    c. Anovulatory cycles
    d. Late ovulation

46. Menorrhagia refers to
    a. Uterine bleeding that occurs at regular intervals < 21 days apart
    b. Prolonged and excessive uterine bleeding occurring at regular intervals
    c. Infrequent uterine bleeding that occurs at intervals > 40 days apart
    d. Uterine bleeding that occurs at irregular but frequent intervals

47. Which of the following is least likely to be included in the differential diagnosis of dysfunctional uterine bleeding for a perimenopausal women?
    a. Neoplasia
    b. Blood dyscrasias
    c. Pregnancy
    d. Vaginal trauma

48. Which one of the following characteristics is not associated with primary amenorrhea?
    a. Irregular menses
    b. Absence of menarche
    c. Lack of pubic hair
    d. Abnormal growth and development

49. The most common cause of secondary amenorrhea is
    a. Oral contraceptives
    b. Polycystic ovaries
    c. Pregnancy
    d. Anovulation

50. What is the first test that should be ordered in a woman who presents with secondary amenorrhea?
    a. Thyroid profile
    b. Prolactin
    c. Pregnancy test
    d. Progestin challenge

Answers

1. c	26. b
2. a	27. a
3. d	28. d
4. d	29. c
5. d	30. a
6. b	31. b
7. c	32. c
8. a	33. c
9. c	34. d
10. c	35. a
11. c	36. d
12. b	37. a
13. a	38. c
14. c	39. c
15. b	40. a
16. d	41. b
17. b	42. d
18. b	43. a
19. b	44. b
20. c	45. c
21. d	46. b
22. d	47. d
23. d	48. a
24. c	49. c
25. d	50. c

Bibliography

Beck, W. W. (Ed.). (1990). *Obstetrics and Gynecology*. Media, PA: Harwal Publishing

Centers for Disease Control (1993). "1993 Sexually Transmitted Diseases Treatment Guidelines" *Morbidity and Mortality Weekly Report*. September 24, *(42)14*

Clarke-Pearson, D. L., & Dawood, M. Y. (1990). *Green's gynecology: Essentials of clinical practice*. Boston: Little, Brown and Company.

Cunningham, F. G., MacDonald, P. C., Gant, N. F., Leveno, K. J., Gilstrap, L. C. (1993). *Williams obstetrics* (19th ed.). Norwalk, CT: Appleton & Lange.

Gompel, C., & Silverberg, S. G. (Eds.). (1994). *Pathology in gynecology and obstetrics* (4th ed.). Philadelphia: J. B. Lippincott.

Harris, J. R., Hellman, S., Henderson, I. C., & Kinne, D. W. (Eds.). (1991). *Breast diseases*. Philadelphia: J. B. Lippincott.

Hatcher, R. A., Trussell, J., Stewart, G. K., Kowal, D., Guest, F., Cates, W., & Policar, M. S. (1994). *Contraceptive technology* (16th rev. ed.). New York: Irvington Publishers.

Herbst, A. L., Mishell, D. R., Stenchever, M. A., & Droegemueller, C. W. (1991). *Comprehensive gynecology* (2nd ed.). St. Louis: Mosby Year Book

Miller, K. E., Logh, D. P., & Folley, A. (1992). Evaluation and follow-up of abnormal Pap smears. *American Family Physician, 45*(1), 143-150.

Moskosky, S. B. (Ed.). (1992). *Ob-Gyn nurse practitioner certification review guide*. Potomac, MD: Health Leadership Associates.

National Cancer Institute Workshop (1989). The 1988 Bethesda system for reporting cervical/vaginal cytological diagnoses. *JAMA, 262*(7), 931-934.

Rakel, R. E. (Ed.). (1993). *Conn's current therapy*. Philadelphia: W. B. Saunders.

Rakel, R. E. (Ed.). (1990). *Textbook of family practice*. Philadelphia: W. B. Saunders.

Sanfilippo, J. S., Muram, D., Dewhurst, J., & Lee, P. A. (Eds.). (1994). *Pediatric and adolescent gynecology*. Philadelphia: W. B. Saunders.

Schroeder, S. A., Tierney, L. M., McPhee, S. J., Papadakis, M. A. & Krupp, M. A. (Eds.). (1992). *Current medical diagnosis and treatment*. Norwalk, CT: Appleton & Lange.

Scott, J. R., DiSaia, P. J., Hammond, C. B., & Spellacy, W. N. (1990). *Danford's obstetrics and gynecology*. Philadelphia: J. B. Lippincott.

Shuler, P. A. (1993). *Breast disease in women and men: A clinicians' handbook*. Durant, OK: Essential Medical Information Systems.

Star, W. L., Shannon, M. T., Sammons, L. N., Lommee, L. L., & Gutierrez, Y. (1990). *Ambulatory Obstetrics: Protocols for Nurse Practitioners/Nurse-Midwives*. San Francisco, CA: School of Nursing, University of California, San Francisco.

Stenchever, M. A. (Ed.). (1992). *Office gynecology*. St. Louis: Mosby Year Book.

Thomas, C. L. (1985). *Taber's Cyclopedic Medical Dictionary*. Philadelphia: F. A. Davis Company.

U.S. Bureau of the Census, (1992). *Statistical Abstract of the United States: 1992* (112th Ed.). pp. 66, 75, Washington, DC.

U.S. Preventive Services Task Force. (1990). Screening for cervical cancer. *American Family Physician, 41*(3), 853-857.

Wilson, J. R., & Carrington, E. R. (Eds.). (1991). *Obstetrics and gynecology* (9th ed.). St. Louis: Mosby Year Book.

Pregnancy, Contraception and Menopause

Pamela A. Shuler

Pregnancy

- Definition: The condition of having a developing embryo or fetus within the uterus

- Incidence

  1. Birth rate, or number of births per 1,000 population, in the U.S. for the year ending 1990 was 16.7

  2. Early diagnosis of pregnancy is essential so that the woman can

     a. Begin prenatal care, be tested for potentially harmful infections/conditions, discontinue use of tobacco, alcohol, street drugs or teratogenic medications

     b. Plan for adoption or termination if pregnancy is unwanted

- Signs and Symptoms

  1. First Trimester (last normal menstrual period [LNMP] to 12th week)

     a. Positive pregnancy test

     b. Amenorrhea/irregular menses

     c. Nausea with or without vomiting

     d. Breast tenderness/tingling

     e. Fatigue

     f. Urinary frequency/urgency

  2. Second Trimester (13th to 27th week)

     a. Braxton-Hicks contractions (16th to 27th week)

     b. Quickening (16th to 20th week)

     c. Increased skin pigmentation

  3. Third Trimester (28th to 40th week)

     a. Braxton-Hicks contractions (more apparent)

- Differential Diagnosis

  1. Ectopic pregnancy

  2. Myomas

  3. Ovarian tumor

  4. Amenorrhea/irregular menses from other origin

5. Weight gain from other origin

6. Urinary tract infection

7. Gastrointestinal problem

8. Gestational trophoblastic disease (including hydatidiform mole)

■ Physical Findings

1. First Trimester (LNMP to 12th week)

   a. Weight gain of about 1 kg (2 lb)

   b. Breast enlargement, vascular engorgement, nipples more erect and areola darkened

   c. Minimal abdominal enlargement; average uterine diameter at 12 weeks = 8 cm/palpable just above symphysis

   d. Softening of the cervix by 6th to 8th week (Goodell's sign)

   e. Vaginal and cervical cyanosis by 6th to 8th week (Chadwick's Sign)

   f. Softening of cervicouterine junction at 6th to 8th week (Hegar's Sign)

   g. Increased cervical/vaginal secretions (white mucoid, known as leukorrhea)

   h. Fetal heart tones audible with doppler by 10th to 12th week

2. Second Trimester (13th to 27th week)

   a. Weight gain of about 5 kg (11 lb)

   b. Striae—breast and/or abdomen

   c. Fundus palpable above symphysis by 14th to 15th week, at umbilicus by 20th to 22nd week

   d. Fetal heart tones audible with fetoscope by 20th week

   e. Uterine souffle

   f. Ballottement (near 20th week)

   g. Fetal outline palpable (after 20th week)

   h. As a general rule, between 20 and 31 weeks of gestation, the fundal height in centimeters equals the gestational age in weeks

3. Third Trimester (28th to 40th week)

   a. Weight gain of about 5 kg (11 lb)

     b. Breasts—secretion of colostrum (28th to 40th week)

     c. Fundus palpable halfway between umbilicus and the xiphoid process by 28th week and at the xiphoid process by 38th week

     d. Lightening (occurs a few weeks prior to labor)

     e. Bloody show (mucus plug)—indicates impending labor

     f. Rupture of membranes (labor within 24 hours; if no labor within 48 hours, induction is indicated)

     g. Labor

        (1) 1st stage of labor—when cervical effacement and dilatation occurs

        (2) 2nd stage of labor—expulsion of fetus

        (3) 3rd stage of labor—separation and expulsion of the placenta

- Factors for a high-risk pregnancy
  1. Maternal age < 16 or > 35 years
  2. Low socioeconomic status
  3. Malnutrition
  4. Substance use
     a. Cigarette smoking
     b. Alcohol
     c. Street drugs
     d. Illicit use of prescription drugs
  5. Environmental toxin exposure
  6. Family or work stress/problems
  7. Family history of mental, physical, genetic disorders
  8. Previous problems with pregnancy/delivery/post partum
  9. Existence of acute or chronic health problems
  10. Lack of prenatal care
- Complications—high-risk pregnancy
  1. General
     a. Excessive vomiting

b. Inadequate or excessive maternal weight gain

c. Anemias

    (1)   Iron deficiency (severe and/or persistent)

    (2)   Megaloblastic (folic acid deficiency)

    (3)   Acquired hemolytic

    (4)   Congenital (sickle cell, hemoglobin SC disease, beta-thalassemia and sickle cell trait)

d. Urinary tract infections (recurrent or persistent cystitis, acute pyelonephritis, asymptomatic bacteriuria)

e. Gestational diabetes

f. Pregnancy induced hypertension (hypertension with proteinuria after 20th week gestation)

g. Multiple gestation

h. Rh isoimmunization (2nd pregnancy)

i. ABO hemolytic disease (2nd pregnancy)

j. Intrauterine growth retardation (IUGR)

k. Infections

    (1)   Sexually transmitted diseases—HIV, herpes, gonorrhea, chlamydia, syphilis, human papillomavirus (HPV)

    (2)   Toxoplasmosis

    (3)   Hepatitis A, B, C, D or E

    (4)   Rubella

    (5)   Tuberculosis

2. First Trimester (LNMP to 12th week) specific

a. Bleeding—25% of pregnancies have 1st trimester bleeding; half will spontaneously abort, the other half remain viable without problems

b. Cramping—if associated with bleeding, increased chance of abortion

3. Second Trimester (13th to 27th week) specific

a. Incompetent cervix—can lead to premature rupture of membranes and/or labor

      b. Premature rupture of membranes—can lead to serious bacterial infections in both mother and fetus

      c. Preterm labor—labor prior to 38th week of gestation

  4. Third Trimester (28th to 40th week) specific

      a. Polyhydramnios

      b. Oligohydramnios

      c. Placenta previa

      d. Abruptio placentae

      e. Fetal distress

      f. Postterm pregnancy (> 42 weeks)

      g. Pre-eclampsia

      h. Eclampsia

■ Common Disorders

  1. Iron deficiency anemia (mild)

  2. Vaginitis—trichimonas, candida, bacterial vaginosis

  3. Cystitis—acute and uncomplicated

■ Common Complaints

  1. Nausea and vomiting

  2. Backache

  3. Varicosities

  4. Hemorrhoids

  5. Constipation and/or bowel irregularity

  6. Heartburn

  7. Food cravings and pica (laundry starch, clay, dirt, ice)

  8. Ptylism (excessive secretion of saliva)

  9. Fatigue

  10. Headache

  11. Vaginal discharge (leukorrhea)

  12. Urinary frequency

  13. Leg cramps

14. Round ligament pain

15. Breathlessness (dyspnea)

16. Edema

- Diagnostic Testing

  1. Urine or blood pregnancy test that detects human chorionic gonadotropin (hCG) produced by placenta

     a. Review sensitivity/specificity of particular test used

     b. hCG peaks approximately 60 to 70 days after fertilization

  2. Ultrasound is used in obstetrics to

     a. Confirm an intrauterine pregnancy—small white gestational ring is evident after 5 weeks of amenorrhea with vaginal probe and 6 weeks with pelvic sonography

     b. Rule out an ectopic pregnancy (vaginal more accurate than transabdominal)

     c. Assess an intrauterine pregnancy—gestational age and uterine size

     d. Investigate uterine bleeding

     e. Evaluate fetal well-being

     f. Visualize fetus during high-risk procedures—amniocentesis, chorionic villi sampling, percutaneous umbilical blood sampling, intrauterine transfusion, insertion of shunts and drainage of fetal cystic mass, ascites or pleural effusion

- Management

  1. Determination of pregnancy "risk status" should occur at the first visit and be re-evaluated at each successive visit

  2. Schedule of prenatal visits for low-risk pregnancy

     a. Up to 28 weeks—every 4 weeks

     b. Up to 36 weeks—every 2 weeks

     c. 36 weeks to delivery—weekly

     d. Additional visits as indicated

  3. First prenatal visit

     a. Expected date of confinement (EDC)—Nägele's rule—9 months plus 7 days from the start of the LNMP

b. History—age, race, occupation, LNMP date and characteristics, EDC calculation, past medical history, reproductive history, contraceptive use (type last used, date discontinued), symptoms with present pregnancy, substance use (tobacco, alcohol, street drugs), current medications, allergies, nutritional and exercise habits, family history of congenital anomalies and inheritable diseases; social history (current living situation, relationship with father of baby, social support system); nutritional history

c. Physical Examination—height, weight, vital signs, general complete physical examination; abdominal and pelvic examinations to include estimation of uterine size (bimanual examination until uterus becomes an abdominal organ, about 12 weeks, then measure fundal height); evaluation of bony pelvis symmetry/adequacy; examination of cervix for infection, bleeding, effacement, dilatation; detection of fetal heart tones if appropriate gestational age; note affect and mood

d. Laboratory Tests—urinalysis and urine culture with sensitivities, CBC, VDRL, rubella titer, blood group, Rh and antibody screening, HBsAg evaluation; cervical cultures for chlamydia and gonorrhea, cultures for herpes genitalis if lesions present; Pap smear; TORCHS panel; HIV testing if indicated or desired; other tests as indicated, e.g., sonogram and 1 hour glucose screen

4. Return visits

a. History—feelings about pregnancy; stressful home/work situations; symptoms including headaches, altered vision, abdominal pain, nausea/vomiting, vaginal bleeding or fluid leakage, dysuria, fetal movement; common discomforts

b. Physical Examination—blood pressure (actual and extent of change), weight (actual and amount of change), edema, fundal height with a centimeter tape measure, fetal heart rate(s), determination of fetal lie, presentation, position, variety and engagement, presenting part/station

c. Procedures/Tests

(1) 9 to 12 weeks—chorionic villous sampling is done when indicated for genetic reasons

(2) 15 to 18 weeks—genetic amniocentesis for women > 35 years if considering abortion as an option; family history of congenital anomalies; history of previous child with

chromosomal, metabolic, neural tube problem

(3) 16 to 18 weeks—maternal serum alpha-fetoprotein (MSAFP) determination in maternal blood to detect neural tube defect

(4) 14 to 24 weeks—ultrasound if EDC unclear

(5) 24 to 28 weeks—screen for gestational diabetes and repeat CBC for all patients; urinalysis and culture if indicated

(6) 28 weeks—Rh immunoglobulin for unsensitized Rh-negative patients

(7) 28 weeks on—ultrasound to evaluate suspected intrauterine growth retardation

(8) 28 to 32 weeks—repeat vaginal examination to confirm presenting part and determine station, measure pelvis, evaluate cervix (CAREFULLY)

(9) 34-36 weeks—repeat CBC if hgb < 11 g/dl or Hct $< 33\%$ at 28 weeks

(10) 36 weeks to delivery—culture active herpes lesions

(11) 38 weeks—culture cervix for group B β-hemolytic streptococci, treat if positive

(12) Postterm— > 41 to 42 weeks

    (a) Obtain ultrasound and perform nonstress tests twice weekly

    (b) Conduct biophysical profile to identify compromised fetus

■ Medical Consultation Guidelines

1. Pre-eclampsia

2. Diabetes mellitus and glucose intolerance of pregnancy

3. Third-trimester bleeding

4. Previous fetal wastage (greater than 16 weeks gestation)

5. Habitual abortions (3 or more under 16 weeks gestation)

6. Known drug abuse

7. Rhesus sensitization or other IgG antibody sensitization

8. Post-maturity at 41 weeks by menstrual dating

9. Hemoglobinopathies

10. Anemia unresponsive to iron/diet therapy

11. Multiple gestation

12. Premature rupture of membranes

13. Suspicion of IUGR

14. High-risk for Pre-term labor

15. Polyhydramnios or oligohydramnios

16. Maternal cardiac, hypertensive or renal disease

17. Recurrent urinary tract infections

18. Abnormal MSAFP

19. Fetal malpresentation after 34 weeks gestation

20. Family or personal history of congenital anomalies or chromosomal abnormalities

21. Positive human immunodeficiency virus (HIV) test

22. Other conditions as indicated

- General Considerations

    1. Emphasize importance of good nutrition, adequate rest, exercise and good hygiene

        a. Mother should gain about 10 to 12 kg (22-27 lb)

        b. A daily caloric increase of 300 kcal throughout pregnancy is recommended

        c. Encourage reduction of caffeine consumption to 0 to 1 cup/day

        d. In general, exercise is not limited (should follow mother's typical regime); however, extreme fatigue should be avoided

        e. Encourage good hygiene, but avoid tub baths in 3rd trimester (increased chance of falls)

        f. Douching is not recommended

        g. Good oral hygiene and dental examinations should continue throughout pregnancy

    2. Review warning signs of potential complications (fever, chills, abominal pain, headaches, blurred vision, vaginal bleeding, decreased fetal movement, premature rupture of membranes)

    3. Education regarding avoidance of

    a. Any medications not prescribed (including over-the-counter medications)

    b. Radiographs (x-rays)

    c. Substance use—tobacco, alcohol, street drugs

    d. Saunas/hot tubs

    e. Cat litter—fecal matter (toxoplasmosis risk)

4. Discuss employment issues (mental stress, physical strain, fatigue, prolonged standing/sitting etc)

5. Review travel plans—no restrictions for low risk pregnancy; should walk every 2 hours

6. Discuss sexual activity

    a. Generally, in low-risk pregnancies, intercourse is not harmful

    b. Avoidance of intercourse is recommended if threat of abortion or preterm labor

7. Encourage enrollment with partner (if applicable) into childbirth preparation classes (7th month)

8. Discuss breastfeeding option (7th month)

9. Discuss future family planning (8th month)

10. Review home environment and anticipated needs prior to bringing baby home (7th to 9th months)

11. Review labor and delivery issues (8th to 9th months)

Ectopic Pregnancy

- Definition: A gestation that occurs outside the endometrial cavity, 98% are tubal

- Etiology/Incidence

1. Exact cause unknown

2. Conditions that prevent or retard passage of fertilized ovum into uterine cavity

    a. Salpingitis

    b. Peritubal adhesions

    c. Developmental abnormalities of tube

      d. Previous tubal surgery

      e. Tumors that distort tube

      f. External migration of ovum

      g. Menstrual reflux

  3. Risk factors

      a. History of previous ectopic pregnancy

      b. History of PID

      c. History of infertility

      d. Pregnant with IUD

      e. Pregnant while using low-dose progestins or postcoital estrogens for contraception

      f. Pregnant after in vitro fertilization

      g. History of DES exposure

  4. Incidence

      a. General population—1 to 2%

      b. Intrauterine device in place—4 to 9%

      c. Previous tubal surgery—5 to 30%

      d. Pelvic inflammatory disease—10 to 15%

      e. Previous ectopic pregnancy—10 to 15%

      f. History of gonorrhea, chlamydia, bacterial vaginosis

  5. Sites—oviduct (95%), ovary, abdomen, cervix

■ Signs and Symptoms

  1. "Great masquerader"—clinical presentation may mimic many abdominal and pelvic conditions

  2. Pelvic pain—usually unilateral

  3. Low back pain

  4. Lower quadrant(s) abdominal pain— usually unilateral

  5. Shoulder pain (if blood in peritoneum)

  6. Amenorrhea or missed menstrual period

  7. Abnormal vaginal bleeding/spotting (usually begins 7 to 14 days after

missed period)

8. Early pregnancy symptoms (nausea, vomiting, malaise etc)

9. Syncopal symptoms—collapse and shock (if ruptured)

10. History of infertility/IUD use

- Differential Diagnosis

   1. Adnexal torsion

   2. Acute appendicitis

   3. Pelvic inflammatory disease

   4. Ruptured corpus luteum cyst

   5. Ruptured ovarian follicle

   6. Urinary calculi

   7. Threatened or inevitable abortion

   8. Hydatidiform mole

   9. Heterotopic (coexistent ectopic and intrauterine) pregnancies—1 in 30,000 pregnancies

- Physical Findings

   1. Tender adnexa with palpable mass/fullness

   2. Uterine softening and mild enlargement

   3. Exquisite cervical motion tenderness

   4. Cul-de-sac fullness

   5. If intraperitoneal bleeding has occurred (leakage from tubal ampulla or ruptured pregnancy)—peritoneal signs such as abdominal distention and mild paralytic ileus may be present; recto vaginal examination may reveal fluid in cul-de-sac

   6. Abdominal and pelvic examinations may be completely unremarkable

   7. Vaginal bleeding may be present

- Diagnostic Tests/Findings

   1. Complete blood count (CBC) may indicate anemia and slight leukocytosis

   2. Urine pregnancy tests for hCG—positive 50% of cases (detects hCG levels of 25+ mIU/mL)

   3. Serum hCG Beta-subunit testing (β-hCG)—positive in 100% of cases

(detects hCG levels of about 0.05 mIU/mL) of serum; allows diagnosis of pregnancy several days after conception

4. Serial testing of serum hCG

   a. Ectopic—level slowly rises or plateaus

   b. Intrauterine—level doubles every 2 days

   c. Spontaneous abortion—level falls

5. Type and Rh (if not already done)

6. Ultrasound

   a. Transabdominal—intrauterine sac visualized at hCG levels of 6000 to 6500 mIU/mL

   b. Vaginal (superior method)—intrauterine sac detected at hCG levels of 1500 to 2000 mIU/mL

7. Culdocentesis (extremely painful, invasive procedure with limited value)—aspiration of the pouch of Douglas confirms hemoperitoneum

8. Laparoscopy (most definitive procedure)—direct visualization of the tubes and ovaries indicates ectopic

9. Endometrial histology (from dilatation and curettage)—decidua without chorionic villi

10. Laparotomy

- Management/Treatment

  1. Physician referral required

  2. Surgical procedures

     a. Unruptured tubal ectopic (operative laparoscopy is often performed over laparotomy since patient morbidity and health care costs are reduced)

        (1) Tubal expression—pregnancy milked from fimbriated end of tube (associated with high recurrence rate)

        (2) Salpingostomy—tube opened, ectopic pregnancy removed, tube closed

        (3) Segmental resection of tube

     b. Large or ruptured tubal ectopic

        (1) Salpingectomy—removal of affected tube

        (2) Removal of adjacent ovary at time of salpingectomy

3. Chemotherapeutic Agents

   a. Methotrexate—injected into ectopic pregnancy or administered systemically

      (1) May be appropriate for certain unruptured tubal or nontubal ectopic pregnancies, such as abdominal, cervical or ovarian

   b. Iron therapy may be necessary during convalescence if patient anemic

   c. D immunoglobulin (RhoGAM) should be given to Rh-negative patients

- General Considerations

   1. Education of patient regarding prognosis of future pregnancies

      a. Conservative surgery for unruptured ectopic

         (1) 70 to 80% chance of conceiving

         (2) 10 to 15% experience another ectopic

      b. Radical surgery (salpingectomy) for ruptured or unruptured ectopic

         (1) 50% chance of conceiving

         (2) 10 to 15% experience another ectopic

      c. Previous ectopic is not a contraindication for future pregnancies; however several precautions are indicated

         (1) Immediate notification of health care provider upon missed period

         (2) Early location of pregnancy with serial testing of serum hCG

         (3) Careful observation with early ultrasound

   2. Include the patient/family as an active participants in the diagnostic and therapeutic plans

   3. Encourage the patient/family to express concerns and fears

   4. Assist patient/family, as appropriate, in meeting physical, psychological, social, cultural, environmental and spiritual needs

   5. Referral to resource agencies as appropriate

Abortion

- Definition: Termination of a pregnancy prior to viability (20 to 24 weeks)

1. Spontaneous—expulsion of products of conception without medical or mechanical intervention

    a. Threatened—presence of vaginal bleeding and uterine cramping without cervical dilation

    b. Inevitable—gross rupture of membranes in the presence of cervical dilatation; bleeding may or may not be profuse

    c. Incomplete—a portion of the products of conception are expelled and a portion are retained in the uterine cavity

    d. Missed—retention of dead products of conception in utero for 4 to 8 weeks or more

    e. Recurrent—three consecutive spontaneous abortions; the following etiologies should be ruled-out

        (1) Cervical incompetence

        (2) Uterine anomalies

        (3) Infection

        (4) Hormonal dysfunction

        (5) Chromosomal aberrations

2. Induced—the purposeful removal of the products of conception

    a. Voluntary—elective abortion performed for a variety of personal, maternal reasons

    b. Therapeutic—induced abortion secondary to medical contraindications to pregnancy, fetal malformation, genetic disease or rape

- Incidence

    1. Approximately 15% of all pregnancies will spontaneously abort

    2. 1.5 million legal pregnancy terminations were performed in the U.S. in 1988

- Signs and Symptoms of spontaneous abortion

    1. Vaginal bleeding (may include clots, tissue)

    2. Bright red, painless vaginal bleeding in second and third trimester, often associated with placenta previa

    3. Cramping abdominal pain

    4. Low back pain

5. Pelvic pressure

6. Dull, midline, suprasymphyseal pain

7. Tenderness over uterus

8. Fatigue, dizziness, light headedness if hemorrhage

9. Gross preterm rupture of membranes

- Differential Diagnosis

  1. First trimester

     a. Threatened abortion

     b. Inevitable abortion

     c. Incomplete abortion

     d. Complete abortion

     e. Missed abortion

     f. Ectopic pregnancy

     g. Molar pregnancy

     h. Cervicitis

     i. Cervical polyp

     j. Anemia

  2. Second and third trimester

     a. Placenta previa

     b. Abruptio placenta

     c. Anemia

     d. Fetal distress

     e. Cervicitis

     f. Molar pregnancy

     g. Cervical intraepithelial neoplasia (CIN)

     h. Cervical polyps

     i. "Bloody show"

- Diagnostic Tests/Findings

  1. Ultrasound scanning for gestational size and evidence of fetal activity

  2. hCG levels (often serial)

3. Complete blood count (identify anemia and/or infection)

4. Pelvic examination to determine uterine size and characteristics of cervix and bleeding (chlamydia and gonorrhea cultures if indicated)

5. Fetal heart tones if appropriate gestational age

6. Coagulation studies if indicated

7. Type, Rh, cross match if indicated

- Management/Treatment

  1. First trimester

     a. Referral to M.D. if passage of clots or tissue; ectopic suspected or molar pregnancy

     b. Bed rest until bleeding subsides

     c. Pelvic rest (no sexual intercourse) until 2 weeks after bleeding stops

     d. Injection of RhoGAM (if more than 12 weeks) or MICRhoGAM (if less than 12 weeks) within 72 hours if patient is Rh negative and has threatened, incomplete or complete abortion or with termination of ectopic pregnancy

     e. Treat anemia and/or cervicitis as appropriate

     f. Consult with M.D. if cervical polyps present

  2. Second and third trimesters

     a. All patients require M.D. consult

     b. Immediate transfer to M.D. if placenta previa, abruptio placenta, maternal shock, molar pregnancy and/or fetal distress

     c. Administer RhoGAM to all Rh negative patients

     d. Treat cervicitis or abnormal Pap smear as indicated

- Legal Status of Induced Abortion

  1. In 1973, induced abortion became legal throughout the U.S.

  2. Since 1973, the maternal mortality rate related to induced abortion has dramatically decreased—current rate is approximately 30/100,000

  3. In 1989, states were given the right to place restrictions on the provision of abortion services

- Pre-Abortion Procedures (Induced)

  1. History

a. Past medical history

b. Current acute or chronic illnesses

c. Pertinent psychological and social history

d. Current medications

e. Allergies to local anesthetics, analgesic agents, antibiotics, and other drugs

f. Current substance use (tobacco, alcohol, street drugs)

g. Recent menstrual history, including LNMP

h. Reproductive history, including prior pregnancies (types of deliveries and complications), sexually transmitted diseases, pelvic inflammatory disease, surgery of cervix or uterus, history of fibroids

i. Contraceptive history and future plans

2. Physical examination

a. Vital signs

b. Heart/lungs

c. Breasts

d. Abdomen

e. Thorough pelvic examination

f. Note affect, mood

3. Diagnostic Tests/Findings

a. Urine pregnancy test

b. Determination of gestational age—limitations are designated by state statutes; most states allow induced abortions up to 24 weeks gestation

c. Hematocrit

d. Rh determination

e. Blood typing

f. STD screening

g. Ultrasound to assess pregnancy length, pelvic architecture and/or fetal position may be necessary

4. Treatments

a. If past history of pelvic inflammatory disease, prophylactic antibiotics prior to procedure are indicated

- Methods of Induced Abortion

    1. Surgical methods

        a. Menstrual extraction—vacuum aspiration performed up to 6 weeks from LNMP

        b. Vacuum curretage—most widely used procedure; may be performed in office through 16 weeks gestation with appropriate emergency back-up

        c. Dilatation and Curettage (D&C)—rarely performed in the U.S.; replaced with vacuum curretage

        d. Dilatation and Evacuation (D&E)—extends D&C and vacuum curretage into 2nd trimester during 13 to 15 weeks gestation; appears to be safest method through 20 weeks

        e. Hysterotomy—requires surgical incision into the uterus to remove fetus and placenta; may be used after failed 2nd trimester abortion or when another need exists to enter pelvic cavity; most authorities agree procedure is outdated as a routine abortion procedure

        f. Hysterectomy—same indications as hysterotomy; also results in sterilization

    2. Medical methods—the following agents may be used for 2nd trimester amnioinfusion procedures

        a. Prostaglandins—suppositories and injections most common agents used in the U.S. after the 15th week

        b. Hypertonic saline

        c. Hypertonic urea

    3. Adjunctive techniques

        a. Laminaria (seaweed)—used to gently/slowly dilate cervix prior to evacuation for 12+ weeks

        b. Synthetic osmotic dilators—lamicel (magnesium sulfate-impregnated sponge) and Dilapan (expanding polymer of polyacrilonitrile) produce faster dilatation than laminaria for 12+ weeks

        c. Oxytocin—Commonly given intravenously as an adjunct to 2nd trimester procedures

■ Post-Abortion Treatment

1. Administer RhoGAM if patient is Rh negative

2. Supply patient with contraceptive supplies or pills

3. Prophylactic antibiotics are prescribed for all patients by many clinics—tetracycline 500 mg orally q.i.d. for 3 to 7 days

4. Analgesic—nonsteroidal anti-inflammatory medication or acetaminophen with codeine is often prescribed for pain control

5. Methylergonovine—may be used in 2nd trimester procedures to decrease risk of hemorrhage

6. Two to three week follow-up to assess healing

7. Social services and/or mental health referrals as indicated

■ Complications of Induced Abortion

1. Most common conditions

   a. Bleeding/hemorrhage

   b. Infection

   c. Retained products of conception

   d. Intrauterine blood clots

   e. Continuing pregnancy

   f. Uterine perforation

2. Rare occurrences

   a. Live-born fetus

   b. Cervical laceration

   c. Uterine rupture

   d. Coagulation defects

   e. Infertility

   f. Embolism

   g. Rh sensitization

   h. Potential for subsequent adverse pregnancy outcome with one or more induced abortions

■ General Considerations

1. Provide a supportive, nonjudgmental setting so that the woman can

explore her feelings concerning pregnancy and abortion

2. Review post abortion danger signs with patient

    a. Fever/chills

    b. Muscular aching

    c. Fatigue

    d. Abdominal pain, cramping or backache unrelieved by pain medication

    e. Tenderness (to pressures) in the abdomen

    f. Prolonged/heavy vaginal bleeding (greater than saturating one pad/hour)

    g. Foul vaginal discharge

    h. Delay (8 weeks or more) in resuming menstrual periods

3. Emphasize importance of contraception usage and review methods as appropriate

4. Same as numbers 2 to 5 in Ectopic Pregnancy Section under General Considerations

Oral Contraceptives (The Pill)

- Prevalence of Use and Efficacy

1. 14 million U.S. women use oral contraceptives (OC) annually

2. Two categories of pills

    a. Combined pills—contain various doses of

        (1) One of two synthetic estrogens—ethinyl estradiol or mestranol

        (2) One of the following progestins—norethindrone, norethindrone acetate, ethynodiol diacetate, norethynodrel, norgestrel, levonorgestrel, desogestrel, gestodene or norgestimate

        (3) Multiphasic combined pills alter the dosage of both the estrogen and progestin components throughout the pill-taking schedule

    b. Progestin-only minipills

        (1) Mechanism of action—changes the endometrium, cervical

mucus, and possibly tubal physiology

(2)　Minipills are not as effective as combination pills

3.　Expected failure rates (perfect user)

a.　Combined pills—0.1% to 3.0% (can approach 5.0% in women less than 22 years)

b.　Progestin-only minipill—0.1% to 13% (higher efficacy rates for lactating women and those > 40 years

4.　Typical failure rate approaches 3% (both types)

5.　Progestin potency—combined and minipills

a.　Norethindrone, norethindrone acetate and ethynodiol diacetate are equivalent

b.　Norgestrel or levonorgestrel have much greater potency

c.　Desogestrel, gestodene, norgestimate have highest selective potency

- Mechanism of Action

1.　Estrogenic effects

a.　Inhibits ovulation by suppression of follicle-stimulating hormone (FSH) and luteinizing hormone (LH)

b.　Inhibits implantation by altering uterine secretions and lining

c.　Accelerates ovum transport

d.　Initiates luteolysis

2.　Progestin effects

a.　Hampers sperm transport (creates thick, cervical mucus) and capacitation

b.　Slows ovum transport and inhibits sperm penetration of ovum

c.　Impedes implantation by suppressing endometrium

d.　Inhibits ovulation, in part, by suppression of LH

- Noncontraceptive Benefits of Combined Pills

1.　Decreases duration and amount of menstrual flow

2.　Minimizes menstrual cramps

3.　Provides some protection against

a.　PID (chlamydia excluded)

  b. Functional ovarian cysts

  c. Ovarian and endometrial cancer

  d. Ectopic pregnancy

  e. Premenstrual syndrome

  f. Osteoporosis (controversial)

  g. Endometriosis

  h. Uterine fibroids

  i. Benign breast disease (fibrocystic and fibroadenomas)

  j. Iron deficiency anemia

  k. Toxic shock

  l. Duodenal ulcer

  m. Pregnancy complication

 4. Acne is improved

 5. Improved enjoyment of sex life (threat of pregnancy minimized)

- Potential Undesirable Effects of Hormones (side effects are very individualized)

 1. Estrogen excess

  a. Increased breast size (ductal and fatty tissue)

  b. Cervical erosion and ectopia

  c. Dysmenorrhea

  d. Leukorrhea

  e. Growth of leiomyomata

  f. Nausea

  g. Stimulation of breast neoplasia

  h. Chloasma

  i. Cerebrovascular accident

  j. Deep vein thrombosis, hemiparesis

  k. Telangiectasias

  l. Thromboembolic disease

  m. Hepatocellular adenomas or cancer

    n. Pulmonary emboli

2. Estrogen excess or progesterone deficiency

    a. Bloating

    b. Dizziness, syncope

    c. Edema

    d. Headache (cyclic)

    e. Irritability

    f. Nausea, vomiting

    g. Weight gain (cyclic)

    h. Dysmenorrhea

    i. Hypermenorrhea, menorrhagia and clotting

3. Estrogen deficiency

    a. Absence of withdrawal bleeding

    b. Bleeding/spotting during pill days 1 to 9

    c. Continuous bleeding/spotting

    d. Flow decrease, hypomenorrhea

    e. Atrophic vaginitis

4. Progesterone excess

    a. Breast tenderness (also estrogen excess)

    b. Flow length decreased

    c. Hypertension

    d. Myocardial infarction

    e. Appetite increase

    f. Depression

    g. Fatigue

    h. Hypoglycemia symptoms

    i. Libido decrease

    j. Weight gain (non-cyclic)

5. Progesterone deficiency

    a. Bleeding/spotting during pill days 10 to 21

    b. Delayed withdrawal bleeding

  6. Androgen excess

    a. Acne

    b. Hirsutism

    c. Libido increase

    d. Oily skin and scalp

    e. Edema

- Risks Associated with low-dose combined ($<$ 50 mcg) pills

  1. Myocardial infarction risk increased if

    a. Estrogen $>$ 50 micrograms (these pills are no longer used)

    b. Smokers over age 35

    c. Cigarette smoker $>$ 15 cigarettes/day

    d. Obese

    e. Sedentary

    f. Diabetic

    g. Hypertensive

    h. Hyperlipidemia

    i. Family history of cardiovascular disease or diabetes

  2. Hypertension risk increase is usually mild and returns to normotensive levels when pills discontinued

  3. Arterial cardiovascular disease risk

    a. Use of levonorgestrel combination pills only increases low-density lipids (LDL), decreases high-density lipids (HDL)

    b. Estrogenic component of current low-dose oral contraceptives does not appear to significantly alter lipoproteins

  2. Cerebrovascular disease risk increased if

    a. Cigarette smoker

    b. Hypertensive

  3. Neoplasia

    a. Breast cancer

(1) Research continues to investigate whether OC use is a risk factor for breast cancer

(2) Majority of current, case-controlled studies have not identified OC use as a risk for the development of breast cancer in any age group or with any specific pill dosage or formulation

(3) Suggestion that there is a slight increased risk in nulliparous long term OC users

b. Cervical cancer

(1) The role that OC use plays in cervical cancer incidence requires further investigation

(2) Differences in sexual practices between OC users and nonusers and relationship of sexual practice to cervical cancer prevents any definitive isolation of the effects of OCs on cervical cancer

(3) Long-term use of OCs has shown, in some studies, an increased risk of preinvasive cervical neoplasia

 c. Endometrial cancer—OC use seems to offer protection against this form of cancer; greatest protective effect with use greater than 3 years

 d. Ovarian cancer

(1) Risk is decreased for women on the pill

(2) Duration of protection is related to length of pill use (more time on the pill leads to increased duration of protection)

(3) Pill users with low parity (four or less) are most protected

e. Liver adenoma and cancer

(1) Development of a benign hepatocellular adenoma (BHA) is rare in long-term pill users

(2) Attributable risk of BHA is about 3 to 4 cases per 100,000 for OC users and increases after 4 years of use

(3) Hepatocellular carcinoma is extremely rare in young women

f. Pituitary adenoma—incidence is not increased with OC use

4. Gallbladder disease

a. Cholelithiasis—OCs do not cause gallstones, but their use may accelerate development of gall bladder disease in susceptible women

5. Glucose metabolism

   a. Glucose tolerance and plasma insulin levels may be adversely affected, primarily with high dose pills

   b. Glucose metabolism returns to normal when OCs are discontinued

   c. Risk is minimized if pill dose is low

- Risks Associated with Taking Minipills

  1. Menstrual Irregularities

     a. Spotting/Breakthrough bleeding

     b. Prolonged cycles

     c. Amenorrhea

  2. More frequent development of functional ovarian cysts

  3. Although the overall incidence of ectopic pregnancy is not increased, when pregnancy occurs it is more likely to be ectopic

- Absolute Contraindications to OCs

  1. Pregnancy

  2. Thrombophlebitis/thromboembolic disorders (past/present)

  3. Stroke or coronary artery disease (past/present)

  4. Breast cancer

  5. Undiagnosed abnormal vaginal bleeding

  6. Estrogen-dependent cancer

  7. Benign or malignant liver tumor (past/present)

  8. Current impaired liver function

  9. Smokers > 35 years

  10. Sickle Cell disease

- Relative Contraindications to OCs—consult with M.D., then monitor closely

  1. Carcinoma in situ

  2. Migraine headaches (especially with neurological symptoms)

  3. Hypertension (from OCs that is uncontrolled)

4. Cardiac, renal, liver dysfunction

5. Hyperlipidemia

6. Diabetes

7. Major depression

8. Recovering from fracture or severe injury

9. Impending surgery or immobility

10. Sickle Cell disease

■ Prescribing Oral Contraceptives—Risk Factor Screening

1. History

   a. Past medical history

   b. Current acute or chronic illnesses

   c. Current medications

   d. Allergies to local anesthetics, analgesic agents, antibiotics, and other drugs

   e. Current substance use (tobacco, alcohol, street drugs)

   f. Recent menstrual history, including LNMP

   g. Reproductive history, including prior pregnancies (types of deliveries and complications), sexually transmitted diseases, pelvic inflammatory disease, surgery of cervix or uterus, conization of cervix, abnormality of uterine shape, history of fibroids, endometriosis

   h. Sexual history—age at coitus, number of partners during past year and number during lifetime, sexual practice

   i. Contraceptive history and future plans/desires

2. Physical examination

   a. Vital signs

   b. Neck/thyroid

   c. Heart/lungs

   d. Breasts

   e. Abdomen

   f. Extremities

      g. Thorough pelvic examination

      h. Rectovaginal examination

  3. Laboratory tests

      a. Hematocrit

      b. VDRL or RPR

      c. Urinalysis

      d. Fasting lipid profile for women 35 years of age or older or those with positive cardiovascular history

      e. Urine pregnancy test if indicated

      f. Pap test

      g. STD screening

      h. Rubella titer (optional)

      i. Fasting blood sugar and lipid panel (optional)

      j. HIV test (optional)

■ Prescribing Oral Contraceptives—General Guidelines

  1. Healthy women without risk factors may continue to use low-dose combination pills until menopause

  2. Women over 35 who smoke cigarettes should not use oral contraceptives but may be minipill candidates after consult

  3. When prescribing oral contraceptives, both the dose and potency of each steroid must be considered

  4. Most women are started on a low-dose, 35 mcg or less, estrogen combined pill or multiphasic pill

  5. Minipills (progestin-only) are often used by

      a. Breastfeeding women

      b. Women who have contraindications to combination pills

      c. Women with history of severe headaches or hypertension on combined pills

■ General Considerations

  1. Review instructions for

      a. Taking the prescribed pill

b. "Missed" pill(s)

2. Encourage the patient to always keep a backup method of birth control, such as foam, condoms, suppositories, diaphragm etc. on hand

3. Emphasize that OCs do not protect against sexually transmitted diseases; encourage condom use

4. Inform the patient that

   a. The majority of minor side effects (nausea, breast tenderness, breakthrough bleeding etc.) diminish with continued pill use (usually after the first 3 to 6 months)

   b. Medications that affect liver metabolism may decrease efficacy of pill (Rifampin, Dilantin, Phenobarbital, Primodine, Tegretol)

   c. The minipill must be taken the same time daily

   d. OCs may potentiate the action of valium, librium, tricyclic antidepressants and theophylline

5. Review danger signals — patient should be told to contact a health care provider if any of the following symptoms develop

   a. Combined Pills

      (1) Abdominal pain (severe)

      (2) Chest pain (severe), cough or shortness of breath

      (3) Headache (severe), dizziness, weakness or numbness

      (4) Eye problems (vision loss or blurring)

      (5) Speech problems

      (6) Severe leg pain (calf or thigh)

   b. Minipills

      (1) Severe abdominal pain — may be due to ovarian cyst or ectopic pregnancy

      (2) Pill taken late — with a 3 hour or more delay in taking pill, use a back-up contraceptive method for 2 days

6. Remind patient that she should also notify health care provider if she develops

   a. Depression

   b. Yellow jaundice

      c. Breast lump

      a. Migraine headaches

      a. Breast discharge/milk

7.   Inform the patient that after stopping the pills, return to fertility may be delayed for two to three months or may occur after missing one to two pills

8.   Inform patient of noncontraceptive benefits and advantages

9.   Review potential undesirable effects

10. Assist patient in evaluating personal "failure risk"

11. Encourage the patient to express her concerns/fears

12. Review and demonstrate breast self-examination

13. Emphasize importance of regular Pap tests

14. Review STD (including AIDS) prevention and transmission

15. Encourage adherence to a well-balanced diet, regular exercise program and stress management plan

Norplant Implants

- History and Description

  1.   Recently approved for use in the U.S.

  2.   Levonorgestrel (35 mg) is contained in 6 slender, flexible, silastic rods measuring 2.4 mm by 34 mm

  3.   Rods are inserted in a fan-like pattern under the skin of the upper arm (local anesthesia is used)

- Mechanism of Action and Efficacy

  1.   Levonorgestrel slowly diffuses through the rods into the patient's system

  2.   Mechanism of progesterone is same as in Minipill (progestin-only oral contraceptives)

  3.   Low failure rate—less than 2%

  4.   System is effective for 5 years

  5.   Effectiveness is correlated to the body weight of the user (if weight is greater than 70 kg or 154 pounds, probability of becoming pregnant

increases during the second year of use)

- Noncontraceptive Benefits of Norplant Implants
    1. Scanty or no menses
    2. Decreased anemia
    3. Decreased menstrual cramps/pain
    4. Suppressed ovulatory pain (mittelschmerz)
    5. Possible reduced risk of endometrial cancer

- Potential Side Effects and Complications
    1. Most women do not have major problems with Norplant
    2. Menstrual irregularities vary widely
    3. Headache, dizziness
    4. Nervousness
    5. Nausea
    6. Dermatitis, acne
    7. Change in appetite, weight gain (usually less than 5 pounds over 5 years)
    8. Breast tenderness or discharge
    9. Dermatitis
    10. Hair loss
    11. Ovarian cysts
    12. Slight visibility of rods beneath skin
    13. Insertion or removal problems
    14. Effects on lipid metabolism and the cardiovascular system are unclear

- Contraindications
    1. Known or suspected pregnancy
    2. Acute liver disease; benign or malignant liver tumors
    3. Undiagnosed abnormal vaginal bleeding
    4. History of thrombophlebitis or thromboembolic disorders
    5. History of heart attack, chest pain due to diagnosed heart disease or coronary-artery disease

6.   History of stroke or cerebrovascular disease

7.   Known or suspected carcinoma of the breast

- Risk Factor Screening

   1.   Complete history, physical examination and laboratory tests (same as for oral contraceptives)

   2.   Patients with the following problems should have a more thorough evaluation prior to Norplant use

   a.   Breast nodules, fibrocystic disease or an abnormal mammogram

   b.   Diabetes

   c.   Elevated cholesterol or triglycerides

   d.   High blood pressure

   e.   Migraine or other headaches

   f.   Epilepsy

   g.   Depression

   h.   Heart or kidney disease

- General Considerations

   1.   Inform the patient that

   a.   The majority of minor side effects (irregular bleeding, nausea, breast tenderness etc.) may diminish during the first 9 to 12 months, although they may not

   b.   Norplant implants become effective within 24 hours of insertion

   c.   Norplant implants should be replaced in 5 years

   d.   Weight gain can reduce effectiveness

   2.   Instruct the patient to

   a.   Avoid bumping the area where the implants were inserted

   b.   Keep insertion area clean and dry for 3 to 4 days after insertion

   3.   Review danger signals—patient should be told to contact a health care provider if any of the following symptoms develop

   a.   Severe lower abdominal pain—ectopic pregnancy is rare but can occur

   b.   Heavy vaginal bleeding

    c. Arm pain

    d. Pus or bleeding at insertion site (possible infection)

    e. Expulsion of an implant

    f. Delayed menstrual periods after a long interval of regular periods

    g. Migraine headaches, repeated very painful headaches, blurred vision

4. Emphasize that the Norplant system does not protect against sexually transmitted diseases; encourage condom use if indicated

5. Thorough education about Norplant

6. Same as numbers 8 to 15 in Oral Contraception under General Considerations

Intrauterine Devices (IUDs)

- Prevalence of Use and Efficacy

  1. Approximately 2% of U.S. women at risk of pregnancy use the IUD

  2. Most types of IUDs have failure rates from 1% to 2%

  3. Current IUDs have a limited life-span

- Types

  1. IUDs currently marketed in the U.S.

      a. Copper T 380A (ParaGard)

         (1) Ten year life-span, but must be changed every 8 years in U.S.

         (2) The most effective IUD ever marketed in the U.S.

         (3) T-shaped plastic frame wrapped with fine copper wire

      b. Progesterone T (Progestasert system)

         (1) 1 year life-span

         (2) Releases 65 mcg/day of levonorgestrel

         (3) Associated with higher incidence of ectopic pregnancy

  2. Some women are still using barium-impregnated plastic devices— Lippes loop and Saf-T-Coil, although these IUDs are no longer on the U.S. market

- Mechanism of Action—the exact mode of action is not completely understood; several theories have been postulated

1. Inhibition of sperm capacitation and survival

2. Ovum transport through the tubes is accelerated

3. Fertilization is inhibited

4. Implantation is prevented due to lysis of blastocyst; inflammatory changes and suppression of the endometrium; increased production of prostaglandins

- Side Effects and Complications

    1. Spotting, bleeding, hemorrhage

        a. Most have an increase in blood loss which is usually minor and uncomplicated; 5 to 15% have IUD removed due to symptoms related to bleeding or spotting

        b. Pregnancy and infection

    2. Anemia

        a. Monitor Hgb/Hct

        b. Iron supplementation may be necessary

        c. If Hgb < 9gm% or Hct < 27% — remove IUD

    3. Cramping/Pain

        a. Dysmenorrhea may accompany IUD use

        b. Rule out pregnancy and infection

        c. Non-steroidal anti-inflammatory agents may be used for pain control

        d. 15 to 40% of IUD removals are related to pain complaints

    4. Uterine perforation, embedding, cervical perforation

        a. Incidence — 1 in 2,500

        b. Occurs most frequently if inserted 48 hrs to 8 weeks postpartum

    5. Infection — pelvic inflammatory disease

        a. Highest rate during first 2 to 6 weeks after insertion

        b. Risk is greatest in women who

            (1) Have past history of PID

            (2) Are nulliparous

         (3)   Have multiple sex partners

  6. Pregnancy

     a. Rate—2 to 3/100 (1/3 related to undetected or partial expulsion)

     b. Spontaneous abortion

         (1)   50% if IUD left in situ

         (2)   20 to 30% if IUD removed early

     c. Ectopic pregnancy

         (1)   5% of pregnancies will be ectopic

         (2)   Progestasert users have 6 to 10 fold higher ectopic rate than copper IUD users

  7. Expulsion of the IUD—2 to 10% spontaneously expel IUD in first year

- Absolute Contraindications

  1. Pregnancy (known or suspected)

  2. Active, recent or recurrent pelvic infection including known or suspected chlamydia, gonorrhea, bacterial vaginosis

  3. Wilson's Disease—inability to metabolize copper

- Strong Relative Contraindications

  1. Risk factors for PID (including multiple sex partners)

  2. Risk factors for HIV infection

  3. History of PID or ectopic pregnancy

  4. Undiagnosed, irregular or abnormal uterine bleeding

  5. Cervical or uterine malignancy (known or suspected)

  6. Unresolved abnormal Pap smear

  7. Abnormal size or shape of uterus (including fibroids that distort cavity)

  8. Previous problems with IUD pregnancies or expulsion

  9. Past history of severe vasovagal reactivity or fainting

  10. Impaired coagulation response

  11. Valvular heart disease (may need prophylactic antibiotics)

  12. Allergy to copper

  13. Impaired ability to check for string

14. Follow-up care and/or emergency treatment difficult to obtain

15. Diabetes

16. Nulliparity

■ Risk Factor Screening

1. Complete history, physical examination and laboratory tests (see section on oral contraception)

2. Additional allergy screening—copper

3. STD cultures, wet mount and Pap smear

■ Insertion

1. Safe anytime in menstrual cycle

   a. Infection and expulsion rates higher when inserted during menses

   b. At midcycle, cervix is dilated as during menses, therefore insertion is facilitated

2. Postpartum IUD insertions—4 to 8 weeks after delivery

3. Insertion via the withdrawal technique (retracting the outer barrel over the plunger) reduces the risk of uterine perforation

4. Prophylactic antibiotics may be used (no consensus exists)

   a. Doxycycline 200 mg orally at time of insertion and 100 mg orally 12 hours later

   b. Breast feeding women—erythromycin 500 mg orally 1 hour prior to insertion and 500 mg orally 6 hours after insertion

■ General Considerations

1. Ensure that patient is an informed IUD user

2. Review instructions for

   a. Checking string

   b. Monitoring periods

   c. Noting infection signs/symptoms

   d. Prophylactic antibiotics

   e. Pain control

   f. STD prevention and risk reduction

3. Review danger signals—patient should be told to contact a health care

provider if any of the following symptoms develop

   a. Period late (pregnancy), abnormal spotting or bleeding

   b. Abdominal pain, pain with intercourse

   c. Infection exposure, abnormal discharge

   d. Not feeling well, fever, chills

   e. String missing, shorter or longer

4. Same as numbers 8 to 15 in Oral Contraception under General Considerations

Diaphragm

- Description and Efficacy

1. Dome-shaped cup

2. Made of latex rubber

3. Flexible, metal spring rim (flat, coil or arcing)

4. Diameters range from 50 to 95 mm

5. Patient must be measured for appropriate size by trained health care provider

6. Failure rates range from 6% to 18% depending upon motivation and care in which diaphragm is used

- Mechanism of Action

1. Inserted into vagina before intercourse

   a. Posterior rim rests in the posterior fornix

   b. Anterior rim fits snugly behind the pubic bone

2. Contraceptive jelly is placed within the dome and around the circumference

3. Contraceptive effect

   a. Dome acts as a barrier, decreases cervical exposure to sperm

   b. Spermicide effect of contraceptive jelly

- Noncontraceptive Benefits and Advantages

1. Some protection against sexually transmitted diseases; however vaginal irritation from nonoxynol-9 could increase HIV susceptibility

2. Protection against cervical HPV and subsequent dysplasia

3. Relatively safe

4. Does not require partner involvement

5. Does not interrupt sex act

6. Intermittent contraception

7. Immediate protection

- Potential Undesirable Effects

   1. Local skin irritation

   2. Vaginal trauma (rare)

   3. Increased risk of urinary tract infection

   4. Risk of toxic shock syndrome (rare)

   5. Possible increased incidence of bacterial vaginosis in frequent users

- Contraindications

   1. Allergy to spermicide, rubber, latex or polyurethane

   2. Abnormalities in vaginal anatomy that interferes with fit or stability

   3. Inability to learn correct insertion technique

   4. History of

      a. Toxic shock syndrome

      b. Repeated urinary tract infections that persist despite diaphragm refitting

- Risk Factor Screening

   1. Complete history, physical examination and laboratory tests (same as for oral contraceptives)

   2. Additional allergy screening

      a. Spermicide

      b. Rubber, latex

      c. Polyurethane

- General Considerations

   1. Review instructions for

      a. Insertion/removal (must be left in 6 hours after intercourse; maximum time left in vagina is 24 hours

b. Repeated intercourse

c. After intercourse

d. Caring for diaphragm (avoid oil-based lubricants and medications); checking for perforations

2. Inform patient if 10 to 20 pound weight gain, diaphragm "fit" should be evaluated

3. Review danger signals for toxic shock syndrome—patient should be told to contact a health care provider if any of the following symptoms develop

a. Sudden high fever

b. Vomiting, diarrhea

c. Dizziness, faintness, weakness

d. Sore throat, aching muscles and joints

e. Rash (like a sunburn)

4. Emphasize importance of

a. Using diaphragm with repeated intercourse

b. Checking diaphragm and supplies prior to intercourse

c. Practicing inserting and removing diaphragm before use

5. Inform patient of noncontraceptive benefits and advantages

6. Inform patient of potential undesirable effects

7. Assist patient in evaluating personal "failure risk"

8. Same as numbers 8 to 15 in Oral Contraception under General Considerations

Vaginal Sponge

- Description and Efficacy

1. Small pillow-shaped polyurethane sponge

2. Contains 1 gram of nonoxynol-9 spermicide

3. The concave dimple side fits over the cervix to decrease chance of dislodgement during intercourse

4. Most common product is the "Today Sponge"

5. Available in one size, over-the-counter (OTC)

     6.   First-year failure rates range from 18% to 36% depending upon motivation and care in use

     7.   Best used with condom

■ Mechanism of Action

     1.   Sponge is moistened with water prior to insertion into the vagina

     2.   Sponge provides continuous protection for 24 hours (must be left in 6 hours after intercourse; maximum time left in vagina is 24 to 30 hours)

     3.   Contraceptive effect

         a. Sponge acts as a barrier, decreases cervical exposure to sperm

         b. Spermicide effect

■ Noncontraceptive Benefits and Advantages

     1.   Same as diaphragm

     2.   Sponge's relationship to HPV, cervical dysplasia and HIV acquisition under investigation

■ Potential Undesirable Effects

     1.   Local skin irritation

     2.   Difficulty removing sponge

     3.   Risk of Toxic Shock Syndrome (rare)

■ Contraindications

     1.   Same as diaphragm

     2.   Full-term delivery within past 6 weeks, recent abortion or miscarriage, vaginal bleeding (including menses)

■ Risk Factor Screening

     1.   None required by health care provider (OTC product)

     2.   If patient seen in clinic, same risk factor screening as for diaphragm

■ General Considerations

     1.   Nurse may not interact with patient if purchased OTC

     2.   If patient seen in clinic, review

         a. Instructions for

            (1)   Insertion/removal

            (2)   Repeated intercourse

(3)   After intercourse

b. Danger signals for toxic shock syndrome (same as listed for diaphragm)

c. Importance of

(1)   Using sponge with repeated intercourse

(2)   Keeping adequate supply of sponges

d. Practicing inserting and removing sponge before use

3.   Same as numbers 8 to 15 in Oral Contraceptives under General Considerations

Vaginal Spermicides

■ Description and Efficacy

1.   Two components

a. Inert base or carrier

b. Spermicidal chemicals

(1)   Nonoxynol-9 (most common)

(2)   Octoxynol

2.   Several types of spermicidal preparations

a. Foams—used alone, with condoms or diaphragm

b. Creams and gels—used alone or with diaphragm (main use)

c. Suppositories—used alone or with condoms

d. Vaginal contraceptive film (VCF)—used alone or with condoms or diaphragm

3.   Products available over-the-counter

4.   First-year failure rates range from 6% to 21% depending upon motivation and care in use

5.   Best used with condom

■ Mechanism of Action

1.   Spermicide chemicals are surfactants that destroy the sperm cell membrane

2.   Foams, creams and gels—inserted in vagina prior to each sex act ($<$ 30 minutes is optimal, but $<$ 1 hour required)

3.   Suppositories—inserted 10 to 15 minutes prior to each sex act; remains

effective no more than 1 hour

4. VCF—inserted on or near cervix, 5 to 15 minutes prior to each sex act; remains effective no more than 1 hour

5. Contraceptive effect—spermicide effect

- Noncontraceptive Benefits and Advantages

1. Potential protection against sexually transmitted diseases; however vaginal irritation from spermicide could increase HIV susceptibility

2. Can be purchased OTC

3. Relatively safe

4. Intermittent contraception

5. Immediate protection

6. Can be used as extra protection with other methods

- Potential Undesirable Effects

1. Local skin irritation

2. Unpleasant taste of spermicide with oral-genital sex

3. Foaming sensation in vagina

4. Incomplete melting and dispersion of suppositories

- Contraindications

1. Allergy to spermicidal or base ingredients

2. Inability to learn correct insertion technique

3. Abnormalities in vaginal anatomy that interferes with appropriate placement or retention of spermicide

- Risk Factor Screening

1. None required by health care provider (OTC product)

2. If patient seen in clinic, same risk factor screening as for diaphragm

- General Considerations

1. Nurse may not interact with patient if purchased OTC

2. If patient seen in clinic, review

   a. Instructions for

      (1) Insertion

      (2) Repeated intercourse

      (3)   After intercourse

   c. Importance of

      (1)   Using spermicide product with repeated intercourse

      (2)   Keeping adequate supply

  3. Same as numbers 8 to 15 in Oral Contraceptives under General Considerations

Depo-Provera

- History and Description

  1. Has been used by > 15 million women worldwide

  2. Recently approved for use in the U.S. (1992)

  3. 150 mg of depo-medroxyprogesterone acetate (DMPA) is administered via deep intramuscular injection every 3 months

- Mechanism of Action and Efficacy

  1. Inhibits ovulation by supressing FSH and LH levels and eliminating the LH surge

  2. Develops shallow and atrophic endometrium

  3. Creates thick cervical mucus which decreases sperm penetration

  4. Low failure rate—$< 1\%$; low body weight appears to increase failure rate (less body fat to store hormone)

  5. Injections are given every 3 months; 2-week "grace period" of contraceptive protections between injections

  6. Reversible method; return to fertility 77% by 12 months and 82% by 24 months (less rapid than Norplant or progestin-only pills)

- Noncontraceptive Benefits

  1. Scanty or no menses

  2. Decreased anemia

  3. Decreased menstrual cramps/pain

  4. Suppressed ovulatory pain (mittelschmerz)

  5. Possible reduced risk of endometrial cancer, ovarian cancer and pelvic inflammatory disease

  6. Management of pain associated with endometriosis

7. Convenient; not related to intercourse

8. Method not evident to partner, family etc.

9. Option for individuals who do not have control over exposure to conception, i.e., mentally or otherwise impaired

10. May be used by breastfeeding women

11. May be used by patients on anti-convulsant medications (DMPA may actually decrease the frequency of seizures)

- Potential Side Effects and Complications

    1. Allergic reactions—anaphylactic and anaphylactoid reactions are RARE, but may occur immediately following Depo-Provera injections

    2. Menstrual irregularities

        a. Vary from woman-to-woman

        b. Prolonged menstrual bleeding

        c. Bleeding or spotting between periods/Amenorrhea

    3. Headache

    4. Nervousness

    5. Decreased libido

    6. Breast discomfort

    7. Depression

    8. Weight gain

    9. May decrease bone density with long-term use; risk is increased if risk factors for osteoporosis exist (estrogen deficiency, cigarette smoking, heredity, etc.)

    10. Lipid changes—high density lipoprotein cholesterol levels fall significantly

    11. Relative risk of breast cancer associated with DMPA use is unclear

- Contraindications

    1. Absolute

        a. Previous allergic reaction to DMPA

        b. Known or suspected pregnancy

        c. Unexplained abnormal vaginal bleeding

2. Relative

    a. Concern over weight gain

    b. Pregnancy planned in near future

■ Risk Factor Screening

1. Complete history, physical examination, laboratory tests (same as for oral contraceptives) and mammogram in age appropriate

2. Pregnancy test if more than 2 weeks between 3 month injections

3. Patients with the following problems should have a more thorough evaluation prior to DMPA use

    a. Breast nodules, fibrocystic disease or an abnormal mammogram

    b. Diabetes

    c. Elevated cholesterol or triglycerides

    d. High blood pressure

    e. Migraine or other headaches

    f. Epilepsy

    g. Depression

    h. Gallbladder, heart or kidney disease

■ Providing Depo-Provera

1. Deep intramuscular injection of 150 mg DMPA is given every 3 months

2. DO NOT MASSAGE INJECTION SITE. (Massage may lower the effectiveness of DMPA)

■ General Considerations

1. Inform the patient that

    a. The majority of minor side effects (irregular bleeding, breast tenderness etc.) may or may not diminish during the first 9 to 12 months

    b. Use a back-up method of birth control during the first 2 weeks following the injection, unless it was administered during the first 5 days of menses, in which case it is immediately effective

    c. If pregnancy is desired, discontinue injections several months prior to planned conception

2. Review danger signals—patient should be told to contact a health care provider if any of the following symptoms develop

   a. Weight gain

   b. Headaches

   c. Heavy bleeding (check for anemia)

   d. Depression

   e. Inability to conceive after discontinued use of injections for 1 year

3. Emphasize that Depo-Provera does not protect against sexually transmitted diseases; encourage condom use

4. Same as numbers 8 to 15 for Oral Contraception under General Considerations

Natural Family Planning

- Description and Efficacy

   1. Entails planning or avoiding pregnancy by abstaining from sexual intercourse during the fertile phase of the menstrual cycle

   2. During the first year of use, married U.S. women experience an average failure rate of 20/100 when practicing periodic abstinence

   3. Menstrual cycle charting is based on observing physiologic changes during the monthly cycle; it can be used to plan or prevent pregnancy

   4. Natural family planning includes the following methods—calendar rhythm, basal body temperature (BBT) measurement, ovulation or Billings (cervical mucus evaluation)

   5. Sympto-thermal refers to combining evaluation of cervical mucus changes with basal body temperature

- Physiologic Principles

   1. Ovulation usually occurs about 14 days prior to the onset of menstruation

   2. Sperm viability is approximately 2 to 7 days

   3. Life span of ova is approximately 72 hours

   4. Pregnancy is unlikely to occur if intercourse is delayed from 4 days prior to and for 3 or 4 days after ovulation

- Noncontraceptive Benefits and Advantages

1. No absolute contraindications

2. Increases body and fertility awareness

3. May be used by breastfeeding women

■ Potential Side Effects and Disadvantages

1. Unintended pregnany

2. No protection against HIV and other STDs

3. Limits sponteneous sexual intercourse during fertile periods

■ Contraindications

1. Irregular menses

2. History of anovulatory cycles

3. Irregular temperature charts

4. Inability to consistently interpret and record length of cycle, cervical mucus characteristics and/or temperature

■ Basic Instructions

1. Calendar method

a. Record the duration of eight menstrual cycles on a calender

b. Determine the length of each cycle (one cycle goes from the first day of one menstrual period through the day before the next period starts)

c. Identify the shortest and longest cycles

d. The earliest day of fertility is determined by subtracting 18 days from the length of the shortest cycle and latest day of fertility is determined by subtracting 11 days from the length of the longest cycle

e. To prevent pregnancy, avoid intercourse or use a back-up method during the fertile period

2. Basal body temperature charting (BBT)

a. BBT refers to the lowest body temperature of a healthy person upon wakening

b. BBT increases 0.4 to 0.8 F degrees due to thermogenic effect of progesterone

c. A drop in BBT may be noted 12 to 24 hours prior to ovulation each month followed by a sustained increase for several days

d. By recording the BBT on designated chart for 3 to 4 consecutive months, it is possible to determine the time of ovulation

e. To prevent pregnancy, avoid intercourse or use a back-up method until temperature has remained elevated for 3 consecutive days

3. Cervical mucus method (ovulation or Billings method)

a. Recognizable cervical mucus changes occur in most ovulating women

b. After menstruation cervical secretions are usually absent or scant; thick, white, yellow or cloudy

c. Discharge then becomes clear, abundant, elastic, thin and slippery a few days prior to ovulation (low saline content and high estrogen level); stretchy characteristic termed spinnbarkeit

d. Intercourse is permitted after menses ends until cervical mucus secretion is detected; abstinence is then required until 4 days after the peak amount of mucus is observed

e. Presence of mittelschmerz may also aid in identifying fertile days

f. Normal lubrication during sexual arousal, as well as, douching, vaginal infections, spermicides, lubricants etc. can interfere with ability to identify mucus changes

4. Sympto-thermal method—combines cervical mucus changes with temperature changes and other symptoms associated with ovulation

- General Considerations

1. Thoroughly review basic female anatomy and the menstrual cycle

2. Provide thorough, clear, verbal and written instructions

3. Encourage expression of fears and concerns

4. Provide information regarding back-up method(s) as appropriate

5. Emphasize lack of protection for HIV and other STDs; encourage use of condoms

Male Condoms

- Description and Efficacy

1. Sheath-like covering

2. Made of rubber (latex) or processed collagenous tissue ("skin")

    a. Lubricants may be added to outer surface

    b. Spermicides may be added to inner and/or outer surface(s)

3. Used alone or with another method for extra protection

4. Condoms differ in size, shape, thickness, color, taste and packaging

5. Products available over-the-counter (OTC)

6. First-year failure rates range from 3% to 12% depending upon motivation and care in use

7. Condom use is increasing due to STD and AIDS awareness

- Mechanism of Action

  1. Prevent sperm from entering vagina (barrier)

  2. Placed on erect penis, prior to any contact with vagina

  3. Penis with condom in place is removed immediately following ejaculation

  4. Contraceptive effect—barrier and sometimes spermicide effect

- Noncontraceptive Benefits and Advantages

  1. Same as for Vaginal Spermicides

  2. Condom users maintain an erection longer

- Potential Undesirable Effects

  1. Less sensation (lubricant improves sensation)

  2. Interruption of foreplay

  3. Condom breakage

  4. Natural "skin" condoms do not provide STD nor HIV protection

- Contraindications

  1. Men who cannot maintain an erection

  2. Allergy to rubber and/or spermicide (men or women)

  3. Lack of responsibility by male partner

- Risk Factor Screening

  1. None required by health care provider (OTC product)

  2. If female patient seen in clinic and partner uses condoms, same risk factor screening as for diaphragm

- General Considerations
    1. Nurse may not interact with patient/partner if purchased OTC
    2. If patient/partner seen in clinic
        a. Review instructions for use
            (1) Latex provides > STD/HIV protection
            (2) Avoid petroleum-based lubricants/products
            (3) Leave 1/2" of empty space in condom tip (decreases risk of condom perforation or tear)
            (4) Lubrication increases sensation and decreases chances of breakage
        c. Emphasize importance of
            (1) Use of condom during intercourse using appropriate technique; spermicide use
            (2) Maintaining adequate supply
    3. Same as numbers 8 to 15 in Oral Contraceptives under General Considerations

Female Sterilization (tubal ligation)

- Description and Efficacy
    1. An intraperitoneal procedure that is usually performed under general anesthesia
    2. Can be performed during cesarean section, after vaginal delivery, after abortion, or as internal procedure
    3. The fallopian tubes are occluded to prevent the sperm and egg from uniting
    4. Several surgical approaches
        a. Laparotomy
        b. Minilaparotomy
        c. Laparoscopy
        d. Colpotomy/culdoscopy
    5. Several types of procedures
        a. Surgical ligation/excision

    b. Fimbriectomy

    c. Fulguration (electrocoagulation)

    d. Mechanical tubal occlusion devices

       (1)   Clips

       (2)   Bands

       (3)   Rings

  6. Failure rates of female sterilization is 1:400

  7. Sterilization should be considered permanent

■ Contraindications

  1. Inability to give informed consent

  2. Indecisive regarding desire for future pregnancies

  3. Failure of patient to meet institutional, state and/or federal sterilization guidelines if applicable

■ Complications

  1. Fatality rates for U.S. approach 3 per 100,000, which is low when compared to maternal mortality rates which are 14 deaths per 100,000 live births

  2. Anesthesia complications (most common)

  3. Infection

  4. Hemorrhage

  5. Uterine perforation

  6. Bladder or intestinal injury

  7. Post-operative pain/discomfort

  8. Sterilization failure

  9. Ectopic pregnancy

    a. Overall risk is decreased, since chance of pregnancy is decreased

    b. If pregnancy occurs, risk of ectopic is 4% to 64%

    c. Studies suggest ectopic pregnancy more likely to follow electrocoagulation procedure than ligation/excision or mechanical occlusion methods

■ Risk Factor Screening

1. Same as listed for Oral Contraception

■ General Considerations

1. Provide a supportive, nonjudgmental setting so that patients can explore feelings concerning voluntary sterilization

2. Emphasize PERMANENCE of procedure

3. Reassure patients that they should feel free to decide against sterilization at any point prior to the procedure

4. Encourage patients to fully discuss sterilization decision with partner or person(s) of choice

5. Fully review procedural

    a. Techniques

    b. Benefits

    c. Risks

    d. Alternatives

6. Encourage patients to ask questions and to express concerns/fears

7. Review preoperative instructions (written)

8. Review postoperative instructions (give in writing)

9. Review postoperative danger signs

    a. Fever (> 100.4 °F)

    b. Dizziness with fainting

    c. Abdominal pain that is persistent or increasing

    d. Bleeding or fluid from incision

10. Review potential complications and danger signs of ectopic pregnancy (see Ectopic Pregnancy section)

11. Provide realistic information regarding chances of reversal upon request

    a. Depends upon procedure performed

    b. 4 cm of healthy fallopian tube must remain

Male Sterilization

■ Description and Efficacy

1. Vasectomy—a simple outpatient procedure that can be performed

quickly, safely and cost-effectively under local anesthesia

2. The vas deferens are incised, each end is then either fulgurated or ligated to prevent passage of sperm

3. Recent surgical modification

    a. Open-ended vasectomy

        (1) Testicular end of vas is left open

        (2) Abdominal end is fulgurated

        (3) Fewer postoperative complications

        (4) Increased failure rate

        (5) Higher success rates for reversal

    b. No-scalpel vasectomy

        (1) Reaches the vas through puncture in scrotum, rather than scalpel incision

        (2) Carries lower complication rate, especially hematomas

4. Failure rate of male sterilization is 1:600

5. Sterilization should be considered permanent

- Contraindications: Same as for Female Sterilization
- Complications

    1. Mortality extremely low—1 death in 300,000 procedures

    2. Hematoma

    3. Infection

    4. Epididymitis

    5. Granuloma

    6. Failure

- Risk Factor Screening

    1. History

        a. Past medical history

        b. Current acute or chronic illnesses

        c. Current medications

        d. Allergies to local anesthetics, analgesic agents, antibiotics, pain medications and other drugs

   e. Current substance use (tobacco, alcohol, street drugs)

   f. Sexual history, including STDs

2. Contraindications

   a. Local skin infection

   b. Varicocele, large hydrocele, inguinal hernia, scar tissue from previous surgery

   c. Special precautions with clotting disorders, diabetes, and recent CAD

3. Physical examination

   a. Vital signs

   b. Head, ears, eyes, nose, throat

   c. Heart/lungs

   d. Abdomen

   e. Musculoskeletal/Neuro

   f. Thorough genital examination

   g. Rectal/prostate

4. Laboratory tests (not usually done)

   a. Hematocrit

   b. Urinalysis

   c. Clotting times

   d. STD screening (optional)

   e. HIV test (optional)

- General Considerations

1. Same as 1 to 8 under Female Sterilization

2. Review postoperative danger signs

   a. Fever (> 100.4 °F)

   b. Bleeding or pus from incision site

   c. Excessive pain or swelling

3. Emphasize need for sperm analysis before method can be relied upon

4. Provide realistic information regarding chances of reversal upon request

Menopause

- Definition: Permanent cessation of menstrual activity either as a normal part of aging or as a result of surgical removal of both ovaries
- Etiology/Incidence
    1. During the climacteric (transitional phase beginning before menopause and continuing after it, during which a woman passes from her reproductive stage)
        a. The number of maturing ovarian follicles gradually decreases
        b. The ovaries no longer respond to pituitary stimulating hormones so estrogen levels drop, but FSH and LH production increases
        c. Fertility declines and menstrual flow diminishes
    2. Menstrual cessation occurs between 45 and 55 years, average is 51 years
    3. Cessation prior to 40 is usually considered premature menopause
    4. Estrogen deficiency increases women's risk for cardiovascular disease and osteoporosis; it is also responsible for the majority of symptoms or problems associated with menopause
- Signs and Symptoms of Estrogen Deficiency
    1. Vulva
        a. Atrophy
        b. Pruritus
        c. Thinning of pubic hair
    2. Vagina
        a. Dyspareunia due to decreased lubrication
        b. Blood-stained discharge
        c. Vaginitis
        d. Dryness
        e. Loss of rugae
        f. Vaginal ph more alkaline

3. Bladder/Urethra

   a. Atrophy

   b. Cystitis

   c. Frequency/urgency

   d. Stress incontinence

4. Uterus

   a. Loss of muscle tone

   b. Possible uterovaginal prolapse

5. Skin

   a. Dryness

   b. Hyperpigmentation/hypopigmentation

   c. Decreased sweat and sebaceous gland activity

6. Cardiovascular

   a. Atherosclerosis

   b. Coronary artery disease

7. Skeleton—osteoporosis

8. Breasts

   a. Size reduction

   b. Loss of tone

9. Neuroendocrine

   a. Vasomotor instability (hot flashes/night sweats)

   b. Sleep disturbances

   c. Psychological disturbances (mood changes, depression, anxiety)

- Differential Diagnosis

   1. May include

      a. Pregnancy

      b. Endometrial cancer if bleeding present

      c. Other causes of

         (1) Vaginitis

         (2) Cystitis

      (3)   Stress incontinence

      (4)   Psychological distress

- Physical Findings

  1. A full history and physical (including blood pressure, breast examination, pelvic examination, Pap smear and mammogram) should be performed

  2. Genitourinary atrophy

  3. Skin—some degree of atrophy and loss of collagen

  4. Kyphosis—if osteoporosis present

  5. See Signs and Symptoms

- Diagnostic Tests/Findings

  1. Pregnancy test—negative (if suspected)

  2. Vaginal cytologic examination (Pap smear)—low estrogen effect with predominantly parabasal cells

  3. Progesterone challenge test—absence of uterine bleeding is considered a negative response

  4. Plasma FSH (> 40 mIu/ml; LH levels also increased)

- Management/Treatment

  1. Diet, exercise, stress management, calcium supplements and hormone replacement therapy (HRT) should be discussed

  2. Minimum daily calcium requirements

     a. Premenopausal and menopausal women on HRT—1,000 mg daily

     b. Postmenopausal women not on HRT—1,500 mg daily

  3. Hormone replacement therapy

     a. Estrogens—Conjugated estrogens, 0.3 to 0.625 mg or estradiol, 0.5 to 1 mg or estrone sulfate, 0.625 mg orally daily; or estradiol (Estraderm) skin patches 0.05 to 0.1 mg (change twice weekly). Estrogen may be taken on days 1 to 25 each month or daily

     b. Progestins—cyclic or continuous with estrogen; prevents endometrial hyperplasia or cancer; not required if patient has had hysterectomy

  4. Contraindications to HRT

    a. Estrogens—known or suspected cancer of the breast, known or suspected estrogen-dependent neoplasia, known or suspected pregnancy, undiagnosed abnormal genital bleeding, past or present history of thrombophlebitis or thromboembolic disorders

    b. Progestogens—past or present history of thrombophlebitis, thromboembolic disorders or cerebral apoplexy, liver dysfunction or disease, known or suspected carcinoma of the breast, undiagnosed vaginal bleeding, missed abortion, pregnancy

- General Considerations

  1. Pharmacological and non-pharmacological options should be thoroughly discussed with the patient prior to establishment of a treatment regimen. The patient's individual symptoms and concerns guide development of the plan

  2. Thoroughly discuss side-effects of HRT if prescribed

  3. Review/teach breast self-examination

  4. Encourage patient to discuss concerns/fears

  5. Emphasize importance of follow-up appointments

     a. Standard physical examination for those on HRT to include annual mammogram, pelvic examination, blood pressure, height measurement

     b. Endometrial examination (vaginal ultrasound and endometrial biopsy) for patients with abnormal vaginal bleeding beyond 3 to 6 months of initiating HRT

  6. Education on the variety of nondrug menopausal symptom relief methods, strategies

  7. Ginseng has estrogen-like effects, thus should be avoided in patients with contraindications to estrogen

- Note: Ambulatory obstetrics: *Protocols for nurse practitioners/nurse midwives* (1990) by W. L. Star, M. T. Shannon, L. N. Sammons, L. L. Lommel & I. Gutierrez and *Contraceptive technology* by R. A. Hatcher, J. Trussell, F. H. Stewart, G. K. Stewart, D. Kowal, F. Guest, W. Cates & M. Policar (1994) served as the primary reference for this chapter.

Questions

Select the best answer

1. Which of the following is not one of the findings in the first trimester of pregnancy?
   a. Goodell's sign
   b. Urinary frequency/urgency
   c. Round ligament pain
   d. Chadwick's sign

2. Which of the following statements is correct regarding the second trimester of pregnancy?
   a. Weight gain is about 11 lb
   b. Fundus palpable halfway between umbilicus and xiphoid process
   c. Fetal heart tones are first audible with doppler
   d. Lightening occurs

3. In making the diagnosis of pregnancy, which of the following conditions should be ruled-out?
   a. Urinary tract infection
   b. Myomas
   c. Gastrointestinal problems
   d. All the above

4. A woman in her 30th week of pregnancy could experience
   a. Her fundus to be at the xiphoid process
   b. Lightening
   c. Secretion of colostrum
   d. Bloody show

5. Which of the following is considered to be a common complaint of pregnancy?
   a. Arthralgia
   b. Varicosities
   c. Cramping
   d. Dysuria

6. Which of the following complications are most likely to be problematic in the first trimester?
   a. Incompetent cervix
   b. Bleeding
   c. Placenta previa
   d. None of the above

7. Which of the following statements is incorrect regarding pregnancy?

   a. Work stress is a risk factor for pregnancy.
   b. Vaginal discharge is a common complaint during pregnancy
   c. Vaginal ultrasound is more sensitive in detecting an ectopic pregnancy than transabdominal methods
   d. Softening of cervix occurs by the 28th week

8. How is the EDC determined using Nägele's rule?
   a. Subtract 7 days and add 9 months from the start of the LNMP
   b. Nine months plus 7 days from the start of the LNMP
   c. Add 9 months from the start of the LNMP
   d. Subtract 7 plus 5 to the last day of the LNMP and count back 3 months

9. Which of the following statements is true regarding diagnostic testing during pregnancy?
   a. At weeks 14 to 24 chorionic villous sampling is done when indicated for genetic reasons
   b. At weeks 16 to 18 alpha-fetoprotein determination in maternal blood
   c. At weeks 15 to 18 screen for gestational diabetes
   d. At 28 weeks, culture cervix for group B β-hemolytic streptococci

10. Which of the following should be avoided during pregnancy?
   a. A daily caloric increase of 300 k cal
   b. Exercise ad lib
   c. Douching
   d. Intercourse during last trimester

11. A woman with an ectopic pregnancy is likely to have which of the following?
   a. Pregnancy located in the ovary
   b. Hypertension
   c. Referred shoulder pain
   d. Fever with nausea and/or vomiting

12. All of the following conditions are thought to increase a woman's chances of having an ectopic pregnancy EXCEPT
   a. Past history of pelvic inflammatory disease
   b. Former pregnancy with IUD
   c. Uterine myoma
   d. Previous ectopic pregnancy

13. What percentage of women with an ectopic pregnancy will have a positive serum Beta hCG test?
   a. 50%
   b. 95%
   c. 75%

d. 100%

14. Treatment of ectopic pregnancy includes
   a. Tubal expression
   b. Salpingectomy
   c. Methotrexate
   d. All of the above

15. Inevitable abortion refers to
   a. Death of the embryo or fetus without expulsion
   b. Gross rupture of membranes in the presence of cervical dilatation
   c. Expulsion of products of conception without medical or mechanical intervention
   d. Presence of bleeding and uterine cramping without cervical dilation

16. All of the following conditions can lead to recurrent abortions except
   a. Chromosomal aberrations
   b. IUD use
   c. Infection
   d. Uterine anomalies

17. Which of the following complications could occur after an induced abortion?
   a. Continuing pregnancy
   b. Cervical laceration
   c. Infertility
   d. All the above

18. Post-abortion danger signs include
   a. Abdominal pain
   b. Nausea and vomiting
   c. Dysuria
   d. Shortness of breath

19. Typical failure rates for combined oral contraceptives approach
   a. 3%
   b. 0.1%
   c. 0.5%
   d. 1%

20. Estrogen in oral contraceptives has all of the following effects except
   a. Acceleration ovum transport
   b. A decrease in HDL and LDL increase
   c. Suppresses FSH and LH
   d. Alteration of endometrial lining

21. A woman taking combined high dose (> 50 mcg estrogen) oral contraceptives has

an increased chance of developing
a. Ovarian cancer
b. Endometrial cancer
c. Breast cancer
d. Myocardial infarction

22. All of the following statements regarding oral contraceptives are correct except
a. Minipills may be taken by breastfeeding women
b. Healthy women who do not smoke may continue to use low-dose combination pills until menopause
c. Provides some protection against STDs
d. Taking combined oral contraceptives provides some protection against PID

23. The Norplant implant system is effective for
a. 5 years
b. 3 years
c. Indefinitely
d. 1 year

24. A woman who is considering using the Norplant system should be counseled regarding
a. Failure rate of 3%
b. Potential menstrual irregularities
c. Risk of developing hypertension
d. Intensification of ovulatory pain

25. The following statements regarding Norplant implants are correct except
a. Nervousness is a potential side effect
b. The majority of minor side effects diminish during the first 3 to 6 months of use
c. Effectiveness correlated to body weight of user
d. Norplant implants become effective within 24 hours of insertion

26. A woman with an IUD presents at the clinic requesting a pregnancy test, which is positive. What percentage of pregnancies spontaneously abort if the IUD is left in situ?
a. 50%
b. 20%
c. 30%
d. 40%

27. IUDs marketed in the U.S. have which of the following similar characteristics?
a. Chance of developing ectopic pregnancy is increased
b. Life-span is 10 years
c. Incidence of uterine perforation is 1 in 2,500

d. Allergy to copper is a contraindication

28. Complications associated with IUD use include all of the following except
    a. Infection
    b. Pregnancy
    c. Dysmenorrhea
    d. Ovarian cyst development

29. When counseling a patient who has an IUD, emphasis should be placed on which of the following statements?
    a. Need to change IUD every 2 to 3 years
    b. Risk factors associated with infection
    c. Risk of developing anemia
    d. Pain control for dysmenorrhea

30. Which of the following statements regarding the diaphragm is correct? The diaphragm
    a. Has a 25% failure rate
    b. Can be used with or without contraceptive jelly/creme
    c. Is an intermittent form of contraception
    d. Is contraindicated if the patient has multiple sex partners

31. The following statements regarding diaphragms are correct except
    a. Diaphragms must be inserted within 1 hour of coitus to be most effective
    b. The dome-shaped cup is made of latex rubber
    c. An increased incidence of urinary tract infections is associated with diaphragm use
    d. There are no absolute contraindications for diaphragm use except latex allergy

32. When counseling a patient who plans to use a diaphragm, which of the following areas regarding toxic shock syndrome (TSS) should be reviewed?
    a. TSS is a rare occurrence with diaphragm users
    b. It may mimic flu-like symptoms (fever, nausea, diarrhea)
    c. TSS may develop if the diaphragm is left in place longer than the recommended time interval
    d. All the above

33. Negative side effects or characteristics associated with the vaginal sponge do not include which of the following?
    a. The sponge may be difficult to remove from the vagina
    b. Local skin irritation may develop secondary to use
    c. It is difficult to know what size to purchase, since it is OTC
    d. It should not be used if the woman is spotting or menstruating

34. First-year failure rates for the vaginal sponge range from

    a. 10%-15%
    b. 18%-36%
    c. 20%-25%
    d. 15%-20%

35. Since the vaginal sponge can be purchased over-the-counter, which of the following circumstances may arise?
    a. The patient may not be as likely to obtain a Pap smear
    b. Incorrect usage secondary to misunderstanding the written instructions
    c. The risk of toxic shock syndrome may not be appreciated and its danger signs may not be recognized
    d. All of the above

36. What is usually responsible for the contraceptive effect of vaginal spermicide?
    a. Benzoyl oxide
    b. Inert base
    c. Nonoxynol-9
    d. None of the above

37. The following statements about vaginal spermicide are correct except
    a. First-year failure rates range from 6% to 21%
    b. Spermicides provide some protection against STDs
    c. The spermicidal product is best inserted into the vagina immediately following coitus
    d. Is more effective if used with another method, i.e., condoms

38. Which of the following is the most common spermicidal chemical used in spermicides?
    a. Nonoxynol-9
    b. Octoxynol
    c. Surfactant
    d. Inert Base

39. The following statements about condoms are correct except
    a. Condom use has decreased over the past 5 years
    b. Latex condoms provide greater STD/HIV protection than "skin" condoms
    c. Spermicides may be added to the inner or outer surfaces
    d. Women may have an allergic to rubber condoms

40. The risk of condom breakage can be reduced by
    a. Using a petroleum-based lubricant
    b. Leaving a 1/2" empty space at tip of condom
    c. Using a condom made from "skin" rather than rubber
    d. Using a condom that is made from thinner rubber

41. The first-year failure rates for condom use range from

a. 1%-5%
b. 3%-12%
c. 5%-10%
d. 3%-18%

42. The most important point to cover when counseling a woman who wants a sterilization is
    a. The failure rate is 1:400
    b. The procedure should be viewed as being permanent
    c. Fatality rates are low, 3 per 100,000 women
    d. The procedural technique

43. A contraindication for female sterilization is
    a. Inability to give informed consent
    b. Past history of ectopic pregnancy
    c. Nulliparity
    d. Young age

44. The most common complication from female sterilization is
    a. Hemorrhage
    b. Infection
    c. Anesthesia complications
    d. Ectopic pregnancy

45. When compared to female sterilization procedures, male procedures
    a. Have slightly lower failure rates
    b. Are more expensive
    c. Have higher mortality rates
    d. Are more complex

46. All of the following conditions are potential complications associated with a vasectomy except
    a. Hematoma
    b. Prostatitis
    c. Epididymitis
    d. Failure

47. Which of the following vasectomy postoperative danger signs should be reported?
    a. Fever < 100 °F
    b. Bleeding at incision site
    c. Mild incisional pain
    d. All of the above

48. Which of the following statements regarding menopause is incorrect?

    a. FSH and LH production increases
    b. Estrogen deficiency is responsible for the majority of symptoms
    c. Progesterone challenge test is positive
    d. Number of maturing follicles gradually decreases

49. The average age a woman experiences menopause is
    a. 45 years
    b. 40 years
    c. 51 years
    d. 55 years

50. Which of the following conditions characterizes the climacteric?
    a. Dyspareunia
    b. Dryness of skin
    c. Sleep disturbances
    d. All the above

51. Depo-provera is used
    a. To treat menopause
    b. As an adjunct in the management of female infertility
    c. As a contraceptive method
    d. To increase ovulation by stimulating FSH and LH levels

52. Depo-provera is administered
    a. By injection
    b. By transdermal method
    c. Through implant method
    d. Orally (50 mg tablets daily); alternated with estrogen 0.625 mg days 1 to 25 for women with intact uterus

53. The greatest problem with the use of natural family planning methods is
    a. Interruption of menstrual cycle with lactating women
    b. Unintended pregnancy
    c. Interference with spontaneous sexual intercourse during fertile period
    d. Obsession with implementing the method effectively

Answers

1.	c	27.	c
2.	a	28.	d
3.	d	29.	b
4.	c	30.	c
5.	b	31.	a
6.	b	32.	d
7.	d	33.	c
8.	b	34.	b
9.	b	35.	d
10.	c	36.	c
11.	c	37.	c
12.	c	38.	a
13.	d	39.	a
14.	d	40.	b
15.	b	41.	b
16.	b	42.	b
17.	d	43.	a
18.	a	44.	c
19.	a	45.	a
20.	b	46.	b
21.	d	47.	b
22.	c	48.	c
23.	a	49.	c
24.	b	50.	d
25.	b	51.	c
26.	a	52.	a
		53.	b

Bibliography

Beck, W. W. (Eds.). (1990). *Obstetrics and gynecology*. Media, PA: Harwal Publishing.

Dickey, R. P. (1993). *Managing contraceptive pill patients*. Durant, OK: Essential Medical Information Systems.

Gambrell, R. D. (1990). *Estrogen replacement therapy*. Durant, OK: Essential Medical Information Systems.

Goldzieher, Joseph W. (1989). *Hormonal contraception: Pills, injections and implants*. Durant, OK: Essential Medical Information Systems.

Hatcher, R. A., Trussell, J., Stewart, F. H., Stewart, G. K., Kowal, D., Guest, F., Cates, W., Policar, M. (1994). *Contraceptive Technology* (16th ed.). New York: Irvington Publishers.

Pritchard, J. A., MacDonald, P. C., & Gant, N. F. (1991). *Williams Obstetrics*. Norwalk, CT: Appleton-Century-Crofts.

Rakel, R. E. (Ed.). (1993). *Conn's current therapy*. Philadelphia: W. B. Saunders Company.

Rakel, R. E. (Ed.). (1990). *Textbook of family practice*. Philadelphia: W. B. Saunders Company.

Schroeder, S. A., Tierney, L. M., McPhee, S. J., Papadakis, M. A., & Krupp, M. A. (Eds.). (1992). *Current medical diagnosis & treatment*. Norwalk, CT: Appleton & Lange.

Scott, J. R., DiSaia, P. J., Hammond, C. B., & Spellacy, W. N. (1990). *Danford's obstetrics and gynecology*. Philadelphia: J. B. Lippincott Company.

Star, W. L., Shannon, M. T., Sammons, L. N., Lommel, L. L., & Gutierrez, Y. (1990). *Ambulatory obstetrics: Protocols for nurse practitioners/nurse midwives*. San Francisco, CA: School of Nursing, University of California, San Francisco.

Thomas, C. L. (1985). *Taber's cyclopedic medical dictionary*. Philadelphia: F. A. Davis Company.

U. S. Bureau of the Census, (1992). *Statistical Abstract of the United States: 1992* (112th Edition). Washington, D.C. pp. 66 and 75.

Musculoskeletal Disorders

Madeline Turkeltaub

Osteoarthritis (OA)

- Definition: Degenerative disorder of movable joints which causes deterioration of articular and new bone formation at joint surfaces.

- Etiology/Incidence
    1. Primary Osteoarthritis—occurs without obvious cause
        a. Frequency
            (1) Ten times more frequent in females than males
            (2) 85% of cases are in people between 55-64 years of age
        b. Familial tendency
        c. Obesity
        d. Postural abnormalities
        e. Joint enlargement
        f. Gait changes
    2. Secondary Osteoarthritis—results from underlying abnormality
        a. Trauma—old fracture
        b. Joint disorders—Gout, Congenital Dysplastic Hip
        c. Avascular necrosis—post trauma, post sepsis, due to use of steroids

- Signs and Symptoms
    1. Pain—stiff in morning or following inactivity, improves within 30 minutes; begins insidiously
    2. Limitation of movement in affected joint
    3. Joints most frequently involved
        a. Weight bearing
        b. Distal interphalangeal joints (DIP), Proximal interphalangeal joints (PIP)
        c. Neck, low back, hip, knee, metatarsophalangeal (MTP)

- Differential Diagnosis
    1. Other rheumatologic conditions, such as
        a. Rheumatoid arthritis

    b. Pseudogout

    c. Reiter's syndrome

    d. Arthritis of chronic ulcerative colitis

- Physical Findings

    1. Hands

        a. Heberden's nodes—enlargement of DIP joints

        b. Bouchard's nodes—equivalent to Heberden's nodes, but in PIP joints

    2. Joints

        a. Localized tenderness

        b. Crepitus on movement

        c. Bony consistency to the enlargement

    3. Neurologic—pain due to pressure on nerves by affected joints

    4. Hips—reduced internal rotation.

- Diagnostic Tests/Findings

    1. Radiogram—four cardinal radiologic features

        a. Unequal loss of joint space

        b. Osteophytes

        c. Juxta-articular sclerosis

        d. Subchondral bone

    2. Synovial fluid aspirate is usually normal

- Management/Treatment

    1. Preserving function and decreasing pain are the goals of treatment

    2. Treating biomechanical factors

        a. Weight loss

        b. Correct uneven leg length with heel wedge

        c. Use canes or crutches to decrease weight bearing on affected joint

        d. Quadriceps setting for knee involvement

        e. Cervical collar for cervical spine pain

        f. Isometric exercises for the abdominal muscles decrease

lumbosacral spine pain

3. Local measures

   a. Ice to improve range of motion (ROM) and exercise performance

   b. Moist heat to decrease muscle spasm and relieve morning stiffness.

4. Medications

   a. Aspirin

   b. Non-steroidal anti-inflammatory drugs (NSAIDS)

   a. Acetaminophen, 500 mg, 3 or 4 times a day

5. Use ASA and NSAIDs intermittently

6. Instruct on side effects of NSAIDs including

   a. Gastrointestinal intolerance

   b. Fluid retention

   c. Platelet abnormalities

   d. Hepatic and renal dysfunction

7. Surgery—refer to physician for procedures, such as fusion or joint replacement

8. Educate regarding body mechanics, muscle strengthening, and range of motion exercises

Rheumatoid Arthritis (RA)

- Definition: Chronic inflammatory disease of any synovial joint and associated tendon sheath

- Etiology/Incidence

  1. Affects 6.5 million Americans

  2. 30% of patients have mild disease with remissions and little deformity

  3. 10% have a single period of active disease with only occasional exacerbations

  4. About one-half of patients have progressive disease

  5. Affects three times as many women as men

  6. Often emerges in young adulthood—peak incidence 20s-30s

  7. Later peak in incidence occurs in 60 to 70 year olds

  8. Other diseases of joints, such as gout and OA may predispose to RA

- Signs and Symptoms

  1. Morning stiffness lasting several hours

  2. Pain—joint pain and/or stiffness develops insidiously over several weeks to months

  3. Fatigue, malaise, weakness, low-grade fever

  4. Proximal interphalangeal (PIP) and metacarpophalangeal (MCP) joints are the most commonly affected

  5. The first ROM loss is full extension

- Differential Diagnosis—joint inflammation is a prominent feature of the following conditions

  1. Ankylosing spondylitis

  2. Rheumatic fever

  3. Systemic lupus erythematosus

  4. Arthritis of inflammatory intestinal disease

  5. Psoriatic arthritis

  6. Reiter's syndrome

- Physical Findings

  1. Soft tissue swelling

     a. Most frequently in MCP joints, wrists and PIP joints

     b. Usually symmetrical

  2. Tenderness and pain on passive motion, usually no erythema

  3. Warmth at site of inflamed joint

  4. Limited range of motion at joint

  5. Permanent deformity in chronic disease

     a. Flexion contractures

     b. Subluxation

     c. Ulnar deviation of fingers at MCP joints

  6. Synovial cysts can be visualized and palpated

     a. Baker's cysts (synovial cysts of the popliteal space) are common in patients with rheumatoid arthritis

- Diagnostic Tests/Findings
    1. Erythrocyte sedimentation rate is elevated
    2. Rheumatoid factor can be isolated in 70-80% of patients with RA
    3. Antinuclear antibodies are present
    4. Radiography findings
        a. Early changes are often limited to periarticular osteoporosis
        b. In time, bony margins of joints show erosion
        c. In late stage, joint space will be narrowed
    5. Joint fluid shows inflammatory changes
    6. CBC—mild to moderate anemia
- Management/Treatment
    1. The goals of treatment are
        a. To relieve pain
        b. To relieve inflammation
        c. To maintain optimal function
        d. To prevent deformity
        e. To educate the patient
    2. Conservative management includes
        a. Education
        b. Rest
        c. Physical therapy
        d. Nonsteroidal anti-inflammatory agents
    3. If conservative management is ineffective, refer to M.D. for intra-articular corticosteroids
    4. If patient is unresponsive, additional medications from the following categories may be added
        a. Antimalarials, e.g., hydrochloroquine sulfate
        b. Gold salts—intramuscular or orally
        c. Corticosteroids (not more than 10 mg of prednisone or equivalent per day)

      d. Cytotoxic agents

  5. Education

      a. Explain what an autoimmune disease is

      b. Stress management and relaxation techniques

  6. Multidisciplinary management

      a. Physical therapy

      b. Occupational therapy

  7. Management plan for daily living

Gout

- Definition: Gout is a metabolic disease associated with abnormal accumulation of urates in the body and characterized by recurring acute arthritis. The classic gouty attack is podagra, involving the big toe.

- Etiology/Incidence

  1. 90% of patients with primary gout are men over 30 years of age

  2. The onset in women is usually age at menopause plus 20 to 30 years

  3. Due to deposition of crystals of monosodium urate (MSU)

  4. Related to either uric acid overproduction or decreased uric acid excretion

  5. Decreased uric acid excretion is the problem in 90% of patients with gout

  6. Rapid fluctuation of serum urate levels may be precipitated by alcohol and food excess; surgery, infection, diuretics or uricosuric drugs

- Signs and Symptoms

  1. Acute onset, frequently monarticular, affecting the first metatarsophalangeal joint, called Podagra

  2. Tophi due to accumulation of urate crystals may be found in ears, hands, feet

  3. Remissions and exacerbations

  4. Involved joint is swollen, tender, warm, red

  5. Temperature elevation to 39 °C

  6. May become chronic with progressive loss and disability

- Differential Diagnosis

  1. Diagnosis may be confirmed based on dramatic response to NSAIDs or colchicine

  2. Acute stage may be confused with cellulitis

  3. Pseudogout presents with similar symptoms but normal serum uric acid

  4. Chronic gout may mimic rheumatoid arthritis

  5. Chronic lead intoxication may result in attacks of gout

  6. See rheumatoid arthritis

- Physical Findings

  1. Limited, painful range of motion in affected joint

  2. Elevated temperature during acute attack

  3. Palpation of tophi in areas indicated above

  4. Affected area hot to touch

- Diagnostic Tests/Findings

  1. Synovial fluid aspirate contains monosodium urate crystals

  2. In later stages of disease, radiograph may show punched-out areas in the bone

  3. Erythrocyte sedimentation rate elevated

  4. White cell count elevated

  5. Uric acid elevated

  6. Hyperuricemia—serum urate > 7.5 mg/dL

- Management/Treatment

  1. Acute attack should be treated first, hyperuricemia later

  2. NSAIDs—indomethacin, 50 mg every 8 hours, continued until symptoms resolve

  3. Colchicine

     a. Most effective during first 24 to 48 hours

     b. Dose—0.5 to 0.6 mg orally, every hour, until pain relieved or GI symptoms occur or maximum dose of 6 mg

  4. Corticosteroids—used for patients who cannot tolerate NSAIDs

  5. Analgesics—codeine or meperidine may be indicated; ASA is

contraindicated

6. Bed rest—for 24 hours after acute attack subsides

7. Diet to maintain daily output of 2000 cc of urine; avoid obesity and prevent dehydration; low purine diet has little effect on blood levels

8. Support is needed during remissions for patient to maintain medical regimen, including

   a. Diet instruction

   b. Prophylactic medication

      (1) Uricosuric drugs—probenecid, 0.5 g/day, with gradual increase to 1 to 2 g/day; avoid use with salicylates

      (2) Allopurinol—100 mg/day for one week initially, then 200 to 300 mg/daily; observe for rash associated with hypersensitivity

9. Comfort may be obtained from cold or hot compresses and elevation of affected area during acute attack.

Osteoporosis

- Definition: Demineralization of bone, resulting in a decrease in bone mass with an otherwise normal structural matrix

- Etiology/Incidence

   1. Most common metabolic bone disease in the U.S.

   2. Clinically evident in middle years and beyond

   3. Affects women more frequently than men, especially postmenopausal women

   4. Caucasians have highest incidence, then orientals, then blacks

   5. Most frequently associated with

      a. Lack of estrogen (postmenopausal or postoophorectomy)

      b. Lack of activity (immobilization)

      c. Malabsorption (postgastrectomy, lactase deficiency)

      d. Vitamin D deficiency

- Signs and Symptoms

   1. Loss of height

   2. Kyphosis

3. Backache

4. Spontaneous fracture or collapse of vertebrae

- Differential Diagnosis: Bone demineralization may also be associated with

  1. Adrenal cortical excess

  2. Hyperthyroidism

  3. Metabolic bone disease, such as hyperparathyroidism and osteomalacia

  4. Myeloma

  5. Metastatic bone disease

- Physical Findings

  1. There may be no specific physical findings, unless a fracture is present

  2. Loss of height is most common

  3. Kyphosis ("dowager's hump") is evident with vertebral compression fractures

- Diagnostic Tests/Findings

  1. Serum calcium, phosphorus and alkaline phosphatase are within normal limits.

  2. Radiography will show osteopenia when bone mass is reduced by 25 to 30%

  3. Lateral radiograph of spine might show

     a. Anterior wedging of thoracic vertebral bodies

     b. Widening intervertebral bodies

  4. Dual-photon absorptiometry more sensitive to bone loss

  5. Additional laboratory tests may be ordered for older patients, including

     a. Albumin (to allow interpretation of serum calcium)

     b. Serum and urine protein electrophoresis (differentiate multiple myeloma)

     c. BUN and creatinine (to rule out chronic renal disease)

- Management/Treatment: Treatment of established osteoporosis must take into consideration the severity of disease, age and coexisting medical problems.

  1. Treatment for acute back pain includes

     a. Rest

     b. Analgesia

     c. External support

     d. Heat

     e. Stool softeners

2. Treatment to prevent osteoporosis includes

     a. Balanced diet—protein not to exceed 20% of total calories; diet counseling to include dietary sources high in calcium and low in fat

     b. Exercise—weight bearing; encourage life style changes related to the importance of exercise; provide active or passive range of motion for bedridden patients

     c. Hormone replacement therapy (HRT) in postmenopausal women or postoophorectomy

          (1) Estrogen and progestin in women with intact uterus

          (2) Estrogen may be used alone in women without uterus

          (3) HRT should be initiated as soon as possible following menopause

     d. Adequate calcium intake 1000 mg daily for women on hormone replacement therapy (HRT); 1500 mg daily for women who are not on HRT. Calcium may be obtained through dietary sources or through calcium supplements

3. Elderly patients must be protected from falls—educate family regarding safe environment

4. Alcohol and smoking should be avoided

5. Regular follow-up with mammogram and pelvic examination for women on HRT

6. Educate teens and young women regarding adequate calcium intake and dangers of excess exercise

Low Back Pain (LBP)

- Definition: Acute, chronic or recurrent pain occurring in the area of the lumbosacral spine and associated musculoskeletal areas

- Etiology/Incidence

1.   80% of the population will experience low back pain sometime during their lifetime

2.   Low back pain from trauma or mechanical causes is most common from 30 to 40 years of age

3.   Most acute neck or back pain is caused by muscle strain and spasm of the paraspinal muscle groups

4.   LBP is a self limited condition

   a.   40% remit in one week

   b.   60 to 80% in three weeks

   c.   90% in two months

- Signs and Symptoms

   1.   Pain

   2.   Numbness

   3.   Weakness

   4.   Bowel and bladder dysfunction

- Differential Diagnosis

   1.   Congenital disorders, e.g., asymmetry

   2.   Tumors involving nerve roots or meninges

   3.   Trauma

      a.   Lumbar strain

      b.   Compression fracture

   4.   Spondylosis and spondylolisthesis

   5.   Metabolic disorders, e.g., osteoporosis

   6.   Arthritis of the spine

   7.   Degenerative diseases

   8.   Herniated nucleus pulposus

   9.   Infections

   10. Mechanical causes, e.g., weak abdominal muscles, pelvic tumors, prostate disease

   11. Psychogenic

- Physical Findings

1. Postural deformity of the spine

2. Gait and heel-and-toe walking will detect weakness of gastrocnemius and tibialis anterior muscles

3. Straight leg raising—pain on early arc is associated with L_5-S_1 disc

4. Flexing thigh on pelvis (femoral stretch test)—associated with L_3 problems

5. Neurologic testing for motor weakness and sensory deficits

6. Local tenderness or spasm on palpation

7. Specific lesion-isolating findings

    a. L_{3-4} disc

        (1) Pain in lower back, hip, anterior leg to great toe

        (2) Numbness in anteromedial thigh and knee

        (3) Weakness in quadriceps leading to atrophy

        (4) Diminished patellar reflex

    b. L_{4-5} disc

        (1) Pain over sacroiliac joint, hip, lateral thigh

        (2) Numbness of lateral leg, web of great toe

        (3) Weakness on dorsiflexion, difficulty walking on heels

        (4) Reflexes usually unchanged

    c. L_5-S_1 disc

        (1) Pain over sacroiliac joint, hip, back of thigh and leg to heel

        (2) Numbness in back of calf and lateral foot to small toe

        (3) Difficulty walking on toes

        (4) Atrophy of gastrocnemius

        (5) Diminished or absent Achilles tendon reflex

- Diagnostic Tests/Findings

    1. Begin with standard radiography—AP, lateral and oblique to determine lumbar alignment, vertebral body side, bone density.

    2. CT Scan—can detect lateral entrapment of spinal nerve roots

    3. MRI—provides early detection of disc degeneration. Can be used in

pregnant women.

■ Management/Treatment: Key elements include

1. Bed rest—length depends on patient's response

2. Analgesia

    a. Salicylates or acetaminophen

    b. Nonsteroidal anti-inflammatory drugs

    c. Occasionally, opiates may be required

3. Muscle relaxants

    a. Limit use to 1 to 2 weeks

    b. Avoid in older patients

4. Patient education

    a. Good body mechanics

    b. Diet

    c. Appropriate exercise

    d. Sleeping posture

5. Corsets

6. Traction

7. Transcutaneous electrical nerve stimulation (TENS)

8. Back and abdominal exercises are indicated for prevention and recurrences. Contraindicated during acute episode

9. Back massage

10. Many times there is a psychosocial overlay—a psychosocial assessment should be conducted for

    a. Stress

    b. Depression

    c. Domestic violence

    d. Inadequate coping ability

    e. Marriage/family problems

11. Encourage limited early return to work

12. Stress management

Bursitis

- Definition: Inflammation of the synovial membrane lining of a bursal sac; There are more than 150 bursae throughout the body
- Etiology/Incidence
    1. Occurs most commonly in middle and old age, following trauma or unaccustomed repetitive use of the part
    2. Infection in a joint space
    3. Inflammation as part of a systemic process, such as rheumatoid arthritis or gout
    4. Most common locations
        a. Subdeltoid
        b. Olecranon
        c. Ischial
        d. Prepatellar
- Signs and Symptoms
    1. Abrupt onset of pain which increases on motion (superficial)
    2. Local tenderness, erythema
    3. Regional tenderness and limited motion (deep bursitis)
- Differential Diagnosis
    1. Rheumatoid arthritis
    2. Gout or pseudogout
    3. Septic arthritis
- Physical Findings
    1. Restriction of movement
    2. Tenderness over rotator cuff
    3. Swelling and redness (prepatellar/olecranon)
- Diagnostic Tests/Findings
    1. Aspirate fluid with an 18 gauge needle and request laboratory analysis
        a. Culture
        b. WBC count—elevation is associated with bacterial infection

      c. RBC count—associated with trauma

      d. Glucose—decreased with bacterial infection

      e. Crystals—associated with microcrystalline bursitis

      f. Mucin clot—poor clot associated with bacterial infection

- Management/Treatment

    1. If bursitis is traumatic

      a. Splint part

      b. Apply heat 30 minutes t.i.d. or q.i.d.

      c. ASA or NSAID—Naproxen 250 mg b.i.d. or t.i.d.

    2. If symptoms recur and fluid reaccumulates inject long acting corticosteroids into bursa

    3. If septic bursitis

      a. Incision and drainage

      b. Parenteral antibiotics

    4. Education regarding care of injured part

      a. Ice for first 24 hours

      b. After swelling is stabilized, warm, moist heat several times daily

Epicondylitis (Tennis Elbow)

- Definition: Inflammation in the region of the lateral epicondyle of the humerus at the origin of the common extensor muscles

- Etiology/Incidence

    1. Specific pathogenesis of tennis elbow is not known

    2. Occurs most frequently in the dominant extremity during mid-life (may be athletic or work related)

- Signs and Symptoms

    1. Pain exacerbated by constant motion of the forearm and twisting motions

    2. Gradual onset of dull pain along lateral aspect of elbow

    3. Point tenderness over the epicondyle

    4. Limited motion

- Differential Diagnosis
    1. Rheumatoid arthritis
    2. Gout
    3. Referred pain from cervical spine disease
- Physical Findings
    1. Burning or aching pain with grasping or lifting
    2. Point tenderness present at or just distal to lateral epicondyle
- Diagnostic Tests/Findings
    1. Radiographs—usually normal or small calcium deposits
- Management/Treatment
    1. Pain relief
        a. Mild analgesics
        b. Rest
        c. Ice to tendon
    2. Tennis elbow band to remove tension on epicondyle
    3. Peri-tendon cortisone injection
    4. For continued pain
        a. Immobilize for 6 to 8 weeks in a long arm cast with 90° elbow flexion
        b. Physical therapy to restore strength and motion when cast is removed
    5. Reinforce an exercise program to condition muscle groups in the forearm and wrist
    6. If associated with a sport, evaluate whether improper technique was responsible for injury

Carpal Tunnel Syndrome

- Definition: Median nerve compression of the wrist beneath the transverse carpal ligament
- Etiology/Incidence
    1. Related to repeated forceful wrist flexion
    2. More common in women

3. Frequently involves dominant hand
4. May be associated with
   a. Pregnancy
   b. Endoneural edema in diabetes mellitus
   c. Thyroid disease
   d. Occupational activities

■ Signs and Symptoms
1. Burning, tingling, numbness sensation along the distribution of the median nerve
2. Pain exacerbated on dorsiflexion of wrist
3. Night pain that interferes with sleep
4. Clumsiness in performing fine hand movements
5. May be uni- or bilateral

■ Differential Diagnosis
1. Compression syndromes of the median nerve
2. Mononeuritis multiplex

■ Physical Findings
1. Decreased two point discrimination on affected side
2. Positive Tinel's sign—sensation of electric shock on percussion of volar aspect of wrist
3. Positive Phalen's sign—pain and/or paresthesias when hands are held in forced flexion for 30 to 60 seconds
4. Decreased sensation and muscle atrophy of thenar eminence

■ Diagnostic Tests/Findings
1. Electromyography
2. Segmental sensory and motor conduction testing

■ Management/Treatment
1. Elevate extremity
2. Splinting hand and forearm
3. Injection of corticosteroids into carpal tunnel, if bursitis is involved

4. Refer to M.D. for surgical intervention

5. Notification of health care provider if symptoms increase

   a. Numbness and tingling persists

   b. Sensation in fingers decreases

6. Take NSAID with food and report any gastric distress

7. Consideration of occupational changes if appropriate

Knee pain

- Definition: Knee pain is due to mechanical, inflammatory and/or degenerative problems

- Etiology/Incidence

  1. Trauma

  2. Most frequently exercise related condition

  3. Tears of medial meniscus are 10 times more common than lateral meniscus

- Signs and Symptoms

  1. Locking—most frequently indicative of meniscal tear or loose bodies

   2. "Giving way" or "buckling"—related to patella dislocation or ligamentous instability

  3. Effusions around knee—associated with hemarthrosis and anterior cruciate ligament; fluid under patella noted on ballottement

  4. Crepitus

- Differential Diagnosis

  1. Single painful knee with minimal edema

     a. Dislocated patella

     b. Degenerative joint disease (DJD)

     c. Prepatellar bursitis

  2. Single edematous knee

     a. Baker's cyst

     b. Torn ligaments

     c. Loose bodies

    d. Meniscal tears

- Physical Findings—the physical examination is confirmatory, following a careful history.

    1. McMurray's test—a palpable or audible click when knee is raised slowly with foot externally rotated. The examiner's hand rests on the joint line. Positive = medial meniscal injuries

    2. Anterior drawer test—positive = anterior cruciate ligament tear

    3. Pain on resisted knee extension

- Diagnostic Tests/Findings

    1. Radiographs of knees—AP and lateral

    2. Laboratory examination would be indicated if arthritis suspected.

- Management/Treatment

    1. Rest, cold pack, immobilization

    2. NSAIDs

    3. ROM of knee, if possible, to prevent stiffness

    4. Quadriceps setting

    5. Aspirate effusion

    6. Review range of motion and muscle strengthening exercises

Ankle Sprain

- Definition: Sprains are associated with stretched, partially torn or completely ruptured ligaments.

- Etiology/Incidence

    1. Lateral sprains to the ankle are the most frequent sports-related injury

    2. Most commonly involved structures include the anterior talofibular and fibulocalcaneal ligaments.

    3. 10% of ankle sprains are injuries to the medial ligament, resulting from pronation and eversion of the ankle

- Signs and Symptoms

    1. Sprains are classified on a grading system of 1 through 3. Signs and symptoms are associated with each grade as follows:

        a. Grade 1—related to a stretched ligament; mild or minimal sprain

    (1)   Mild localized tenderness

    (2)   Normal range of motion

    (3)   No functional disability

  b. Grade 2—characterized by incomplete or partial rupture of ligament fibers

    (1)   Moderate to severe pain with weight bearing; difficulty in walking

    (2)   Abnormal range of motion

    (3)   Swelling and local ecchymosis

    (4)   Pain immediately after injury

  c. Grade 3—complete disruption of ligament

    (1)   Ambulation is impossible

    (2)   Resists any motion of the foot

    (3)   Marked pain, edema, hemorrhage

    (4)   Egg-shaped swelling within 2 hours of injury

- Differential Diagnosis

  1. Avulsion fractures of the malleoli or tarsal bones

  2. Epiphyseal fractures in young patients

  3. Fracture of the calcaneus

  4. Fracture of the base of the fifth metatarsal

  5. Injury to the bifurcate ligament

- Physical Findings: Drawer sign determines anterior talofibulor rupture—tibia is stablized with one hand with foot in neutral and plantar flexed position, force applied to heel with the other hand, if positive anterior displacement of talus occurs

- Diagnostic Tests/Findings

  1. Radiograph of the ankle to detect fractures

  2. Arthrography of ankle—determines site and extent of ligamentous injury

  3. MRI

- Management/Treatment: Treatment depends upon the degree of injury

1. General treatment
   a. Rest
   b. Ice—15 to 20 minutes every 1 to 2 hours for 72 hours, then begin contrast baths
   c. Compression
   d. Elevation
   e. Non-weight bearing
   f. NSAIDs for 10 to 14 days
   g. Begin ROM when asymptomatic
   h. Refer grade 3 sprains for casting
2. Rehabilitation may begin on the first day after the injury and is individualized.
   a. ROM
   b. Achilles tendon stretching
   c. Isometrics
   d. Manual resistance exercises
   e. Build up ankle strength after healing to prevent subsequent injury

Muscle Strain

- Definition: Overuse of muscle tendons, resulting in inflammation, often associated with repetitive motion. Does not include disruption of tissue
- Etiology/Incidence: Strains occur during mild stress by overusing muscle groups not usually used
- Signs and Symptoms: Pain after overuse or injury
- Differential Diagnosis
  1. Sprain
  2. Fracture
- Physical Findings
  1. Pain on range of motion
  2. Edema
  3. Ecchymosis

4. Pain of muscle strain resolves after 1 to 2 days.

■ Diagnostic Tests/Findings: Usually none indicated unless symptoms persist or to rule out suspected fracture

■ Management/Treatment

1. Rest of affected part with assistive devices, if needed

2. Ice t.i.d. for 20 minutes

3. Compression

4. Elevation

5. Analgesics

6. NSAIDs

7. Education efforts focus on prevention

8. Increase awareness of repetitive motion

9. Identify possible changes which will decrease stress on the extremity

10. Emphasize warm up and stretching before any activity—occupational or sports related

Questions

Select the best answer

1. Mr. Johnson, age 55, has developed a slight limp and pain in his right leg which is worse when first getting out of bed. These complaints are most frequently associated with

   a. Rheumatoid arthritis
   b. Osteoarthritis
   c. Gout
   d. Osteoporosis

2. On history, Mr. Johnson indicated that he had suffered a fracture of his right leg in a car accident 10 years ago. Based on this history, it is likely that his present symptoms are

   a. Unrelated
   b. Related to infection
   c. Secondary to the trauma
   d. Associated with obesity

3. On physical examination, enlargement of an 83 year old patient's distal interphalangeal joints is noted. Enlargement of these joints is known as

   a. Heberden's nodes
   b. Bouchard's nodes
   c. Tinel's sign
   d. Tenosynovitis

4. Most frequently, synovial fluid aspirate to diagnose osteoarthritis

   a. Is high in protein
   b. Has a poor mucin clot
   c. Is normal
   d. Has WBCs

5. Osteoarthritis is often associated with

   a. Systemic symptoms of disease
   b. Restricted joint motion
   c. Elevated temperature
   d. Inflammation of the proximal interphalangeal joints

6. Which of the following is not a radiological feature of osteoarthritis?

   a. Unequal loss of joint space

    b. Subchondral bone

    c. Osteophytes

    d. Osteoporosis

7. Applications of ice to arthritic joints is more frequently done to

    a. Decrease muscle spasm

    b. Improve range of motion

    c. Numb the affected extremity

    d. Reposition the joint

8. Rheumatoid arthritis is associated with

    a. Remissions and exacerbations

    b. Weight bearing joints

    c. Obesity

    d. High purine diet

9. Nonsteroidal anti-inflammatory medications are frequently used in the treatment of musculoskeletal conditions. It is important to remind a patient to

    a. Take antacids one hour after taking NSAID

    b. Exercise at least one-half hour after taking medication

    c. Take the medication at least one time per day

    d. Take NSAIDs with food

10. The incidence of rheumatoid arthritis peaks

    a. Between 20 and 30

    b. Between 60 and 70

    c. Between 30 and 60

    d. Both a and b

11. Mrs. Franklin has been complaining of fatigue and painful, hot, swollen PIP joints. Mrs. Franklin's symptoms occurred six months ago, and recurred one week ago. It would not be unusual for a CBC to show

    a. Positive rheumatoid factor

    b. Mild to moderate anemia

    c. Elevated hematocrit

    d. Elevated WBC

12. The joints most commonly affected by rheumatoid arthritis are the

    a. Proximal interphalangeal and metacarpophalangeal joints

    b. Distal interphalangeal joints

    c. Spinous processes

    d. Elbow and shoulder

13. When diagnosing rheumatoid arthritis, all of the following are potential differential diagnoses, except

    a. Reiter's syndrome
    b. Psoriasis
    c. Rheumatic fever
    d. Ankylosing spondylitis

14. The goals of treatment for rheumatoid arthritis include all of the following, except

    a. Pain relief
    b. Independence
    c. Prevention of deformity
    d. Creating dependence on medication

15. Which category of medication is not currently used for the treatment of rheumatoid arthritis?

    a. Antimalarials
    b. Gold salts
    c. Antibiotics
    d. Cytotoxic agents

16. Podagra is an example of

    a. Pseudogout
    b. Gout
    c. Osteosarcoma
    d. Septic arthritis

17. Tophi associated with gout are often found in

    a. Ear lobes
    b. Kidneys
    c. Fingernails
    d. Ankle and knee joints

18. Mr. Adams, age 55, has a history of chronic exposure to lead. He presents with pain and swelling of his left foot. These facts are both associated with

    a. Rheumatoid arthritis
    b. Gout
    c. Fracture
    d. Osteoarthritis

19. The most common metabolic bone disease in the U.S. is

    a. Rickets
    b. Scurvy

c. Osteomyelitis

d. Osteoporosis

20. When providing dietary counseling for a patient at risk for osteoporosis, it would be best to recommend

a. Baked potato and one ounce of sour cream

b. A dish of ice cream with whipped cream

c. A glass of skim milk and an apple

d. Spinach salad with oil and vinegar

21. When a patient with gout experiences mild pain, the medication which is indicated is

a. ASA

b. NSAIDs

c. Allopurinol

d. Probenecid

22. Mr. Jones, age 27, is complaining of acute onset lower back pain after helping to move a refrigerator. His pain is on the right and shoots down the back of his thigh. The intervertebral space most likely affected is

a. L_4-L_5

b. L_5-S_1

c. L_3-L_4

d. T_{10}-L_1

23. Mr. Jones's pain persists for one week. He has been treated with bedrest and NSAIDs with minimal relief. The first diagnostic test to be ordered is

a. Anteroposterior and lateral x-ray of the spine

b. MRI

c. CT scan

d. Spinal tap

24. A scan would be indicated for a patient with back pain, when

a. Severe neurological deficits are detected

b. Pain persists for more than 2 days

c. NSAIDs do not relieve pain.

d. Muscle atrophy is noted

25. Aspirate from a joint space affected by bursitis may be indicative of a bacterial infection, when

a. WBCs are decreased

b. Glucose is decreased

c. RBCs are increased

    d. Glucose is increased

26. Tennis elbow is a type of

    a. Tenosynovitis
    b. Rheumatic disease
    c. Epicondylitis
    d. Osteoarthritis

27. Mrs. Thomas was seen, complaining of pain and point tenderness in the area of her elbow which has increased since one week ago, following a day of gardening. A physical finding which differentiates the diagnosis of "tennis elbow" is

    a. A limited range of motion
    b. Burning or aching pain with lifting
    c. Inability to pronate arm
    d. Inability to push down against resistance

28. Positive Tinel's and Phalen's signs are associated with

    a. Carpal Tunnel Syndrome
    b. Torn medial meniscus
    c. Baker's cyst
    d. Epicondylitis

29. "Loose bodies" in the knee would result in the following symptom

    a. Inflammation
    b. "Click" on extension
    c. "Locking"
    d. Instability

30. Mrs. Abbott, age 32, "turned" her ankle when stepping off a curb. She immediately experienced pain on weight bearing and had limited range of motion on examination. The most likely diagnosis is

    a. Muscle strain
    b. Grade 2 ankle sprain
    c. Fractured calcaneus
    d. Grade 3 ankle sprain

Answers

1. b
2. c
3. a
4. c
5. b
6. d
7. b
8. a
9. d
10. d
11. b
12. a
13. b
14. d
15. c
16. b
17. a
18. b
19. d
20. c
21. b
22. b
23. a
24. a
25. b
26. c
27. b
28. a
29. c
30. b

Bibliography

Abrams, W. B., & Berkow, R. (Eds.). (1990). *The Merck manual of geriatrics.* Rahway, NJ: Merck & Co.

Andreoli, T. E., Carpenter, C. J., Plum, F., & Smith, Jr., L. H. (1990). *Cecil: Essentials of medicine.* Philadelphia: W. B. Saunders.

Barker, L. R., Burton, J. R., & Zieve, P. D. (Eds.). (1991). *Principles of ambulatory medicine.* Baltimore: Williams & Wilkins.

Burn, L. (1992). Backache in general practice. *The Practitioner, 236,* 1084-1087.

Goldstein, T. S. (1991). *Geriatric orthopedics.* Rockville, MD: Aspen Publishers.

Greenough, C. G. (1992). Assessment of outcome in patients with low-back pain. *Spine, 17*(1), 36-41.

Hales, T. R. (1992). Defining carpal tunnel syndrome. *American Journal of Public Health, 82*(3), 466-467.

Macfarlane, D. (1992). Osteoarthritis. *The Practitioner, 236,* 1061-1065.

Mowat, A. (1992). Soft tissue injuries. *The Practitioner, 236,* 1068-1073.

Sapira, J. D. (1990). *The art and science of bedside diagnosis.* Baltimore: Urban & Schwartzenberg.

Schroeder, S., Krupp, M. A., Tierney, Jr., L. M., & McPhee, S. J. (Eds.). (1991). *Current medical diagnosis and treatment.* Norwalk, CT: Appleton & Lange.

Silverman, S. L. (1990). Corticosteroid-induced osteoporosis: Assessment, prevention and treatment. *The Journal of Musculoskeletal Medicine, 7*(6), 14-27.

Stanley, K. L. (1991). Ankle sprains are always more than "just a sprain." *Post Graduate Medicine, 89*(1), 251-255.

Sturrock, R. (1992). Rheumatoid arthritis. *The Practitioner, 236,* 1077-1082.

Thompson, J. A., & Phelps, T. H. (1990). Repetitive strain injuries. *Postgraduate Medicine, 88*(8), 143-149.

Wilkerson, L. A. (1992). Ankle injuries in athletes. In M. M. Mellion (Ed.), *Primary care* (pp. 377-392). Philadelphia: W. B. Saunders.

Neurological Disorders

Marilyn W. Edmunds

Headaches

- Definition: Pain in the head
- Etiology/Incidence
    1. Studies show that 80 to 90% of the normal adult population reports recurrent headaches; 30 to 50% of this population has severe or disabling headaches at times; headaches rank as one of the 10 most common presenting symptoms in general practice
    2. Headaches are classified into four major groups
        a. Tension or muscle contraction headache
            (1) Exact etiology unknown
                (a) Electromyographic studies have shown no sustained muscle contraction in tender muscles nor change in blood flow to muscles (Posner, 1992)
                (b) Contraction of cervical muscles as manifestation of emotional stress may be major contributing factor
            (2) Probably most common headache in adults (90% incidence)
        b. Vascular (8% incidence)
            (1) Due to sequential changes affecting intracranial and extracranial arteries; initial stage of vasoconstriction produces brain ischemia, then vasodilation producing throbbing pain
            (2) Categories
                (a) Classic migraine with aura (10% of migraine headache episodes)
                (b) Common migraine without aura (25% incidence)
                (c) Cluster—most common in thin, cigarette-smoking men; less common than migraine
                (d) Hypertensive—occurs only in patients with very severe or episodic hypertension
                (e) Other
                    (i) Cerebral aneurysm
                    (ii) Subarachnoid hemorrhage
                    (iii) Increased intracranial pressure

    c. Traction/inflammation (2% incidence)

        (1) Disease of the bones of the cranium

        (2) Referred pain from eyes, sinuses, teeth, temporomandibular joint (TMJ), ears, back

        (3) Meningeal irritation

        (4) Temporal arteritis

    d. Miscellaneous

        (1) Tumor—incidence increases with age

        (2) Post-traumatic—increasing numbers each year due to greater societal violence

        (3) Hydrocephalus

        (4) Drugs—indomethacin, nalidixic acid, bactrim, oral contraceptives, vasodilators

■ Signs and Symptoms

    1. Headaches have in common, pain located in the head, but the presentation and accompanying symptoms help determine etiology

    2. Careful history taking often more helpful in diagnosis than physical examination or laboratory studies

    3. Prodromal symptoms may be present— flashing lights, "spots" before the eyes

    4. See Table 1 for common signs and symptoms

Table 1
Common Findings in Headaches

Type of Headache	Signs and Symptoms
Muscle contraction 1. Intermittent 2. Continuous daily	Most common in females Responds to OTC analgesics Often with accompanying depression and/or anxiety states
Vascular	Migraine have 3:2 ratio of women to men; 20-50% positive family history; onset 15-25 usually; recurrence is hallmark; several/year; less frequent and severe with age; triggered with menses, oral contraceptives, menopause, relaxation, some chemicals, e.g., alcohol, chocolate, cheeses, wines, foods with tyramine/MSG
1. Classic migraine	Classic has premonitory sensory, motor or visual disturbances; paresthesia, temporary paralysis, photophobia, irritability, nausea, confusion, arm pain or numbness
2. Common migraine	Recurrent headaches often severe; unilateral pain; usually associated with malaise, nausea, vomiting and photophobia
3. Cluster	Grouped headaches over days/weeks; sudden stabbing, burning pain in eye, orbit, cheek on one side; severe unilateral pain with rhinorrhea, nasal congestion, perspiration; agitation often pronounced
4. Hypertensive	Occurs on awakening, daily, occipital, severe often pulsatile
5. Cerebral aneurysm	Gradual, continuous, increasingly intense headache and less responsive to analgesics; coughing or sneezing may aggravate headache
6. Subarachnoid hemorrhage	Sudden, continuous pain, occipital, radiating down neck and back; severity increases with neuro signs of nuchal rigidity, fever, dizziness, vertigo, vomiting, drowsiness
Traction/inflammation 1. Disease of bones of the cranium	Pain present on palpation
2. Referred pain from eyes, sinuses, teeth, TMJ, ears	Sinus pain is dull, aching, nonpulsatile, with feeling of pressure in frontal or sub-maxillary area and behind eyes; local tenderness on palpation, worse when leaning forrward EENT disease produces constant pain, usually in the area of disease as well as in the head; pain is dull and severe
3. Meningeal irritation	Continuous headache, increasing in severity, with neurologic signs, cervical rigidity,
4. Temporal arteritis	See in 5-6th decade; episodic pain which lasts weeks; unilateral but spreading bilaterally; dull pain but may throb; tender nodules overlying arteries; increased ESR, fever, vertigo, vomiting, drowsiness; may also see Peau d'orange skin facies, telangiectasis; medical emergency as patient may lose vision permanently
5. Increased intracranial pressure	Neurological symptoms and intensity of pain parallels the extent of increased pressure
Miscellaneous 1. Tumor	Simultaneous onset of headache and focal neurological signs/symptoms or a change in mental status. Pain usually worse in a.m., unilateral, deep, steady, aching, dull pain; may awaken patient from sleep or be present on awakening
2. Post-traumatic	Within 24 hours develop dull, constant, general aching or cephalic discomfort that may wax and wane through the day; worsens over days/weeks; resolves over weeks or months
3. Hydrocephalus	Slow onset, insidious dull pain; progressive neurologic symptoms paralleling extent of pressure
4. Drugs	Related to time of drug ingestion; variable drugs lead to variable symptoms

■ Differential Diagnosis

1. Almost any disease which originates in the head or neck area may present with a headache

2. Attention should be focused upon deciding whether problem represents a benign headache or a symptom of another disease process, such as Transient ischemic attack (TIA), Cerebrovascular accident (CVA), high blood pressure (HBP), brain tumor, etc.

■ Physical Findings

1. May have normal physical examination

2. Physical abnormalities may only be present during headache

3. See Table 1 for related physical findings associated with different types of headaches

■ Diagnostic Tests/Findings

1. Baseline evaluation

   a. Complete blood count—infections, anemia

   b. Chemistry profile—metabolic problems

   c. VDRL/RPR—syphilis

   d. CT head scan or MRI head scan—only if necessary to rule out tumor, vascular lesions, hemorrhage

2. Selected studies

   a. Sedimentation rate—may be elevated in temporal arteritis, infection, malignancy

   b. Cerebral angiography—rule out vascular lesions

   c. Sinus radiographic films—rule out sinusitis

   d. Cervical spine radiographs—rule out radiculopathy

   e. Biopsy—stenotic area in temporal arteritis

   f. Arteriography—segmental stenosis

■ Management/Treatment

1. Appropriate treatment can only be prescribed once the etiology of the headache has been determined

2. As most headaches result from minor vascular problems or congestion, an initial approach for vague, recurrent headache is very conservative

treatment with analgesics or decongestants. If the complaint of headache is atypical, extremely severe, or fails to respond to more conservative treatment, extensive diagnostic evaluation and referral should be undertaken

3. Standard therapy for the major categories of headache include those listed in Table 2

Table 2
Treatment of Headaches

Type of Headache	Treatment approach
Muscle contraction	
1. Intermittent	Responds to OTC analgesic, massage, stress management, acupuncture, deep breathing, physical exercise
2. Continuous daily	Often responds to antidepressants
Vascular	
1. Classic migraine	Goal is to avoid trigger factors
	Avoid tyramine, chocolate, alcohol, MSG, caffeine, estrogen
2. Common migraine	Structured day, avoid long periods of sleep
	Stress management
	PREVENTIVE THERAPY:
	Calcium channel blockers
	Diltiazem—30-90 mg q.i.d.
	Nifedipine—10-20 mg t.i.d.
	Verapamil HCl—80 mg q.i.d.
	Beta blockers
	Atenolol—to-100 mg daily
	Metoprolol tartrate—50-100 mg daily
	Nadolol—40-160 mg daily
	Propranolol—drug of choice 20-250 mg/day in divided doses
	Tricyclic antidepressants
	Amitriptyline HCl—25-150 mg at bedtime
	Doxepin—75-100 mg at bedtime
	Nonsteroidal anti-inflammatory drugs
	Naproxen sodium—250-500 mg b.i.d.
	Ibuprofen—200-800 mg. q.i.d.
	Ergotamine tartrate—various preparations and dosages
	Miscellaneous drugs
	Antiplatelet aggregation drugs
	Aspirin 650 mg b.i.d.
	Dipyridamole Clonidine—0.1 mg b.i.d. or t.i.d. (in migraines triggered by foods)
	Cyproheptadine—4-12 mg daily
	Methysergide Maleate—4-8 mg daily (for severe intractable headaches)

Table 2
Treatment of Headaches

Type of Headache	Treatment approach
	ABORTIVE THERAPY:

	Rest in a darkened room during attacks
	Sumatriptan, drug of choice; 6 mg injected subcutaneously
	Ergotamine tartrate
	    2 mg at onset, plus one mg every half hour, maximum 6 mg/day
	    or 12 mg/week. IM or subcutaneous: 0.5-1.5 mg to 3 mg weekly.
	    Often used with analgesics
	Dihydroergotamine mesylate—1 mg IM at onset and 1 mg every hour
	    to maximum 3 mg daily and 5 mg weekly (*Facts and Comparisons*, 1993)
	Aspirin 600 mg every 4 hours
	Ibuprofen 600 mg q.i.d.
	Acetaminophen 600 mg every 4 hours
	Biofeedback

	PROPHYLACTIC THERAPY:
3. Cluster	Methysergide (drug of choice) 2 mg t.i.d. or q.i.d. Indomethacin—25-50 mg t.i.d. Prednisone—adjunct Lithium carbonate—300 mg t.i.d.
	ABORTIVE THERAPY:

	Ergotamine tartrate: oral, SL, IM, SQ
	    2 mg SL at onset and 1 mg every half hour to maximum 6 mg/day or
	    12 mg/week. IM or SQ 0.5—1.5 mg to maximum 3 mg/week
	Dihydroergotamine mesylate—1 mg IM at onset and 1 mg every hour to
	    maximum of 3 mg/day and 5 mg/week (*Facts and Comparisons, 1993*)
	Oxygen therapy for 5 minutes

4. Hypertensive	Physician referral Antihypertensive therapy
5. Other: a. Cerebral aneurysm b. Subarachnoid hemorrhage	Referral for surgery Referral

Traction/inflammation
1. Disease of bones
    of the cranium
2. Referred pain
3. Meningeal irritation
4. Temporal arteritis
	Referral
	
	Referral to dentist, EENT
	Referral
	Referral
	Steroids for at least six months:
	Prednisone 40-60 mg/day initially tapered to 10-15 per day as Erythrocyte
	    sedimentation rate (ESR) falls.

Miscellaneous 1. Tumor 2. Post-traumatic 3. Hydrocephalus 4. Drugs	Referral—monitor patient course on follow-up Accurate and precise documentation; blood levels; substitution or withdrawal of drug

■ General Considerations

1. Clues to headaches which are of significance include

   a. Any headache that becomes more continuous and intense, or becomes less responsive to analgesics

   b. Any headache that awakens a patient, decreasing after patient has been up for several hours

   c. Coughing, sneezing, straining, which aggravates persistent headache

   d. Anorexia, nausea, vomiting, which may accompany headache

   e. Complaints of significant, intense, new type of headache which has not been experienced previously

   f. Any sudden onset of headaches, especially in 50(+) year-olds

   g. Any severe, sudden onset of headache

2. Patients who present with significant headaches should be discussed with, or referred to, a specialist

3. Patient education is important in order to avoid precipitating factors, to avoid under- or over-medication, and to gain patient compliance

4. Reassure patient that most headaches are *not* symptoms of severe disease

Transient Ischemic Attacks (TIA)

■ Definition

1. Neurologic abnormalities of sudden onset and brief duration

2. Reflects dysfunction in internal carotid-middle cerebral or vertebral-basilar arterial system

3. Usually lasts less than 30 minutes but may last up to 24 hours; most TIAs resolve within an hour

■ Incidence/Etiology

1. Caused by atherosclerotic plaques leading to cerebral emboli and temporarily interrupting cerebral oxygenation; may also be caused by decreased blood flow

2. More common in men; middle-aged and elderly

3. Incidence increases with age

■ Signs and Symptoms

1. Carotid middle-cerebral

   a. Transient hemiparesis

   b. Temporary memory loss

   c. Temporary loss of vision in one eye

   d. Aphasia

2. Vertebral-basilar arterial TIA

   a. Dysarthria

   b. Diplopia

   c. Vertigo

   d. Dysphagia

   e. Unilaterial or bilateral weakness and paresthesias of the extremities

   f. Ataxia

- Physical Findings (possible in either type of TIA)

   1. Neurological examination may be normal; deep tendon reflexes may be increased for 24 hours following TIA

   2. Carotid bruit

   3. Retinal emboli may be present

   4. Atherosclerotic changes on funduscopic examination

   5. Absence or reduction of peripheral pulses in neck

- Differential Diagnosis

   1. CVA

   2. Focal epileptic seizure disorder

   3. Intracranial tumor

   4. Migraine

   5. Subdural hematoma

- Diagnostic Tests/Findings

   1. Ultrasonography or arteriography can confirm presence of stenosis and identification of involved artery

   2. CT head scan—may reveal evidence of brain tumor, CVA

- Management/Treatment

1. Underlying factors indentified first

2. Aspirin therapy in place of/or trial therapy prior to starting anticoagulants for patients with occasional TIAs

3. Antiplatelet agents, anticoagulants in those prone to cardiogenic emboli

4. Discourage use of tobacco in all forms

5. Decision needs to be made regarding how extensive a work-up should be undertaken; may represent a single event rather than a precursor to CVA

6. Reassurance to patients and family very important

Trigeminal Neuralgia (Tic Douloureux)

- Definition: Disorder of the trigeminal nerve producing sudden, lightening-like paroxysms of pain lasting seconds to minutes in the distribution of one or more divisions of the trigeminal nerve

- Etiology/Incidence

  1. In many patients no identifiable cause can be found

  2. May be caused by compression of trigeminal nerve root at entry point into brainstem

  3. Relatively common cranial nerve disorder affecting approximately 2% of the population

  4. More common in women and usually begins in the 5th or 6th decade

- Signs and Symptoms

  1. Pain occurs as brief, lightening-like stabs, which can be precipitated by touching a trigger zone

  2. Talking, eating, hot or cold blasts of air on face, brushing the teeth can serve as triggers

  3. Pain rarely lasts longer than seconds, but can occur in clusters so that patients may report pain of several hours duration

  4. Spontaneous remissions and exacerbations are common; between paroxysms of pain, patient is asymptomatic

- Differential Diagnosis

  1. Neoplasm of brainstem

  2. Vascular malformation of brainstem

3. Trauma

4. Postherpetic pain

- Physical Findings: No clinical or pathologic findings occur with trigeminal neuralgia, thus a finding of sensory abnormality or cranial nerve dysfunction requires prompt investigation for structural disease of the nervous system

- Diagnostic Tests/Findings: None indicated unless underlying disease suspected

- Management/Treatment

    1. Carbamazepine (Tegretol) is drug of choice

        a. 400 to 800 mg/day; initial dose is usually 100 mg b.i.d.

        b. Side effects include dizziness, sedation, aplastic anemia, thrombocytopenia, leukocytosis, hepatitis

    2. Phenytoin (Dilantin)—also effective but less so than carbamazepine

        a. 300 to 600 mg/day

        b. Side effects include agranulocytosis, leukopenia, aplastic anemia, hepatitis, gingival hyperplasia

    3. Surgical interventions

        a. Creating lesions of gasserian ganglion (by radiofrequency or glycerol injections); most widely applied surgical therapy; may result in partial numbness of the face

        b. Microvascular decompression—80% efficacy rate; pain may recur

        c. Purpose of above operations is to relieve pain with little or no loss of sensation

    4. Patient education

        a. Awareness of triggers

        b. Side effects and administration of medication

        c. Compliance with laboratory evaluations

Seizure Disorder

- Definition: Recurrent, spontaneous, transient paroxysms of abnormal brain activity

- Etiology/Incidence

    1. Cause may be unknown

2. Metabolic disturbances that cause seizures include acidosis, electrolyte imbalance, hypoglycemia, hypoxia, alcohol and barbiturate withdrawal

3. Extracranial causes are heart, lung, liver, kidney disorders

4. Other causes—CNS infections; convulsive or toxic agents; cerebral hypoxia; brain lesions

5. Epileptic seizures can be a natural reaction to physiologic stress or transient systemic injury, or can indicate an epileptic disorder

6. Alcohol withdrawal is probably the most common cause of new onset seizure in adults

7. Most common cause of seizure acivity in known epileptic is noncompliance with treatment regimen

- Signs and Symptoms: Depend upon degree of maturity of nervous system, location of the initial abnormal electrical discharges, manner in which these discharges spread

1. Partial seizures (focal, local)

    a. Simple partial seizures

        (1) No loss of consciousness; rarely last more than a minute

        (2) Jacksonian march movements

        (3) Speech arrest or vocalizations

        (4) Localized paresthesias or numbness

        (5) Nausea, vague light-headedness

        (6) Dreamy states; time distortion

    b. Complex partial seizures

        (1) Onset may consist of a variety of auras, e.g., unusual smell, intense emotions, sensory illusions

        (2) Impaired consciousness ranging from amnesia for ictal event to behavioral unresponsiveness

        (3) May begin with a stare at time consciousness impaired

        (4) Automatisms, e.g., lip smacking, chewing, swallowing, sucking are common

        (5) Sometimes thrashing movements of the extremities occur

        (6) Can severely disrupt daily life

2. Secondary generalized partial seizures—simple or complex seizures can progress to generalized seizures with loss of consciousness and often with convulsive motor activity

3. Primary generalized seizures

    a. Absence seizures (petit mal)

        (1) Onset usually in children (6 to 14 years of age); occasionally appear for first time in older adults

        (2) Loss of consciousness; usually lasts 5 to 30 seconds; begins and ends abruptly; seizures may be so brief as to be inapparent

        (3) Eye or muscle flutterings may occur; patient suddenly stops any activity and resumes it following attack

    b. Tonic-clonic (grand mal)

        (1) Usually preceded by aura and arrest of activity

        (2) Typically begins with a sudden cry followed by loss of consciousness

        (3) Tonic, then clonic contractions of muscles of extremities; trunk and head follow

        (4) Urinary and fecal incontinence may occur

        (5) Attack usually lasts 2 to 5 minutes

        (6) Postictal state may last 20 to 60 minutes with deep sleep, headache, muscle soreness

- Differential Diagnosis

    1. Syncope; breath-holding spells

    2. Hypoglycemia

    3. Psychomimetic drug use

    4. TIA

    5. Migraine

    6. Paroxysmal vertigo

    7. Psychogenic seizures

    8. Schizophrenia

- Physical Findings

    1. Many physical examinations will reveal negative findings between

seizures; however, evidence of systemic diseases can also be found and requires intensive investigation

2. Asymmetry in size of hands, feet and face may indicate abnormality in one cerebral hemisphere

3. Clumsiness, hyperreflexia and marked impairment suggest secondary rather than primary seizure disorder

4. Focal neurologic findings and changes in mental status are indicative of partial epilepsy

- Diagnostic Tests/Findings

1. No diagnostic hematologic or chemical laboratory tracers for epilepsy

2. Skull films—fracture or calcification

3. CT head scan—tumor, hemorrhage, edema, CVA

4. Electroencephalogram—seizure activity

    a. General or focal epileptiform activity

    b. Asymmetry of basic rhythms

    c. Focal slow waves

    d. Diffuse slowing of waves

    e. EEG may be normal when patient is asymptomatic

5. Lumbar puncture—infectious processes

6. 24-hour electroencephalogram—document seizure activity

7. Psychometric studies—verify existence of focal or diffuse brain disturbance

8. Serum prolactin—after tonic-clonic or complex partial seizure, serum prolactin rises 2 to 3 times above upper limits of normal in more than 80% of cases and remains elevated for 10 to 60 minutes following the seizure

- Management/Treatment

1. Neurology referral

2. CBC, liver function tests, BUN and urinalysis prior to antiepileptic drug therapy to establish baseline levels

3. Pharmacologic therapy principles

    a. Many antiepileptic drugs available; best to become familiar with and use few that are most effective for various seizure types

   b. Therapy is based upon

      (1)   Obtaining accurate diagnosis of seizure type or epileptic syndrome

      (2)   Selecting most appropriate drug

      (3)   Monitoring drug serum levels with patient's response and toxicity levels

4.   Drugs (See Table 3)

   a. Carbamazepine (Tegretol)—principal uses in tonic-clonic, partial

      (1)   Give 600 to 1200 mg/day

      (2)   Major side effects—nausea, ataxia, blurred vision, lethargy, hepatotoxicity, fluid retention

   b. Phenytoin sodium (Dilantin)—principal uses in tonic-clonic, partial

      (1)   Give 300 to 400 mg/day (3 to 5 mg/kg)

      (2)   Major side effects—ataxia, dysarthria, lethargy, blood dyscrasias, osteomalacia, hirsutism, gingival hyperplasia, coarsening of features

   c. Diazepam (Valium)

      (1)   Acute emergency management

      (2)   Give 5 to 10 mg IV initially; may be repeated if necessary at 10- to 15-minute intervals up to a maximum of 30 mg

      (3)   Administer IV very slowly or may result in respiratory arrest

   d. Primidone (Mysoline)—principal uses in tonic-clonic, partial

      (1)   Give 750 to 1000 mg/day (10 to 25 mg/kg/day)

      (2)   Major side effects—sedation, nystagmus, mood changes, ataxia

   e. Valproate (Depakene)—principal uses in absence, myoclonic, tonic-clonic, partial

      (1)   Give 750 to 1250 mg/day (30 to 60 mg/kg/day)

      (2)   Major side effects—GI distress, drowsiness, ataxia, alopecia, tremor, blood changes, weight gain

   f. Phenobarbital (Luminal)—principal uses in tonic-clonic, partial

      (1)   Give 60 to 120 mg/day (1 to 5 mg/kg); enhances metabolism

of other drugs via liver enzyme induction

    (2)   Major side effects—sedation, nystagmus, confusion, mood changes, ataxia

Table 3
Drugs of choice in treating seizure disorders

Seizure Category	Drug of Choice	Alternatives
Tonic-clonic and partial	Carbamazepine Phenobarbital	Valproate Phenytoin Primidone
Absence	Ethosuximide Valproate	Clonazepam
Myoclonic	Valproate Clonazepam	Phenytoin Phenobarbital
Simple partial and complex, and secondary generalized partial seizures	Carbamazepine Phenytoin	Valproate Phenobarbital Primidone
Mixed forms	Valproate	Carbamazepine Phenobarbital

(*Facts and Comparisons, 1993*)

5.   Instructions in practicing good general health habits, e.g., proper diet, adequate rest and exercise

6.   Instructions in identification of events or situations that precipitate seizures

■ General Considerations

1.   Eyewitness account of seizure activity helpful in diagnosis

2.   Consult on initial treatment and length of treatment with physician

3.   Medications

    a. Start drugs slowly and increase levels gradually to avoid toxicity

    b. Start with one drug; monitor for effect or toxicity before adding other drugs

    c. Select the simplest regimen possible

    d. Monitor blood levels in problem cases

    e. Withdraw medications gradually

    f. Educate patient about medications and common adverse effects

4. Suspect compliance problems in treatment failures

5. Counsel patient in denial; EEG may be normal; may have difficulty convincing patient of seriousness of problem

Parkinson's Disease

- Definition: Slowly progressive, degenerative central nervous system disorder characterized by bradykinesia, muscular rigidity, resting tremors, postural instability; one subtype characterized by tremor and the other by postural instability and gait difficulty

- Etiology/Incidence

  1. Due to injury or impairment of dopamine-producing cells of the substantia nigra in midbrain; specific etiology still unknown

  2. Suspected causes include

     a. Viral infections, e.g., encephalitis

     b. Chemical intoxication, e.g., carbon monoxide, manganese, methanol, ethanol

     c. Drugs—neuroleptics (antipsychotic, antiemetic), reserpine, lithium

     d. Genetic factors

     e. Vascular—multi-infarct, hypotensive shock

     f. Multiple-system degenerations, e.g., Alzheimer's disease

  3. Affects about 1% of the population 65 years of age and older; men affected more frequently than women

- Signs and Symptoms

  1. Gradual and insidious onset

  2. Resting tremor and bradykinesia most typical Parkinsonian signs and most significant in diagnostic process

  3. Generalized slowness in movements

  4. Lack of facial expression (masked facies); staring expression due to diminished blinking

  5. Impaired swallowing; monotonous speech

  6. Difficulty with repetitive and simultaneous movements

  7. Shuffling gait with short steps

  8. Freezing—sudden and unpredictable inability to move (most disabling

of all symptoms)

- ■ Differential Diagnosis
    1. Benign essential tremor
    2. Progressive supranuclear palsy
    3. Depression
    4. Dementia
    5. MPTP—induced parkinsonism
    6. Chronic manganese poisoning
- ■ Physical Findings
    1. Tremors—affects handwriting initially and leads to "pill rolling" movement; tremors can involve diaphragm, tongue, lips and jaw
    2. Rigidity—increased resistance to passive motion of limbs
    3. Sensory examination—usually normal
    4. Muscle strength may be diminished
    5. Ability to perform rapid successive movements is impaired
    6. Reflexes—normally present, but may be difficult to elicit because of marked tremors or rigidity
    7. Stooped posture; short, shuffling gait
    8. Loss of automatic movements, e.g., blinking, swinging of arms while walking, swallowing of saliva, self expression with hand and facial movements
- ■ Diagnostic Tests/Findings: None specific
- ■ Management/Treatment
    1. Pharmacologic (varies with the stage of the disease and predominant manifestations)
        a. Deprenyl, a monoamine oxidase B inhibitor—may slow progression of illness; 5 mg b.i.d.
        b. Carbidopa/levodopa (Sinemet)—optimum daily dose must be determined by careful titration in each patient; required once significant disability is present
            (1) Available in ratios (carbidopa to levodopa) of 1:4 to 1:10; best to use lowest dose possible to achieve therapeutic response,

and reduce side effects

    (2)   Contraindicated in patients with melanoma

  b. Selegiline (Eldepryl)—indicated as an adjunct in patients being treated with carbidopa/levodopa who exhibit poor response to this therapy

    (1)   10 mg daily (5 mg at breakfast and lunch)

    (2)   May need to decrease dose of Sinemet when adding Eldepryl

  c. Centrally acting anticholinergics primarily to relieve tremor

    (1)   Used in early stages and later to supplement levodopa

      (a) Benztropine (Cogentin)—0.5 to 1 mg t.i.d.

      (b) Trihexphenidyl (Artane)—2 to 5 mg t.i.d.

    (2)   Start with lowest dose possible and increase as tolerated

    (3)   Causes confusion, delerium, and impaired thermoregulation in the elderly

  d. Ergot alkaloids

    (1)   Most traditional use comes in later stages of disease when response to levodopa diminishes

    (2)   Useful at all stages of illness

    (3)   Bromocriptine (Parlodel)—1.25 mg b.i.d. (starting dose); when used alone in mild disease 15 to 30 mg daily is often effective

    (4)   Pergolide (Permax)—0.05 mg b.i.d. (starting dose); as sole therapy in mild disease 2.6 mg daily can be efficacious

2. Nonpharmacologic

  a. Exercise program

  b. Physical therapy

  c. Emotional support in meeting the stress of the illness

  d. Patient education

    (1)   Disease process

    (2)   Medication administration and adverse reactions

    (3)   Fall prevention strategies

    (4)   Dietary instructions—malnutrition and constipation can be

serious consequences of inadequate nutrition

    d. Referral to American Parkinson's Disease Association

Multiple Sclerosis

- Definition: A slowly progressive central nervous system disease characterized by chronic inflammation, demyelination, and gliosis (scarring) leading to a variety of neurological signs and symptoms

- Etiology/Incidence

  1. Cause is unknown but an immunologic abnormality is suspected; perhaps triggered by a viral infection in a genetically susceptible host

  2. Strong genetic predisposition

  3. Incidence is approximately 60 per 100,000 population; somewhat higher in women

  4. Age at onset generally is from 20 to 50 years

- Signs and Symptoms

  1. Manifestations are variable and range from a benign illness to an incapacitating illness

  2. Insidious onset

  3. Common early symptoms include

      a. Weakness in one or more of the extremities, trunk, one side of face

      b. Visual disturbances

      c. Slight stiffness or unusual fatigability of a limb, minor gait disturbances

      d. Difficulties with bladder control

  4. Early symptoms may precede diagnosis of disease by months or years

  5. Excess heat may exaggerate symptoms

  6. Sexual dysfunction

  7. Although intellectual functioning remains generally intact except in later stages, emotional stability may be affected

  8. Characterized by remissions and exacerbations

- Differential Diagnosis

  1. Cerebral infarctions

2. Cervical cord compression

3. Systemic lupus erythematosus

4. Amyotrophic lateral sclerosis

5. Drug intoxication

6. Lyme disease

7. Meningovascular syphilis

■ Physical Findings

1. Mental—apathy; emotional lability; scanning speech (slow enunciation with tendency of hesitation)

2. Cranial nerves

   a. In addition to signs of optic neuritis (partial blindness and pain in the eye), one or more ocular signs may be present

      (1) Partial optic nerve atrophy with temporal pallor

      (2) Changes in visual fields

      (3) Transient ophthalmoplegia with diplopia

      (4) Nystagmus

      (5) Occasional unilateral facial numbness

3. Motor

   a. Deep reflexes generally increased

   b. Babinski's sign and clonus often present

   c. Superficial reflexes, especially upper and lower abdominals are diminished or absent

   d. Muscular weakness

   e. In later stages spasticity and cerebellar ataxia may be present resulting in total disability

4. Sensory—paresthesias, numbness and blunting of sensation may occur

5. Charcot's triad (nystagmus, intention tremor, and scanning speech)— present in advanced disease

6. Course of disease is varied and unpredictable

   a. At first, months and years may separate episodes

   b. Life span is not usually shortened

       c. Disability due to progressive paraplegia or quadriplegia

   7. Diagnosis is based upon deduction from clinical and laboratory features

       a. Numerous diagnostic formulas have been proposed (Hauser, 1994)

       b. Firm diagnosis usually cannot be made during first attack

       c. A history of remissions and exacerbations and clinical evidence of CNS lesions in more than one area is highly conclusive (Silberberg, 1992, p. 2198)

- Diagnostic Tests/Findings

   1. No one specific test exists to confirm diagnosis

   2. CSF—abnormalities consist of mononuclear cell pleocytosis, elevation in total Ig and presence of oligoclonal Ig

   3. MRI—may show many plaques (most useful imaging method available)

   4. CT scans—lesions may be visible on contrast-enhanced scans; may reveal ventricular enlargement

   5. Evoked potentials—may be abnormal early in disease (pattern-shift, brainstem auditory and somatosensory)

- Management/Treatment

   1. May consist of arresting disease process or symptomatic management

   2. No specific therapy

   3. Acute bouts of neurologic dysfunction may be treated with ACTH or other corticosteroids; remain cornerstone of therapy, though efficacy is limited and chronic use entails considerable risk

   4. Chronic fatigue often responds to amantadine

   5. Spasticity and flexor spasms can be alleviated with baclofen or diazepam

   6. Bladder dysfunction

       a. Imipramine, oxybutynin chloride or propantheline—to stimulate urination

       b. Long-term urinary bacterial suppressant therapy

       c. Bethanecol for urinary retention secondary to bladder hyporeflexia

   7. Constipation—stool softeners and laxatives and assurance that lack of a daily bowel movement can be normal

   8. Painful paresthesias and dysesthesias, though usually transient, can be

relieved with carbamazepine, diazepam or phenytoin

9. High-protein, high fiber diet with vitamin supplements

10. Assist patient to adjust to illness

11. Instructions how to avoid factors which precipitate exacerbations

12. Maximize self-care; keep patient active and maximally functional

13. Sexual dysfunction in males may be treated by penile implants or erections may be achieved through the use of papaverine and phentolamine injections

Confusion

- Definition: Disturbed orientation in regard to time, place, or person; sometimes associated with a change in mental status

- Etiology/Incidence

    1. Results from a widespread reduction in cerebral metabolism and an upset in neurotransmission processes

    2. Secondary effect of many diseases

        a. Congestive heart failure

        b. Infections

        c. Pulmonary insufficiency

        d. Hepatic insufficiency

        e. Cancer

        f. Dehydration

        g. Nutritional deficiency, hypokalemia

        h. Burns and multiple trauma

        i. Hypoglycemia

        j. Uremia

        k. CVA or TIA

        l. Withdrawal from alcohol

        m. Sedatives/hypnotics

        n. Miscellaneous hearing and visual disturbances

        o. Drug interactions

    3. Very common, increases with age

- Signs and Symptoms
  1. Apathy and drowsiness may be prominent
  2. Disorientation most marked for time, less for place
  3. Acute confusion, usually short term, reversible; characterized by sudden cognitive impairment with fluctuation in affect, behavior and attention
  4. Chronic confusion is a consequence of progressive cerebral deterioration, combined with physical dependence (Calkins, Ford & Katz, 1992)
  5. Patient's friends or family often bring patient in for evaluation

- Differential Diagnosis
  1. Functional psychosis
  2. Dementia
  3. Drug intoxication
  4. Delerium

- Physical Findings
  1. May have normal examination
  2. May have findings suggestive of underlying disease, (e.g., elevated temperature)
  3. Focal neurologic findings may be present

- Diagnostic Tests/Findings
  1. Deterioration on mental status examinations
  2. Perform tests to rule out underlying disease

- Management/Treatment
  1. Diagnosis of underlying cause or causes
  2. Assure adequate hydration and nutrition—dehydration may be precipitating cause
  3. Medications should be carefully evaluated, eliminated or reduced as possible; check for drug interactions
  4. Assess for age-related drug metabolism changes; dosage adjustment may solve problem
  5. Consult with family
  6. Assess activity of daily living (ADL) functioning

- General Considerations
  1. May see elderly patients with "sundowner's syndrome" who become disoriented when it gets dark and have trouble staying oriented in unfamiliar surroundings
  2. Reassure family that symptoms often wax and wane, transient in nature
  3. Often cause for institutionalization if problem not resolved
  4. Provide reassuring, supportive care that assists the patient in re-establishing orientation
  5. Increase socialization opportunities
  6. Evaluate environment for safety hazards
  7. Educate family

Delirium

- Definition: A condition of short duration, characterized by extreme changes in attention, orientation, perception, intellectual function and affect; may be associated with agitation
- Etiology/Incidence
  1. Etiology: Caused by a variety of conditions resulting in derangement of cerebral metabolism
     a. Systemic infections
     b. Poisoning
     c. Drug intoxication/withdrawal
     d. Seizures
     e. Head trauma
     f. Metabolic disturbances, e.g., hypoxia, hypoglycemia, fluid, electrolyte imbalances
  2. Common in hospitalized elderly (Lipowski, 1989; Foreman & Grabowski, 1992)
- Signs and Symptoms
  1. Disorientation to time, place, or person and memory impairment
  2. Perceptual delusions
  3. Visual hallucinations

4. Reduced ability to pay attention to external stimuli

5. Rambling, irrelevant, or incoherent speech

6. Insomnia

7. Symptoms frequently become worse at nightfall

- Differential Diagnosis

  1. Functional psychoses

  2. Dementia

- Physical Findings

  1. Altered level of consciousness

  2. Other possible findings

     a. Elevated temperature

     b. Multifocal myoclonus

     c. Asterixis—flapping tremor

     d. Papilledema

     e. Focal neurologic findings

     f. Tachycardia, sweating, dilated pupils, elevated blood pressure

- Diagnostic Tests/Findings

  1. Toxicology screen—drug intoxication identification

  2. Diagnostic and laboratory tests specific to suspected underlying disorder

  3. EEG—generalized slowing of background activity in delirium

- Management/Treatment

  1. Physician referral/collaborative management

  2. Depending upon severity

     a. Fluids

     b. Monitor electrolytes

     c. Prophylactic thiamine and other B-complex vitamins

     d. Severe agitation treated with IV diazepam

     e. Less severe agitation

        (1) Reassurance

        (2) Oral haloperidol—drug therapy in elderly "start low, go slow"

- General Considerations
    1. Provide orientation measures
    2. Help patient maintain a sense of body integrity
    3. Provide sense of personal continuity and identity
    4. Environmental modifications

Dementia

- Definition: Organic mental syndrome characterized by impairment in short- and long-term memory with impairment in at least one other aspect of intellectual function, such as abstract thinking, judgment, aphasia, or personality
- Etiology/Incidence
    1. Etiology
        a. Reversible causes
            (1) Intoxication
            (2) Infections
            (3) Metabolic disorders
            (4) Nutritional disorders
            (5) Vascular plroblems
            (6) Space occupying lesions
            (7) Normal-pressure hydrocephalus
            (8) Depression
        b. Irreversible causes
            (1) Alzheimer's disease (most common)
            (2) Multi-infarct disease
            (3) Jakob-Creutzfelt
            (4) Pick's disease
            (5) Parkinson's disease
            (6) Huntington's disease
            (7) AIDS
            (8) Down's syndrome

           (9)   Korsakoff's syndrome

  2.   Estimated to affect 3 to 5% of individuals older than 65 years, increasing to about 20% after the age of 80 years (Cassel, Reisenberg, Sorenson & Walsh 1990)

- Signs and Symptoms

  1.   May vary in order, intensity and duration

  2.   Memory impairment

     a. First and most prominent symptom

     b. Initially, memory limitations related to most recent events

     c. In later stages, long-term memory is affected, and recognition of close family members beomes limited and finally absent

  3.   Personality changes (early changes may go unnoticed)

  4.   Sleep disturbances (may occur in early and late stages)

  5.   Impairment in abstract thinking (progressive from subtle to extreme)

  6.   Impairment in judgment (early stages may go unnoticed)

  7.   Aphasia—loss of power of expression by speech, writing, signs (usually later)

  8.   Apraxia—inability to carry out familiar purposeful movements (later)

  9.   Agnosia—loss of power to recognize sensory stimuli (later)

  10. Social isolation (progressive, subtle at first)

- Differential Diagnosis

  1.   Depression

  2.   Delirium

  3.   Pseudodementia

  4.   Personality disorders

  5.   Progressive degenerative disorders

- Physical Findings

  1.   Physical findings may be absent in early stages of dementia, except for those associated with underlying pathology (see Etiology/Incidence)

  2.   Although physical findings may be absent in the early stages, both patient and family observations are critical to the appropriate diagnosis

    a. In some patients cognitive dysfunction may be preceded by modifications in usual behavior and emotional responses

    b. Habits deteriorate and patient becomes slovenly, dirty and eventually incontinent

    c. Coexisting neurologic features depend on the distribution and nature of brain lesions, and in turn, on the etiology; may be marked in some syndromes and, in others, such as senile dementia, may be absent despite widespread atrophic process

    d. Since dementia is sometimes secondary to a treatable condition, comprehensive investigation is imperative unless cause is obvious

    e. Affect becomes more and more shallow and unstable as condition worsens and leads to severe blunting

- Diagnostic Tests/Findings

1. Mental status examination: Use of published, reliable mental status tests to provide baseline for subsequent evaluations (Walker, 1993); will show mild to severe impairment in intellectual functioning in one or more of the following areas

    a. Memory

    b. Orientation

    c. Recall and calculations

    d. Aphasia, apraxia

    e. Visual spatial skills

    f. Judgement

    g. Abstract thinking

    h. Level of consciousness and cooperation

2. Blessed Dementia Scale—high correlation with neuritic plaque counts in Alzheimer's disease (AD)

3. Mattis Dementia Rating Scale—correlates well with functional capacity of AD patients

4. Laboratory Tests—See Table 4

Table 4
Diagnostic Tests and Significance in Dementia

Test	Significance
CBC	Anemia, infection, hematologic disorders
T3,T4, TSH	Thyroid disease
BUN, creatinine Creatinine clearance	Kidney impairment
Iron studies	Iron deficiency anemia
ALT (formerly SGPT); AST (formerly SGOT) Direct/indirect bilirubin Albumin/protein Alkaline phosphatase	Liver dysfunction
Serum and urine calcium, phosphorus	Parathyroid disease
Total protein-albumin	Malnutrition
Drug levels	Overdosage
HIV	AIDS
Chest radiograph	Heart or lung disease, cancer
Urinalysis	Infection, diabetes, renal disease
ECG	Arrhythmia, heart disease
EEG	Normal or nonspecific findings; may be slow in organic dementia
Lumbar puncture	CNS infections, tertiary syphilis, vasculitis, normal pressure hydrocephalus (NPH)
CT scan, head	Intracranial mass lesions, subdural hematoma, NPH, multi-infarct dementia
MRI brain scan	Tumor, abscess, hydrocephalus, multi-infarct dementia or AV malformation

- ■ Management/Treatment
    1. Treat underlying disease or disorder
    2. Maximize functional abilities; orientation strategies (clock, calendar, pictures)
    3. Modify environment to compensate for deficits and ensure safety
    4. Manage behavioral problems with psychosocial and behavioral strategies
    5. Discontinue nonessential medications
    6. Promote mobility

7. Maintain in home setting as long as possible; structured day

8. Help family cope with illness and caretaking responsibilities (Walker, 1993); family therapy

9. If pharmacological treatment is required for control of agitation or hallucination, drug treatment should be used cautiously

   a. Haloperidol—drug of choice for controlling agitation

   b. Short-acting benzodiazepines (oxazepam or lorazepam)—useful in treating behavioral agitation, but not as useful as low-dose neuroleptics

   c. Tricyclic antidepressants (Nortriptyline or Desipramine); selective serotonin re-uptake inhibitors (Fluoxetine, Sertraline)—for treatment of depression (Thompson-Heisterman, Neese, Abraham, 1994)

10. Incontinence management

11. Anticipate legal and ethical decisions

12. Respite services

13. Home care services

14. Senior citizen or day care centers

15. Support group contacts, such as those provided by Alzheimer's Disease and Related Disorders Foundation

Questions

Select the best answer.

1. The most common type of headache is the

    a. Vascular headache
    b. Traction/inflammation headache
    c. Headache of miscellaneous causes
    d. Tension or muscle contraction headache

2. The throbbing pulsations associated with migraine headaches are thought to be due to

    a. Intracranial and extracranial constriction of cranial arteries
    b. Ischemia of the brain
    c. Vasoconstriction of cranial arteries followed by vasodilitation
    d. Vasodilitation of cranial arteries followed by vasoconstriction

3. Cluster headaches are seen most commonly in

    a. Women with a ratio of 3:2
    b. Middle aged, thin, cigarette smoking men
    c. Young men ages 20-35
    d. Middle aged, anxious, women

4. Sudden stabbing or burning pain in the left orbit is reported by Mr. Jeans, a 47-year-old man. He reports that the pain is severe, and he is anxiously pacing the office while waiting to be examined. He reports that he had the same problem yesterday at the same time. Based only on this information, you might conclude the patient has

    a. Common migraine headache
    b. Sinusitis
    c. Cluster headache
    d. Cranial mass

5. Mr. Brown, a 67-year-old male, comes in with a severe temporal headache. Pain has been dull in nature but gradually increasing in intensity for the last week. Pain started in left temporal area and then spread to the right. He reports feeling sore lumps in the area of his forehead which hurt. Based on this information, what one laboratory test would you most likely order?

    a. CBC
    b. CT scan
    c. ECG
    d. Erythrocyte sedimentation rate

6. Mr. Black, a 73-year-old carpenter reports onset of constant headache 2 weeks ago, which is not relieved by analgesics. At the same time, he developed some feelings of numbness in his left hand and family reports several episodes of confusion. Pain has awakened him twice. This pattern makes you highly suspicious of

    a. Initial onset Alzheimer's disease
    b. First infarct in multi-infarct dementia
    c. Partial seizure disorder
    d. Possible tumor

7. A seizure with no loss of consciousness, of less than a minute duration with localized numbness, is called a

    a. Simple partial seizure
    b. Complex partial seizure
    c. Absence seizure
    d. Grand mal seizure

8. After tonic-clonic or complex partial seizures, which hormone can be found elevated for 10-60 minutes?

    a. Serotonin
    b. Prolactin
    c. Androgen
    d. Estrogen

9. The drug of choice in simple, complex partial seizures, and tonic-clonic seizures is

    a. Diazepam
    b. Primidone
    c. Carbamazepine
    d. Valproate

10. Phenytoin sodium (Dilantin) is often used alone or as adjunctive therapy in tonic-clonic (grand mal) seizures. What regular preventive care should be provided with long-term use of this drug?

    a. Eye examinations
    b. Ear examinations
    c. Dental examinations
    d. Prostate examinations

11. In which age group is onset of petit mal or absence seizures most common?

    a. Infants
    b. School-age children

    c. Elderly

    d. Middle-age

12. Disturbed orientation with regard to time, place or person and sometimes associated with a change in mental status

    a. Delirium

    b. Confusion

    c. Depression

    d. Senility

13. Mrs. Moss, a 72-year-old, is brought into the hospital in a confused state which began suddenly 2 days ago. She failed to recognize her family, could not communicate when she wanted to eat or go to the bathroom, and seemed to be constantly irritated and unable to sleep for more than an hour or so. She is now nervously picking at her hospital gown. You would conclude that Mrs. Moss has

    a. Dementia

    b. Depression

    c. Delirium

    d. Schizophrenia

14. Mr. Hawkes, age 82, has a sudden onset of confusion. His family has been contemplating moving him to a nursing home because he has become incontinent, does not eat or drink, has a mild temperature, and has become difficult to handle. Underlying causes of his confusion might be

    a. Dehydration

    b. Diabetes

    c. TIA

    d. Depression

15. Basic rules in giving medication to the elderly include

    a. Use dosage, based upon their weight

    b. Use pediatric dosage because they have less body fat to bind medication

    c. Start low and go slowly with increases

    d. Start with half adult dose and increase to normal dose over 2 days

16. Organic mental syndrome characterized by impairment in short- and long-term memory with impairment in at least one other aspect of intellectual function

    a. Dementia

    b. Delirium

    c. Cerebral atrophy

    d. Pick's disease

17. Reversible causes of dementia are

    a. Multi-infarct disease and Pick's disease
    b. Infections and AIDS
    c. Intoxication and infections
    d. Parkinson's disease and AIDS

18. Mr. Harper is a 73-year-old white male with diabetes. He experienced a 20-minute episode of monocular blindness, left-sided weakness, and some slurred speech. The most likely diagnosis is

    a. Hypoglycemia
    b. TIA
    c. Stroke
    d. Trigeminal neuralgia

19. The physical finding most likely to be found on physical examination is

    a. Facial paresthesia
    b. Deficits in cranial nerves 2,3,4,6
    c. Loss of deep tendon reflexes
    d. Carotid bruit

20. Mrs. Green is talking to her daughter when she suddenly stops, gazes into space, her eyes become glassy, and she does not blink. She utters some uninelligible sounds, makes smacking movements with her lips and seems confused. This is an example of

    a. Complex, partial seizure
    b. Tonic/clonic seizure
    c. Absence or petit mal seizure
    d. Jacksonian seizure

21. The term apraxia means

    a. Irrational fear of leaving the familiar setting of home
    b. Psychomotor defect in which one is unable to properly use a known object
    c. Inability to smell
    d. Lack of sensory/perceptive ability to recognize impressions from one or more of the senses

22. Mrs. Lynn was diagnosed recently with Alzheimer's disease. One of the most obvious behaviors the family might expect to see in the next few months is

    a. Memory loss for recent events
    b. Dissolution of personality

   c. Inability to feed herself

   d. Hostile behavior

23. The prompt diagnosis of temporal arteritis is important because

   a. It is expensive to evaluate and treat

   b. It is correlated with tumor development

   c. Failure to promptly treat may lead to permanent vision loss

   d. Narcotics are not helpful in reducing pain

24. Jerry James, a known epileptic, is brought into the emergency room following a grand mal seizure. This is the second time this month that he has been brought in by ambulance for evaluation. What is the most common cause of seizure activity in a known epileptic?

   a. Incorrect medication

   b. Worsening of electrical disruption in the brain

   c. Failure to take antiepileptic medication

   d. Increase in seizure triggers

25. A 38-year-old female comes in with the complaint of experiencing severe frontal headache, for several days, worse on awakening, slight fever, and worse when bending over. She has these headaches each spring and fall. You suspect she has

   a. Cluster headaches

   b. Sinusitis

   c. TMJ pain from clenching teeth during sleep

   d. Mastoiditis

26. Mr. Brown has noticed lately that it seems his hands shake for no apparent reason and that it takes him more time to dress in the morning for work. He thinks that perhaps he should be considering retirement since he just celebrated his 65th birthday, although he could work until 70 years of age at his current job. These symptoms would probably be indicative of

   a. Benign essential tumor

   b. Alcohol withdrawal

   c. Bell's palsy

   d. Parkinson's disease

27. Automatic movements which usually disappear eventually in an individual with Parkinson's disease are

   a. Those associated with repetitive and simultaneous movements

   b. Those associated with dressing and hygiene

   c. Those associated with swinging of arms while walking

   d. Those associated with throwing a ball

28. The patient with trigeminal neuralgia presents with

    a. Flaccid muscles of the neck
    b. Dysphasia and respiratory symptoms
    c. Paroxysms of excruciating facial pain
    d. Paralysis of face, usually unilateral

29. Drug of choice for the treatment of trigeminal neuralgia is

    a. Phenytoin
    b. Levodopa
    c. Carbidopa/levodopa
    d. Carbamazepine

30. Trina Smith, a beautiful woman in her mid-forties, is seen in your office for the first time with complaints of weakness in her right leg, which feels "tired" at the end of the day. She also says she feels dizzy occasionally. Prior to the onset of these vague symptoms, she has been very healthy. Your reaction at this time would be to

    a. Refer her to a neurologist immediately
    b. Work her up for essential (primary) hypertension
    c. Suspect Multiple Sclerosis
    d. Suspect seizure disorder, absence or petit mal

31. Multiple Sclerosis is characterized by

    a. Multiple psychosomatic complaints
    b. Shuffling gait and pill-rolling movement of fingers
    c. Blank facies and emotional lability
    d. Remissions and exacerbations

Answers

1. d
2. c
3. b
4. c
5. d
6. d
7. a
8. b
9. c
10. c
11. b
12. b
13. c
14. a
15. c
16. a
17. c
18. b
19. d
20. a
21. b
22. a
23. c
24. c
25. b
26. d
27. c
28. c
29. d
30. c
31. d

Bibliography

Abrams, W. B., & Berkow, R. (Eds.). (1991). *The Merck manual of geriatrics*. Rahway, NJ: Merck & Co. Inc.

American Psychiatric Association. (1987). Organic mental disorders. In diagnostic and statistical manual of mental disorders (3rd ed., rev.), (pp. 101-128). Washington, DC: American Psychiatric Association.

Barker, L. R., Burton, J. R., & Zieve, P. D. (1991). *Principles of ambulatory medicine* (3rd ed.). Baltimore: Williams and Wilkins.

Bates, B. (1991). *A guide to physical examination and history taking* (5th ed.). Philadelphia: J. B. Lippincott.

Calkins, E., Ford, A. B., & Katz, P. R. (Eds.). (1992). *Practice of geriatrics* (2nd ed.). Philadelphia: W. B. Saunders

Cassel, C. K., Riesenberg, D. E., Sorensen, L. B., & Walsh, J. R. (1990). *Geriatric medicine* (2nd ed). New York: Springer-Verlag.

Ebersole, P., & Hess, P. (1990). *Toward healthy aging*. St. Louis: C. V. Mosby Company.

Edmunds, M. (1991). *Introduction to clinical pharmacology*. St. Louis: Mosby Yearbook.

Foreman, M. D., & Grabowski, R. (1992). Diagnostic dilemma: Cognitive impairment in the elderly. *Journal of Gerontological Nursing*, 18(9), 5-12.

Gallo, J. J., Reichel, W., & Andersen, L. (1988). *Handbook of geriatric assessment*. Rockville, Maryland: An Aspen Publication.

Hauser, S. L. (1994). Multiple sclerosis and other demyelinating diseases. In K. J. Isselbacher, E. Braunwald, J. D. Wilson, J. B. Martin, A. S. Fauci & D. L. Kasper (Eds.), *Harrison's principles of internal medicine* (13th ed.), (pp. 2287-2295). NY: McGraw-Hill.

Kane-Carlsen, P. A. (1990). Transient ischemic attacks: Clinical features, pathophysiology and management. *Nurse Practitioner*, 15(7), 9-14.

Lipowski, Z. J. (1989). Delirium in the elderly patient. *New England Journal of Medicine*, 320(9), 578-582.

Olin, B. R. (Ed). (1993). *Facts and comparisons*. St. Louis: J. B. Lippincott.

Posner, J. B. (1992). Headache and other head pain. In J. B. Wyngaarden, L. H. Smith

& J. C. Bennett (Eds.), *Cecil textbook of medicine* (19th ed.), (pp. 2117-2123). Philadelphia: W. B. Saunders.

Reichel, W. (1989). *Clinical aspects of aging* (3rd ed.). Baltimore: Williams & Wilkins.

Silberberg, D. H. (1992). The demyelinating diseases. In J. B. Wyngaarden, L. H. Smith & J. C. Bennett (Eds.), *Cecil textbook of medicine* (19th ed.), (pp. 2196-2202). Philadelphia: W. B. Saunders.

Thompson-Heisterman, A., Neese, J. B., & Abraham, I. L. (1994). Organic mental disorders. In C. Houseman (Ed.). *Psychiatric certification review guide for the generalist and clinical specialist in adult, child and adolescent psychiatric and mental health nursing* (pp 369-407). Potomac, MD: Health Leadership Associates.

Walker, L. S. (1993). Psychosocial problems. In C. A. Kopac & V. L. Millonig (Eds.), *Gerontological nursing certification review guide for the generalist, clinical specialist, nurse practitioner* (pp. 363-424). Potomac, MD: Health Leadership Associates.

Wilson, J. D., Braunwald, E., Isselbacher, K. J., Petersdorf, R. G., Martin, J. B., Fauci, A. S., & Root, R. K. (1991). *Harrison's principles of internal medicine* (12th ed.). New York: McGraw-Hill.

Psychosocial Disorders

Sister Maria Salerno

Depression (Major)

- Definition: An affective state characterized by feelings of sadness, guilt, low self-esteem, and often related to a loss. The loss may or may not be recent. The term is used to denote a mood, a normal emotion in times of crisis or other life events, as well as a full clinical syndrome called "major depression." Depression is commonly categorized as

  1. Adjustment Disorder (with depressed mood)

     a. Associated with an identifiable psychosocial event (stressor)

     b. Short-term

     c. Often self-limiting

     d. Treated with crisis intervention or short-term psychotherapy

     e. Lasts as long as the stressor does or until a new level of adaptation is reached

     f. May be a normal emotion with feelings of sadness, disappointment, despair, frustration, or unhappiness

     g. May be a normal grief or bereavement state appropriately following a loss

  2. Major Depression—an enduring life mood, a persistent state of dysphoric emotions, thinking, and feeling which does not pass or fade away

     a. Primary can not be ascribed to another illness or drugs

     b. Secondary can be ascribed to another illness or drugs, e.g.,

        (1) Substance abuse (alcoholism most common cause)

        (2) Anxiety disorders

        (3) Antihypertensives

        (4) Hypothyroidism

        (5) Heart disease

        (6) Disfigurement

  3. Dysthymic Disorder

     a. Milder than Major Depression

     b. Often associated with chronic drug use

    c. More chronic (Usually two years or more)

    d. Lacks somatic signs of depression

  4. Bipolar Disorder-recurrent episodes of depression interspersed with bouts of mania.

    a. Heredity a strong factor

    b. Tricyclic antidepressants (TCA) often precipitate a manic response called "hypomania"

    c. Early onset, usually before age 30

    d. Incidence in Blacks and Whites similar

    e. Incidence is similar in males and females

■ Etiology/Incidence

  1. Psychosocial and/or biochemical causes for depression have been theorized.

    a. Psychosocial

      (1) Psychoanalytical

        (a) Anger turned inward

        (b) Regression to a less mature stage of functioning

      (2) Environmental

        (a) Stressful life events

        (b) Changes or inadequacies in social support

      (3) Psychodynamic

        (a) Personality development
          (i) Passive/dependent
          (ii) Obsessive/compulsive

        (b) Effects of past relationships and developmental tasks on coping styles, particularly use of defense mechanisms.
          (i) Denial
          (ii) Suppression
          (iii) Sublimation

      (4) Cognitive

        (a) Self-reinforcing habit of unrealistic negative ideas

        (b) Recent or past style of thinking and relating

(c) Learned "helplessness"

b. Biochemical

(1) Catecholamine

(a) Poorly functioning neurotransmitter

(b) Primarily dopamine, norepinephrine, epinephrine, and serotonin

(2) Endocrine

(a) Cortisol

(b) Thyroid releasing hormone

2. Incidence

a. Depressive illness most common mental health problem seen in general practice

b. Estimated 9 to 16 million Americans suffer from depressive illness, yet fewer than a third will receive treatment

c. Twice as many women as men with major depression worldwide

d. Lifetime risk for developing depressive illness

(1) 20% for females

(2) 10% for males

e. Major depression can occur in any age group

(1) Adolescents and the elderly at higher risk

(2) Other risk factors

(a) Family history of depressive illness, alcoholism, or major medical illness

(b) Prior depressive episode

(c) Being post partum

(d) Unanticipated or prolonged stress

b. Major depression has a 50 to 85% recurrence rate within three to nine years

■ Signs and symptoms

1. Somatic (may be misidentified as normal changes in the elderly)

a. Lack of energy, fatigue, malaise

b. Slowing down of body processes

  (1) Amenorrhea

  (2) Constipation

  (3) Dysphagia

  (4) Psychomotor retardation

c. Changes in eating habits

  (1) Hypophagia

  (2) Hyperphagia

  (3) Anorexia

d. Loss of sexual interest or impotence

e. Aggravation of any physical pathology

f. Pains of undetermined etiology in a variety of anatomical sites

g. Sleep disorders

  (1) Early morning awakenings with painful ruminations

  (2) Anxiety insomnia (difficulty falling asleep)

  (3) Hypersomnia (12 to 16 hours/day)

2. Emotional

a. Loss or lack of pleasure

b. Loss of sense of humor

c. Self-dislike

d. Sadness

e. Crying spells

f. Changes in emotional attachment

g. Masked anger, irritability

h. Hypersensitivity

i. Anxiety about ability to cope

j. Increased tension, e.g., agitation, restlessness

k. Feelings of hopelessness/helplessness

3. Cognitive

a. Low self-esteem

b. Loss in perceptual ability

c. Difficulty in concentration

d. Errors in thinking

    (1) Cause of failure within self or personalization

    (2) Course of events unchanging

    (3) Tendency to be global and generalize

    (4) Paranoid delusions

    (5) Magnification and minimization

4. Motivational

    a. Passivity/indifference/apathy (sometimes viewed as lack of cooperation with medical regimen)

    b. Procrastination

    c. Dependence (may even be an aggressive dependence)

    d. Social withdrawal

    e. Paralysis of will

    f. Escape wishes (ultimate escape-death)

■ Differential Diagnosis

1. Since depression may be a manifestation of many illnesses the differential diagnosis must include a thorough search for factors or organic diseases which may be responsible for symptom manifestation including

    a. Infections

    b. Neurological neoplasms

    c. Endocrine disorders

    d. Nutritional deficiencies

    e. Electrolyte disturbances

2. Differentiate major depression from other mental disorders, e.g., schizophrenia, dementia, adjustment disorder with depressed mood

3. Diagnosis of clinical depression requires presence of a dysphoric mood and 4 of 8 of these symptoms to be present every day for at least two weeks:

    a. Increased or decreased appetite

    b. Anxiety insomnia or early morning awakening after 2 to 4 hours sleep.

    c. Reduced activity level

    d. Reduced interest for usually pleasurable activities

    e. Tired, "worn out", or restless

    f. Guilt about incongruent or insignificant things or events

    g. Decreased concentration

    h. Recurrent thoughts about or wishes for death

4. Mnemonic device to recall major symptoms: IN SAD CAGES

    a. *In*terest

    b. *S*leep

    c. *A*ppetite

    d. *D*epressed mood

    e. *C*oncentration

    f. *A*ctivity

    g. *G*uilt

    h. *E*nergy

    i. *S*uicide

■ Physical Findings

1. General—may show lack of personal grooming and hygiene, inattention to dress, slouched posture, slowed speech and movements, long pauses in response to questions, tearfulness. Weight may be less than or more than ideal for body size

2. Mental Status—poor concentration, decreased memory, indecision, pessimism

■ Diagnostic Tests/Findings

1. Initial Tests

    a. CBC—normal

    b. Urinalysis—normal

    c. EKG—normal

    d. Chest radiograph—normal

      e. Glucose—normal

      f. SMA-12—normal

      g. Thyroid function—normal

      h. VDRL—normal

      i. Stool occult—negative

      j. Drug levels—no indication of substance abuse

      k. Arterial blood gases—normal

2. Depression screening instruments— scores indicative of depression

    a. Beck Depression Inventory

    b. Yesavage Geriatric Depression Scale

    c. Zung Self-Rating Depression Scale

3. Special Tests (primarily used in psychiatric and research settings)

    a. TSH response to TRF may be decreased

    b. Dexamethasone-suppression test (DST) used to distinguish between major and minor depression

    c. EEG sleep profile—may show reduction in REM sleep

    d. Platelet Monoamine oxidase (MAO) activity—increased

    e. Biogenic amines (norepinephrine, serotonin)—increased levels

■ Management/Treatment

1. Mild depression

    a. Structured monitoring with weekly appointments with phone contact for backup

    b. Use therapeutic communication skills to

      (1) Encourage verbalization, clarification of feelings and fears, as well as relationship of feelings to specific events if known

      (2) Assess and discuss losses that have occurred and their meaning

      (3) Help correct cognitive errors in thinking

    c. Use crisis or social skills models to teach and promote more effective coping strategies

      (1) Help client recognize need for and identify alternative coping

methods

    (2)   Encourage interaction with other people

    (3)   Encourage planned, regular physical activity

    (4)   Teach relaxation techniques

    (5)   Provide client with anticipatory guidance regarding feelings and usual course of the problem, e.g., gradual improvement and abatement of symptoms

  d. Provide consistency and caring, avoiding a judgmental or blaming attitude

  e. Reinforce positive behaviors

  f. Avoid actions or response that could be interpreted as punishment

  g. Consult with physician or psychiatrist regarding psychotherapy and use of antidepressants. Both have been shown to be of help in mild depression. See tables 1 and 2

2. Moderate to severe depression

  a. Hospitalization of those thought to

    (1)   Be a potential danger to self or others; unable to meet basic needs; suicidal ideation or behavior

    (2)   Have impaired cognition or judgment

    (3)   Need skilled observation for diagnosis, assessment, or monitoring of therapy

    (4)   Have inadequate social supports for outpatient treatment

  b. Antidepressant and/or antianxiety medications; most appropriate initial therapy for reasonably healthy individual; see Table 1 and Table 2

    (1)   Those with delusions, hallucinations, profound psychomotor retardation less responsive

    (2)   Only 65% have complete remission with any one drug

    (3)   Secondary amines (desipramine and nortriptyline)

    (4)   Treatment with tricyclics, tetracyclics, and secondary amines usually begins with 25 to 75 mg/day given at bedtime. Exceptions—protriptyline 5 to 15 mg, nortyptiline 25 to 50 mg

        (a)   Reduce starting dose by 50% in elderly or infirm

        (b)   Increase 25 mg increments every 2 to 4 days; weekly in older patients

        (c)   Avoid simultaneous use of other drugs; if impossible close monitoring required

        (d)   Improvement after two weeks of therapeutic dose; maximum benefit 4 to 8 weeks

        (e)   TCA blood levels if no response after two weeks of therapeutic dose; may be a problem of noncompliance or rapid metabolism

        (f)   Treatment continues 3 to 6 months; after two months on therapeutic dose taper by 25 to 50 mg increments per week prior to discontinuation to avoid withdrawal symptoms (nausea, dizziness, headache, increased perspiration and salivation, photophobia, systolic hypertension)

        (g)   Dispensed in small amounts; 10 day supply can be lethal dose

  c. Psychotherapy

  d. Electroconvulsive therapy (ECT)

    (1)   More rapid improvement than with pharmacologic agents

    (2)   Indicated for severely depressed or suicidal persons for whom pharmacologic agents are contraindicated or ineffective

    (3)   Barbiturates and muscle relaxants used prior to the procedure

    (4)   Confusion, headache, temporary amnesia lasting one to two weeks are common side effects in about 40%; may be clinically apparent up to one month

    (5)   Avoided in persons with brain tumor, recent (3 months) MI, CVA, or perforated viscus repair

Table 1
Antidepressants

Drug Trade Name	Average Daily Dose (mg)a	Anticholinergic Effect	Sedative Effect	Cardiac Conduction Effect	Ortho-Static Hypertension
Tricyclics					
Tertiary amines					
Amitriptyline (Elavil)	50-150	+4	+4	+4	+3
Doxipin (Sinequan, Adapin)	75-150	+3	+4	+2	+2
Imipramine (Tofranil)	50-200	+3	+3	+4	+4
Secondary Amines					
Desipramine (Norpramin; Pertofrane)	75-200	+1	+1	+3	+3
Nortriptyline (Aventyl; Pamelor)	75-100	+3	+3	+3	+1
Protriptyline (Vivactil)	15-40	+3	+1	+4	+2
MAO Inhibitors					
Isocarboxazid (Marplan)	10-30	0	+1	+1	+3
Phenelzine (Nardil)	15-30	0	+1	+1	+3
Tranylcypromine (Parnate)	20-30	0	+1	+1	+2
Tetracyclics					
Amoxapine (Asendin)	200-300	+3	+2	+2	+2
Maprotiline (Ludiomil)	75-150	+2	+3	+3	+2
Other:					
Fluoxetine (Prozac)	40-60	0	0	+1	0
Alprazolama b (Xanax)	.75-4	0	0	0	0
Trazadone (Desyrel)	150-200	0	+4	+1	+4
Lithium carbonate	600-1800 to establish serum level 0.8-1.5 mEq/L initially; maintenance 0.6-1.2 mEq/L, not to exceed 2.0 mEq/L				

a—Lower average doses than these will be seen in elderly and higher in those hospitalized with severe or treatment resisant depression

b—Only benzodiazepine approved for depression

Table 2.
Antidepressants and AntiAnxiety Medications Contraindications and Precautions

Drug Group	Contraindications	Precautions
Antidepressants		
Tricyclics	Acute MI, hypersensitivity; concurrent administration of MAO Inhibitors	In patients with urinary retention; prostatic hypertrophy; narrow angle glaucoma, convulsive disorders; cardiovascular disease; thyroid disease; pregnant patients
MAO inhibitors	Hypertension, cardiovascular disease, headaches, liver disease or advanced renal disease, concurrent use of a tricyclic; schizophrenia	Safety during pregnancy not established; avoid fermented foods, pickles, cheeses, red wine, beer, fava beans, raisins, chocolate; cold remedies, weight reduction meds, e.g., anything with tyramine
Lithium Carbonate	Significant renal disease, dietary salt restriction; cardiovascular disease; brain damage	Use caution with pregnant patients; elderly; patient who is breast feeding; persons with thyroid disease; mild renal and cardiovascular disease; epilepsy
Antianxiety Drugs		
Benzodiazepines	Glaucoma, hypersensitivity	Use caution if hx of allergies; psychological addiction to these drugs; hepatic or renal impairment; lower dose for elderly or breast feeding mothers
Carbamazepine	Severe renal, cardiovascular, or liver disease.	Use with caution if liver, renal disease, or blood dyscrasias
Fluoxetine	Do not administer with MAO inhibitors or with tryptophane supplements	Caution in persons with history of seizures; impaired renal or hepatic function; mania or hypomania; in pregnant or nursing women; in the elderly

3. Diagnostic Considerations

   a. Assess degree of problem related to daily functioning

   b. Refer those with evidence of

      (1) Hallucinations

      (2) Delusions

      (3) Loss of contact with reality

      (4) Psychotic behaviors

      (5) Suicidal thoughts, wishes, or tendencies (See section on suicide)

      (6) An unidentifiable cause for depression

      (7) Diagnosed or suspected moderate to severe depression

4. Client Education

    a. Disease course, expected outcomes, and usual treatment modalities

    b. Purpose, dosage, side effects of medication

        (1) Improvement in symptoms not evident for 3 to 4 weeks

        (2) Importance of adhering to prescribed pharmacologic regimen; avoid abrupt discontinuation of medications

        (3) Caution against concomitant use of over the counter preparations

        (4) Interactions with food or other medications; see Table 2

5. Persons with major depression should be followed at least weekly for first 6 to 8 weeks, preferably by a mental health professional for medication adjustment and brief psychotherapeutic support

6. Persons known to be on antidepressants or receiving care for depression, who are being seen for other reasons should be routinely checked for

    a. Suicidal feelings, plans, intentions, risks

    b. Tremor, blurred vision, dry mouth, tachycardia, postural hypotension

Suicide

■ Definition

1. The intentional taking of one's own life

2. Usually described as

    a. Attempted—unsuccessful conscious attempt to take one's own life

    b. Threatened—verbal or physical indication of intent for self-destruction

    c. Ideation—thoughts or behaviors indicating conscious intent for self-destruction

■ Etiology/Incidence

1. Often a manifestation or complication of depressive illness or anxiety states

2. Between 5 and 15% of depressed patients commit suicide

3. Risk factors include

    a. Sudden crisis or loss

    b. Destructive coping mechanisms

    c. Few or no significant others

    d. Poor social or personal resources

    e. Past suicide attempts or family history of suicide

    f. Previous psychotic problems

    g. Unstable life style

    h. Specific plan

4.   Eight of 10 persons who state an intent to commit suicide do so; risk for depressed patients is greatest during the first month of treatment when the individual begins to feel better and has more energy

5.   In the U.S. women attempt suicide more often, but men are three times as likely to succeed. In elderly, suicide among males outnumber those among women

6.   Adolescents and white males over the age of 45 have a higher incidence rate

7.   In adolescents increased risk has been associated with

    a. Extreme parental control or permissiveness

    b. Loss of communication with parents and teacher

    c. Hostility and difficulty in school or with the law

    d. Lack of social supports (peers, social, work, and school)

- Signs and Symptoms

1.   Feelings of worthlessness and/or helplessness

2.   Preoccupation with a dead relative or friend

3.   Excessive denial, indignation, or anger in response to being questioned about suicide

4.   Verbalization of a plan or rehearsal of a plan

5.   Sudden mood elevation in a depressed patient often accompanied by more energy and calmer, more placid manner

6.   Giving possessions away

7.   Setting affairs in order

8.   Making a will

9. Presence of hallucinations or delusions

10. Intuition on the part of the health professional

11. In adolescents these may be more prominent

    a. Taking excessive risks

    b. Self-destructive behaviors, e.g., drug abuse, accident proneness

    c. Negative self-concept

    d. Expression of wish to die

    e. Withdrawal from family and persons

    f. Increased interest and companionship with animal/pets

- Differential Diagnosis: All depressed clients need to be asked about suicide. If client does not volunteer information ask directly about thoughts of taking their own life. Also ask direct questions to elicit information about a plan, its lethality, and any mental or actual rehearsals of the plan. Risk is highest if planned in 24 hours; low or moderate if planned for a later time

- Physical Findings

  1. There are no specific physical findings, however those of depression may be evident.

     a. General Appearance—unkempt appearance, slumped or stooped posture, slow speech pattern, lack of expression or dejected look or agitation, hostility, tremulousness

     b. Mental Status—disorientation, poor concentration, agitation hallucinations or delusions

  2. Old scars or evidence of injury from past attempts or high risk behaviors

- Diagnostic Tests/Findings: There are no specific laboratory tests. See Diagnostic Tests/Findings in section on Depression

- Management/Treatment

  1. Treatment will usually include hospitalization with psychotherapy, antidepressant medications, and/or ECT. See previous section on Management and Treatment of Depression

  2. If a client is deemed suicidal or if there is concern about the client's potential for suicide do not leave the client alone but obtain immediate psychiatric consultation

Anxiety

- Definition

    1. An unpleasant feeling of dread, apprehension, foreboding, or tension resulting from an unexpected threat to one's feelings of self-esteem or well-being

    2. Major categories

        a. Generalized Anxiety disorder—unrealistic or excessive anxiety and worry about life circumstance

        b. Panic Disorders (Phobias)—unfounded morbid dread of seemingly harmless object or situation

        c. Obsessive compulsive disorder (OCD)— repetitive thoughts (obsession) that a person is unable to control; urge to perform an act that cannot be resisted without great difficulty (compulsion)

        d. Post-traumatic stress disorder (PSD)—delayed (at least 6 months) anxiety after a severe trauma often perceived as a threat to physical integrity or self-concept; intrusive thoughts, flashbacks, and nightmares form the symptomatic triad

- Etiology/Incidence

    1. Various theories related to etiology include

        a. Psychodynamic

            (1) Freudian—conflict between id and superego; ego not strong enough to resolve the conflict

            (2) Sullivanian—fear of disapproval from mother figure; conditional love leads to fragile ego, lack of self-confidence, lack of self-esteem, fear of failure

            (3) Dollar and Miller—learned response to innate drive to avoid pain; anxiety the result of two competing drives or goals

        b. Biologic

            (1) Genetic influence with high family incidence

            (2) Autonomic nervous system response-fight or flight mechanism

        c. Family dynamics

            (1) Individual with dysfunctional behavior is representative of

           family system problems

    (2)   Carrier of problems resulting from disrupted interrelationships

2. Incidence

    a. Anxiety disorders occur in 10 to 15% of clients seen in health care settings

    b. Panic disorders

       (1)   Occur more frequently in women than in men

       (2)   Onset usually in late teens or early adulthood

       (3)   More common in those who have had an early traumatic event, e.g., the death of a parent

    c. Obsessive compulsive disorder

       (1)   Most often seen in adolescence and early adulthood

       (2)   Males and females affected equally

       (3)   More frequent in upper middle class and in persons with higher levels of intellectual functioning

■ Signs and Symptoms

1. Generalized Anxiety and Panic attacks

    a. A feeling of tightness in the throat

    b. Difficulty breathing; feelings of suffocation

    c. Palpitations

    d. Chest tightness or pain

    e. Tachypnea, tachycardia

    f. Gastric distress or discomfort

    g. Nausea

    h. Diarrhea

    i. Feeling of weakness in lower limbs

    j. Tingling, numbness of extremities

    k. Feeling of light-headedness

    l. Dryness of the mouth

    m. Feeling of something caught in the throat

n. Cold sweaty hands

o. Feelings of loss of control; irritability; impatience

p. Motor tension—shakiness, jitteriness, trembling, restlessness

q. Anxiety insomnia, difficulty falling asleep

r. Symptoms of panic generally develop suddenly and have been related to mitral valve prolapse

2. OCD

a. Recurrent, persistent thoughts, ideas or images experienced as intrusive

b. Repetitious, purposeful, intentional behavior which are distressing, time consuming, or interfere with functioning

3. PTSD

a. Intrusive thoughts, flashbacks, nightmares related to the traumatic event

b. Poor impulse control, unpredictability, and/or aggressiveness

c. Avoidance symptoms

(1) Avoids reminders of event

(2) Memory difficulty

(3) Detachment and restricted affect

d. Hyperarousal symptoms

(1) Hypervigilance

(2) Insomnia

(3) Irritability, poor concentration

- Differential Diagnosis

1. Rule out other causes of symptoms

a. Other mental health disorders; drug abuse, withdrawal, or intoxication

b. Endocrine, cardiac, or neurologic problems, e.g.

(1) Thyrotoxicosis

(2) Hypoglycemia

(3) Acute hypoxia

(4) Pheochromocytoma

(5) Seizure disorder

c. Side effects of chemical agents or medications, e.g., caffeine, nicotine, antihistamines, tricyclics

■ Physical Findings

1. Between attacks may all be within normal limits

2. During an attack

   a. General appearance—looks worried, frightened, restless

   b. Vital signs—tachycardia, increased respirations, elevated B.P.

   c. Integumentary—pallor, flushed face, cold clammy hands

   d. Gastrointestinal—possible loss of bowel or bladder control

   e. Mental status—hypervigilence; easy distractibility; poor concentration

   f. Motor tension—shakiness, jitteriness

■ Diagnostic Tests/Findings.

1. Serum drug analysis—negative

2. Thyroid function tests—normal

3. Serum glucose—normal

4. EKG—normal

■ Management/Treatment

1. Cognitive behavioral therapy more effective for generalized anxiety than for panic attacks

   a. Assess usual coping mechanisms, life style, social supports

   b. Establish a trusting, warm, empathetic, respectful relationship

   c. Assist client to identify and describe emotional and physical feelings and to identify the relationship between them

   d. Identify patient behaviors that cause anxiety in the health care provider, once a relationship is established

   e. Use supportive confrontation as needed

   f. Keep focus of responsibility on the client

   g. Encourage use of and teach or refer for relaxation techniques, biofeedback, and meditation

2. Consult with physician regarding use of antianxiety medications. See Tables 2 and 3

   a. Benzodiazepines most widely used

      (1) Therapeutic doses usually do not result in physiologic dependence

      (2) May be misused to "boost" effects of methadone

   b. Antihistamines for those with COPD or potential for abuse of benzodiazepines

   c. Beta Adrenergic Blockers, e.g., propranolol more effective in reducing marked autonomic symptoms (tachycardia, palpations, breathlessness)

   d. Tricyclics and MAO inhibitors good for panic attacks but not for generalized anxiety

3. Refer to psychiatric mental health professional for counseling and more specific therapy

4. Obtain consult regarding testing for other physical or emotional disorders

5. Patient Education

   a. Disease course, expected outcome

      (1) Reassurance that anxiety rarely evolves into a more serious disorder

      (2) Reassurance that symptoms can be alleviated with appropriate therapy

      (3) Condition is temporary and with appropriate therapy and time source of anxiety may be alleviated

      (4) Dosage, side effects, expected action of pharmacologic agents

   b. Chart attacks—date, time, situation, level of anxiety or symptoms on a scale of 0 to 10

Table 3
AntiAnxiety Medication

Generic	Trade Name	Average daily dose*
Benzodiazepines (Longer acting)		
Chlordiazepoxide	Librium	15-40 mg
Clorazepate dipotassium	Tranxene	15-60 mg
Diazepam	Valium	4-40 mg
Halazepan	Paxipam	60-160 mg
Benzodiazepines (Shorter acting)		
Alprazolam	Xanax	0.75-1.5 mg
Lorazepam	Ativan	2-6 mg
Oxazepam	Serax	30-60 mg
Nonbenzodiazepines		
Buspirone	Buspar	20-30 mg
Hydroxyzine	Vistaril, Atarax	30-300 mg
Meprobamate	Equanil, Miltown	400-2000 mg
For control of aggression/and mania		
Carbamazepine	Tegretol	100-200 mg initially Increase to 400-1600 mg until serum level is 8-12 µg/ml

*Divided in 2 to 4 portions per day. Elderly would have lower averages and treatment resistent patients might have much higher averages than those shown.

Alcoholism

- Definition
    1. Recurrent use of alcohol to the extent it significantly interferes with the individuals physical, social, and/or emotional life
    2. Characterized by preoccupation with the drug, loss of control over its use, physical dependence, and tolerance
- Etiology/Incidence
    1. Multifactorial and poorly understood; several etiologic theories have been developed
        a. Psychological
            (1) Retarded ego, weak super ego
            (2) Fixed in lower level of psychosocial development

        (a) Dependent personality with poor impulse control

        (b) Low frustration tolerance

        (c) Low self-esteem

    b. Biologic

        (1) Physiologic changes in enzymes, genes, brain chemistry, hormones cause the disorder

        (2) May be familial, inherited or acquired

  2. About 1 in 12 persons have serious problems related to alcohol use

    a. Children of alcoholics are 4 times as likely to develop alcoholism as children of non-alcoholics

    b. Three times as many men as women are alcoholics and they are more likely to develop the problem early in life

    c. Although the average age of onset is 25 to 35 years of age, recent reports indicate a growing incidence among adolescents

■ Signs and Symptoms

  1. Definite (Level I)

    a. Blackouts

    b. Alcoholic hepatitis

    c. Withdrawal symptoms—hallucinations; fine tremors of face, tongue and hands; disorientation; seizures

    d. Memory loss, confabulation

    e. Nystagmus

    f. Prior exhibition of signs and symptoms of levels II and III

  2. Probable (Level II)

    a. Previous diagnosis of

        (1) Cirrhosis

        (2) Pancreatitis without cholelithiasis

    b. Loss of control over alcohol intake

    c. Numbness of hands and feet

    d. Increased incidence of infection

    e. Weight loss

  f. Forgetfulness

  g. Trauma from accidents or altercations—cigarette burns, healed fractures

  h. Hypothermic injuries

  i. Attempted suicide

  j. Symptoms of associated diseases; see Table 4

 3. Possible (Level III)

  a. Blurred or dim vision

  b. Nocturnal diuresis

  c. Anxiety or depression

  d. Impotence

  e. Symptoms of associated diseases; see Table 4

  f. History of chronic gastritis, anemia, clotting disorders, marital discord or loss of significant relationships (job, family, friends)

Table 4.
Conditions Commonly Associated With Substance Abuse

1.	Frequent upper respiratory infection
2.	Slowly healing skin ulcers
3.	Recurrent vaginal infections
4.	Hepatitis
5.	Sexually Transmited Disease
6.	Mononucleosis
7.	Malnutrition
8.	HIV Infection
9.	Pancreatitis
10.	Tuberculosis

- Differential Diagnosis: Determine level of alcoholism and look for concurrent abuse of other substances

- Physical Findings

 1. Definite (Level I)

  a. General Appearance—fearful, anxious, stuporous, hyperactive, or incoherent

  b. Vital Signs—mild fever, tachycardia, increased or labile BP

    c. Integumentary—flushed face and/or palms, spider nevi, angiomas on face, numerous scars, ecchymotic areas; generalized tissue edema, and dry, dull hair

    d. HEENT—pupil constriction, nystagmus, parotid adenopathy, inflamed buccal cavity, alcoholic odor to breath, fissures at corners of mouth

    e. Cardiovascular—tachycardia; dysrhythmias; weak, irregular peripheral pulses

    f. Abdomen—gastric distention, ascites, enlarged liver, tenderness

    g. Musculoskeletal—muscle wasting, healed or new fractures

    h. Neurological—memory loss, confabulation, hallucinations, disorientation, fine motor tremors, unsteady ataxic gait

2. Probable (Level II) and Possible (Level III)

    a. General Appearance—no major abnormalities

    b. Vital signs—normal or possible tachycardia, hypertension, and cardiac dysrhythmias

    c. Integumentary—unexplained ecchymosis

    d. HEENT—parotid adenopathy, angiomas

    e. Abdomen—hepatomegaly, tenderness

    f. Neurological—hyperreflexia; unsteady walk, ataxia (Wernicke-Korsakoff Syndrome)

■ Diagnostic Tests/Findings

1. Blood alcohol/drug levels—may or may not be severely elevated depending on amount and time of consumption

    a. 300 mg/100 ml at anytime = definite diagnosis

    b. 100 mg/ml on routine exam = definite diagnosis

    c. 150 mg/ml without evidence of intoxication = alcohol tolerance

2. CBC—increased or depressed white count; microcytic, hypochromic or macrocytic, megaloblastic anemia; decreased platelets

3. Blood glucose—hyper or hypoglycemia

4. Electrolytes—hypokalemia and hypomagnesia

5. Liver Function—SGOT, SGPT, and amylase elevated

6. Prothrombin Time—prolonged

7. Urinalysis—infection, ketones

8. Nutritional—albumin and total protein decreased, folic acid low

9. Chest radiograph—enlarged heart, right lower lobe pneumonia

10. ECG—Dysrhythmias, cardiac myopathies, ischemic heart disease

■ Management/Treatment

1. Use history and physical evidence to determine early, middle or late stages. CAGE screening test may help (40 open ended questions related to drinking patterns) (Pokorny, Miller & Kaplan, 1972; Buck, Shaw, Cleary, Delbanco & Aronson, 1987)

2. Complete an addiction severity assessment tool to determine problem severity profile, e.g., MAST (Michigan Alcohol Screening Test)

3. Consult with physician regarding treatment and possible need for detoxification

4. Confront client with diagnosis "Alcoholism"

5. Do not use nebulous statements, e.g., "We think you might have a drinking problem" or "You need to cut down on your drinking"

6. Tell the client it is a disease and treatable

7. Tell the client it is not his/her fault but he/she IS responsible for accepting treatment and the goal of therapy is abstinence

8. Describe treatment options

9. Make appropriate referral for treatment and follow-up

    a. Alcoholics Anonymous (most successful)

    b. Behavioral approaches

    c. Rational emotive psychotherapy

    d. Psychodrama

10. Provide family members with information on alcoholism and encourage involvement in Al Anon (for families of alcoholics) and/or Ala-Teen and Ala-Tots (for teenagers and young children of alcoholics)

■ General Considerations

1. Many treatment programs will not accept pregnant women

2. Alcoholic women have a higher incidence of suicide attempts than

both alcoholic men and the female population as a whole; see section on suicide

3. Females, even with less alcohol consumption are more likely to develop liver disease than men

4. Alcohol use by pregnant women is the leading cause of mental retardation

5. Women's drinking and drug problems are often viewed as less serious than men's and are more frequently misdiagnosed

6. If seeing a patient who was referred for treatment of alcoholism reinforce participation in treatment and use of any agreed upon treatment aids

7. Avoid compounding the problems or hindering recovery by prescribing sedatives or other depressants (cross tolerance)

Table 5
Commonly Abused Drugs

Generic or Trade Name	Street/Slang name
Depressants	
Codeine	School boy
Meperidine HCL (Demerol)	Demies
Hydromorphone HCL (Dilaudid)	Little D
Heroin	H; horse; junk; downtown; hard stuff; scag; white stuff
Methadone HCL	Meth; dollies
Morphine	M; Miss Emma; morph
Opium	Black stuff; Blue Velvet
Methaqualone (Qualude)	Ludes; 714s; Qs; Soapers
Pentobarbital	Downers; yellow jackets
Amobarbital/secobarbital (comb.),	Blues; red hearts; purple
Phenobarbital	hearts; reds; F40s; rainbows
Benzodiazepines (Librium, Valium)	Tanks, downs
Stimulants	
Cocaine	Coke; snow; flake; toot; uptown; crack; blow
Dextroamphetamines;	Bennies; black beauties; copilots
Methamphetamines (Benzedrine)	Dexies; speed; meth; crank
Biphetamine (Desoxyn; Dexedrine)	Crystal; uppers
Hallucinogens	
Lysergic acid diethylamide	LSD; acid
Mescaline (peyote)	Buttons; cactus; mesc.
Myristicin	Nutmeg
Dimethyltryptamine	DMT, STP
Psilocybin	Magic mushroom
Phencyclidine HCL	PCP; angel dust; DOA

Psychoactive Substance Abuse

- Definition
  1. Misuse of any substance capable of producing altered state of consciousness and/or euphoria
  2. Addiction or compulsive use includes
     a. Psychologic craving
     b. Physiologic dependence (withdrawal symptoms with discontinuance)
     c. Tolerance (need for larger and larger doses to produce desired effect)
- Etiology/Incidence
  1. As with alcohol abuse, several theories have been developed to explain the cause of substance abuse. They include
     a. Psychologic
        (1) Failure to complete developmental tasks
        (2) Underdeveloped ego
        (3) Dependent personality
        (4) Poor impulse control
        (5) Ego breakdown with subsequent drug use as a coping mechanism
     b. Biologic hereditary/genetic factors
        (1) Neurotransmitter deficiency
        (2) Enzyme deficiency
     c. Family Dynamics
        (1) Dysfunctional family system
        (2) Absent parent
        (3) Tyrannical or weak ineffective parent
        (4) Negative role models
        (5) Drugs used for stress relief
        (6) Cultural perceptions of drug abuse

2. Incidence
   a. Drug use is the leading cause of death among teens
   b. 26% of female and 24% of males between the age of 12 to 17 years have used an illicit drug
   c. More than 1 million women on legal psychoactive drugs
   d. 66% of psychoactive drugs are prescribed for women
   e. Most commonly used substances alone or in combination; see Table 5
      (1) Depressants—benzodiazepines, barbiturates, opiates, morphine, heroin, alcohol, sedatives, hypnotics, and minor tranquilizers
         (a) Most widely used and abused drugs
         (b) Often prescribed for anxiety, depression, or sleep disorders
      (2) Stimulants (amphetamines, cocaine, caffeine, tobacco)
         (a) Most commonly abused stimulants other than caffeine and nicotine are amphetamine and cocaine
         (b) Twice as many males as females use stimulants primarily in the 21 to 44 year age range
      (3) Hallucinogens (Lysergic acid diethylamide, LSD; myristicene, nutmeg; dimethyltryptamine, DMT; psilocybin, magic mushroom; phencyclidine, PCP or angel dust; mescaline, peyote; cannabis, hashish and marijuana; and chemically related substances)

■ Signs and Symptoms
   1. Depressants
      a. Nausea/vomiting
      b. Myalgia, deep bone or muscle pain (methadone abusers)
      c. Rhinorrhea, sneezing, excessive lacrimation
      d. Headache
      e. Miosis
      f. Euphoria
      g. Apathy, dysphoria, depression

h. Drowsiness, psychomotor retardation, slurred speech

i. Impaired attention, memory, social judgment (disinhibition)

j. Ataxia, tremors, lack of coordination

k. Mood swings, aggression, combativeness; loss of impulse control

l. Auditory hallucinations, paranoia

m. Fever, perspiration (with withdrawal)

2. Stimulants

a. Restlessness, irritability, anxiety, confusion, aggression

b. Tachycardia, cardiac arrhythmia, chest pain (cocaine), increased blood pressure

c. Elation, grandiosity

d. Perspiration or chills

e. Hyper or hypothermia

f. Abdominal pain, nausea/vomiting, diarrhea/frequent urination

g. Insomnia

h. Paranoia, hallucinations (visual and tactile with cocaine)

i. Dilated pupils

3. Hallucinogenics

a. Dilated pupils, vertical and horizontal nystagmus

b. Flushed skin

c. Increased pulse and BP

d. Marked anxiety; panic paranoia

e. Hallucinations, visual and sensory distortions

f. Rapid, severe mood changes, hostility, aggression, violence

g. Depression, suicidal thoughts

h. Grandiosity, euphoria

i. Tremors

j. Flashbacks

k. Insensitivity to pain

■ Differential Diagnosis

1. Poly abuse is common and may present with intoxication, overdose, and/or in various stages of withdrawal

2. Rule out other disorders that may account for presenting signs and symptoms, e.g.

    a. Seizure disorders

    b. Hypo or hyperthyroidism, thyroid storm

    c. Hyper or hypoglycemia

    d. Schizophrenia, mania

    e. Head injury

- Physical Findings: In addition to drug specific signs, some general physical findings might include

    1. General appearance—unkempt, poor hygiene

    2. Vital signs—temperature elevation, increased or decreased BP, tachycardia, tachypnea

    3. Integumentary—bruises, burns, needle marks, infections, cellulitis, ulcerations

    4. HEENT—changes in pupil size, reaction to light, and extraocular movements; poor oral hygiene, puncture wounds under the tongue, pharyngitis, inflammation and or erosion of the nasal mucosa

    5. Abdomen—tenderness, organomegaly

    6. Cardiovascular—dysrhythmia

    7. Neuromuscular—incoordination; decreased pain perception (PCP); alterations and distortions in consciousness, attention, sensory perceptions

- Diagnostic Tests/Findings

    1. CBC—leukocytosis; anemia

    2. Urine and Drug screens—positive for abused substance(s)

    3. If associated diseases are present other alterations will be noted, e.g., abnormal liver enzymes, thyroid function tests, or glucose levels

- Management/Treatment

    1. Depressant Abuse

        a. Identify drugs taken, when taken, and route of administration if possible

    b. Assess level of consciousness

    c. Evaluate for evidence of head trauma

    d. Refer to physician, emergency room, or drug detoxification unit if acute overdose or intoxication is noted

    e. In the meantime provide quiet, lighted room and do not leave patient alone

    f. Monitor vital signs

    g. In consultation with physician determine need for starting an IV

2. Stimulant Abuse

    a. In cases of intoxication, overdose, or withdrawal refer to physician or emergency room

    b. In the meantime provide quiet area with reduced stimuli and high staff profile; aggressive behavior is associated with amphetamine use.

    c. Monitor cardiac rate and rhythm; ventricular arrhythmia/cardiac arrest may occur with toxic levels of cocaine

    d. Persons experiencing stimulant withdrawal may be suicidal as a result of profound CNS rebound depression; use suicide precautions until patient is transferred to emergency room or detoxification unit

    e. For nonemergency cases refer to drug rehabilitation unit

3. Hallucinogenic Abuse

    a. Hallucinogenics do not have a withdrawal syndrome and do not require detoxification as such

    b. Refer patients with psychotic symptoms to the psychiatric unit

    c. Protect client and others from injury

        (1) Darkened, quiet, non-threatening environment to decrease the likelihood of confusion, fear, and violent behavior

        (2) Speak in a soft, non-threatening voice

            (a) If LSD has been taken provide reassurance verbally and by touch and orient the individual ("talking down")

            (b) If PCP intoxication is present do not attempt "talking

down" it will increase the patient's agitation and tendency for violent behavior

    (3)   Suspiciousness and paranoia, visual and auditory hallucinations, and agitation make suicide or accidental injury a likely possibility. Take precautions early

    (4)   If frightened and hallucinating avoid the use of physical restraints, however, use of restraints with PCP users may be necessary for the safety of self and others; PCP is an anesthetic and alters thinking; persons on PCP are a danger to themselves as well as to others

- General Considerations

  1. Primary role is diagnosis and referral

  2. Consult with physician on medication use

    a. Period of drug free observation usually recommended

    b. To control psychotic and assaultive behaviors Haloperidol (Haldol) may be given

    c. To reduce muscle spasm and restlessness diazepam (valium) is used

    d. Phenothiazine neuroleptics should be avoided in patients on PCP because of the possibility of potentiating the anticholinergic effects of PCP

    e. Vitamin C tablets (ascorbic acid) or cranberry juice may be used to acidify the urine and promote excretion of PCP

  3. Many treatment programs will not accept pregnant women

  4. Many treatment programs do not provide child care or other alternatives for woman and can be a significant barrier to help

  5. Alcoholics Anonymous, Al-Anon will also accept other substance abusers. Family members should be given information on Al Anon and Ala-Teen even if patient refuses treatment

  6. Narcotics Anonymous (substance abusers) and Nar-Anon (families of substance abusers) groups are available in some areas

Questions

Select the best answer.

1. Which of the following is associated with higher risk for major depression?

   a. Being male
   b. Having had a traumatic experience in the last six months
   c. Being middle aged
   d. Having a family history of alcoholism

2. Which is true of Major Depression?

   a. Majority of patients will have a reoccurrence
   b. It may be a normal grief reaction
   c. It is often self-limiting
   d. It is more strongly associated with chronic drug use than other depressive states

3. Dysthymic Disorder is distinguished from Major Depression by which of the following?

   a. It usually first manifests itself in old age
   b. It is rarely associated with drug use
   c. It lacks the physical signs of Major Depression
   d. It is rarely chronic

4. Post-traumatic Stress Syndrome is marked by which triad of findings?

   a. Intrusive thoughts, nightmares, flashbacks
   b. Tendency to globalize, psychomotor retardation, hypersomnia
   c. Weight loss, feelings of helplessness, irritability
   d. Indifference, decreased concentration, hyperphagia

5. Mrs. S. is a 65 year old who comes in complaining of feeling depressed. She would like a prescription to make her feel better. Her husband died three weeks ago.

   The data you have at this point indicates

   a. Her problem is a normal grief reaction, but will require surveillance
   b. Diagnostic tests will not be needed
   c. Pharmacologic intervention would not be warranted
   d. Major depression is a possibility

6. Your next step would be to

   a. Refer her for psychologic evaluation

b. Prescribe antidepressants

c. Obtain additional information

d. Reassure her that the problem is self limiting

7. In a patient of this age it would be important to remember that

a. Somatic signs may be overlooked as normal changes

b. Elderly may require higher doses of antidepressants for therapeutic effect

c. Previously undiagnosed Bipolar disorder is probable

d. Tricyclics may cause "hypomania"

8 With further exploration you determine that Mrs. S. has had intermittent episodes of anorexia, difficulty sleeping, has been feeling tired and listless. She has had to force herself to go out with her friends, although she did enjoy her grandson's birthday party a week ago. She denies any thoughts of harming herself. Routine physical and lab work are unremarkable.

The most likely diagnosis for this patient is

a. Adjustment disorder with depressed mood

b. Primary major depression

c. Dysthymic disorder

d. Bipolar disorder

9 Mrs. S. tells you that she can't help thinking that her husband might not have died if she had done things differently.

Which response would be most appropriate?

a. Telling her that these thoughts will decrease in a few weeks

b. Encourage her to elaborate on these thoughts

c. Tell her a psychologist or psychiatrist will best help her with her guilt

d. Suggest an antidepressant will correct this kind of thinking

10. A 17 year-old male student comes into the student health service complaining of weight loss, fatigue, anorexia. He states that the symptoms began about a month-ago after he broke up with his girl-friend. He has difficulty sleeping and says he wakes up thinking about her. He says that since she left him he just doesn't enjoy going out anymore and has been spending most of his free time in his room. His affect is flat and he shows little expression as he relates his problem. The physical examination is within normal limits.

You suspect depression to be his problem. Your next step would be to

a. Prescribe an antianxiety medication

b. Find out how he has coped with losses in the past

c. Explain that this is a temporary situation and will probably clear up in another couple of weeks

    d. Ask him directly about feelings or thoughts of harming himself

11. Which factors in the available data might lead you to suspect that he might be suicidal?

    a. Weight loss, fatigue, anorexia
    b. Insomnia, loss of pleasure, social withdrawal
    c. Age, gender, emotional loss, signs of depression
    d. Intrusive thoughts, flat affect, with normal physical exam

12. Upon further questioning he admits to suicidal ideation. Knowing which of the following would be most helpful in assessing his suicide risk?

    a. Whether there have been any suicides in his family
    b. If he rooms alone or has a roommate
    c. If his family lives nearby
    d. If he has a plan for suicide in the next 24 hours
    e. If he uses marijuana or alcohol

13. This patient has a roommate, but his family lives in another state and he denies substance abuse, or definite plan or time for suicide. What would be the best action at this point?

    a. Consult with a physician regarding psychotherapy and antidepressants
    b. Consult with a physician and arrange for hospitalization
    c. Give him a prescription for antidepressants and arrange to have him stay with his family for a week
    d. Give him a prescription for antidepressants, call his roommate, and have them both check with you in 24 hours

14. A 38 year old married male comes to the clinic asking for an AIDS test. He has been awakening at night with sweating and his heart pounding. He has read in *Time* magazine that night sweats were a sign of AIDS and a few years ago he had to have a transfusion after a car accident. He would also like to have a radiograph of his throat as he feels like there's something stuck in it and wonders if it might be cancer. At times he feels like he's losing control. He denies IV drug use or high risk sexual activities. He denies marital or work problems. In fact, he just got a promotion two weeks ago and he and his wife have bought a new home.

What other information would be most helpful to you in your diagnosis?

    a. How long has he had these symptoms
    b. Whether he has nightmares
    c. If anyone in his family has had a major mental health problem
    d. If he has a prolapsed heart valve

15. If he denies nightmares and has had the symptoms for about two weeks and the

physical findings are normal, you should

a. Order a barium swallow
b. Refer to a gastroenterologist
c. Consider a post traumatic stress syndrome as the probable diagnosis
d. Consider situational anxiety as the probable diagnosis

16. Benzodiazepines are used in anxiety disorders. They are

a. Contraindicated in glaucoma
b. Not helpful for short term use in situational anxiety
c. Usually physiologically addicting
d. As effective as beta blockers for control of palpitations

17. The most common mental health problem seen in general practice is

a. Anxiety
b. Depression
c. Alcoholism
d. Schizophrenia

18. Which of these symptoms is least characteristic of anxiety?

a. Sleep disorder
b. Decreased concentration
c. Irritability
d. Indifference

19. Which of the following would least likely be a cause of anxiety symptoms?

a. Thyrotoxicosis
b. Hyperglycemia
c. Hormone-releasing tumor
d. Prolapsed mitral valve

20. Tricyclics are not used for Bipolar disorders because

a. They may precipitate mania
b. They cause liver dysfunction
c. They may lead to physiologic dependance
d. They may cause a hypertensive crisis

21. Mrs. J. is a 65 year old widow who completed a series of ECT treatments a week ago with positive results. Both she and her daughter are concerned that she continues to experience a significant memory loss.

You could be most helpful by

a. Reporting the problem to her psychiatrist
b. Allow her to ventilate her feelings without any comment regarding the memory

loss
c. Explain that the loss is temporary and full memory will return
d. Inform her that many individuals of her age begin to experience memory loss

22. Mr. P. is a 45 year old divorced male who comes in for a physical exam required for a new job. During the interview he reveals previous hospitalization for pancreatitis and long term self-medication for gastritis. His physical exam is normal except for slight tenderness in the RUQ. A CBC reveals macrocytic, megaloblastic anemia.

Which diagnostic test would be most helpful at this point?

a. ECG and electrolytes
b. Liver function, B_{12} and Folic acid levels, and electrolytes
c. Chest radiograph and ultrasound of the gallbladder
d. Blood albumin levels and bone marrow studies

23. Ms. Z, a 35 year old female, comes into the clinic demanding to be seen immediately. She is agitated and complaining loudly of police brutality. She states that she was unjustly jailed overnight because of a misunderstanding and that she was shackled for more than three hours causing bruises on her wrists and ankles. Upon further elaboration she states the police altered a blood test and said her blood alcohol level was 300.

This information alone indicates

a. Paranoid ideation
b. Alcoholism
c. Need for legal services referral
d. The patient may have a drinking problem

24. Non-compliance with medication is a concern in outpatient treatment of patients with mental health problems. Which of the following would be least helpful in promoting medication regimen compliance?

a. Client involvement in treatment decision making
b. Providing the client with information about expected action and side effects of the medications
c. Arranging follow-up visits with whatever staff are available
d. Maintaining telephone communication with the patient to monitor effects and response to medication

25. One of the most effective treatments for alcoholism is

a. Psychoanalysis
b. Active participation in A.A.
c. Aversion therapy with Antabuse

    d. Active participation in Al-Anon

26. Ms. C is brought to the emergency room from a party by her friends. She is stuporous, confused, and has pinpoint pupils.

These signs are consistent with

    a. PCP intoxication
    b. Heroin use
    c. LSD
    d. Amphetamine withdrawal

27. A 23 year old male comes to the clinic to obtain treatment for a cut on his arm he received in a street fight. His face is badly bruised from a previous fight. He is unkempt and shows evidence of poor personal hygiene. He has a history of alcohol abuse. At present he is tachycardic and has an elevated blood pressure. His pupils are dilated and he is slightly diaphoretic. He complains of chest pain.

These signs are consistent with

    a. Acute alcohol intoxication
    b. Chronic heroin use
    c. Recent use of hallucinogenics
    d. Recent use of cocaine

28. A young male adult is brought into the emergency room by the police. He is highly agitated and hostile and verbally abusive and threatening. He has several lacerations and bruises he sustained in a fight at a disco where he "tore the place apart."

You should

    a. Suspect police brutality
    b. Suspect LSD use
    c. Try to talk the patient down and keep him oriented
    d. Be prepared to administer Haldol

29. Which of the following IS NOT associated with physiologic dependance?

    a. Heroin
    b. Phenobarbital
    c. LSD
    d. Amphetamines

30. Mark is an 18 year old brought to the student health clinic complaining of chest pain and palpitations. He is highly anxious and perspiring. His roommate states he thinks he took some kind of drug.

In addition to myocardial infarction (MI) these symptoms could indicate intoxication or overdose of which of the following?

a. Heroin
b. Alcohol
c. PCP
d. Cocaine

31. Your first action in this case should be to

a. Arrange for emergency room transfer
b. Prepare for cardiopulmonary support
c. Draw blood gasses
d. Do nothing until he is seen by a physician

32. To enhance the excretion of PCP from the body give

a. Haloperidol
b. Ascorbic acid
c. Valium
d. A phenothiazine

33. Which pharmacologic agent is contraindicated in persons on PCP?

a. Valium
b. Phenothiazine
c. Haloperidol
d. Ascorbic Acid

34. CNS rebound is seen in withdrawal of

a. Depressants
b. Stimulants
c. Hallucinogenics
d. Alcohol

35. Aggressive behavior can be seen with abuse of which of the following?

a. Amphetamines
b. Depressants
c. Hallucinogenics
d. Any psychoactive substance

Answers

1. d
2. a
3. c
4. a
5. d
6. c
7. a
8. a
9. b
10. d
11. c
12. d
13. b
14. a
15. d
16. a
17. b
18. d
19. b
20. a
21. c
22. b
23. b
24. c
25. b
26. b
27. d
28. d
29. c
30. d
31. b
32. b
33. b
34. b
35. d

Bibliography

American Psychiatric Association (APA). (1987). *Diagnostic and statistical manual of mental disorders* (3rd. ed. rev.). Washington, D.C. Authors,

Buck, B., Shaw, S., Cleary, P., Delbanco, T. L., & Aronson, M.D. (1987). Screening for alcohol abuse using the CAGE questionnaire. *American Journal of Medicine, 82,* 231-235.

Citrone, L. (1994). Management of depression. *Postgraduate medicine,* 95(1), 132-143.

Coleman, D. (1991). Cardiovascular effects of cocaine abuse. *Journal of the American Academy of Nurse Practitioners, 3*(3), 105-109.

Chychula, N. M., & Okore, C. (1990). The cocaine epidemic, treatment options for cocaine dependence. *Nurse Practitioner. 15*(8), 33-40.

Chychula, N. M., & Okore, C. (1990). The cocaine epidemic: A comprehensive review of use, abuse, and dependence. *Nurse Practitioner. 15*(7), 31-39.

Doenge, M., Townsend, M., & Moorhouse, M. (1989). *Psychiatric care plans: Guidelines for client care.* Philadelphia: F. A. Davis.

Federici, C. M., & Tommasini, N. (1992). The assessment and management of panic disorder. *Nurse Practitioner, 17*(3), 20-34.

Meyo, S. L. (1990). Post-Traumatic stress disorder: An overview of three etiologic variables and psychopharmacologic treatment. *Nurse Practitioner. 15*(8), 41-45.

Meyo, S. L., (1990). The use of antidepressant medications: A guide for the primary care nurse practitioner. *Journal of the American Academy of Nurse Practitioners, 2*(2), 153-159.

National Council On Alcoholism And Drug Dependence, Inc. (1990). *NCADD fact sheet: Alcoholism, other drug addictions and related problems among women.* Washington, DC: National Council On Alcoholism and Drug Dependence.

Oswald, L. (1989) Cocaine addiction: The hidden dimension. *Archives of Psychiatric Nursing, 3*(3), 134-141.

Perry, M. V., & Anderson, G. L. (1992). Assessment and treatment strategies for depressive disorders commonly encountered in primary care settings. *Nurse Practitioner, 17*(6), 25-36.

Pokorny, A., Miller, B. A., & Kaplan, H. B. (1972) The brief MAST: A shortened version of the Michigan alcoholism screening test. *American Journal of Psychiatry, 129*, 342-345.

Starling, B., & Martin, A. C. (1990). Adult survivors of parental alcoholism: Implications for primary care. *Nurse Practitioner, 15*(7), 16-24.

Care of the Aging Adult

Catharine Kopac

Demographics of Older Adults

- Population statistics (Profile of Older Americans, 1993)
    1. Persons 65 years or older numbered 32.3 million
        a. 12.7% of U.S.—1 in every 8 Americans
        b. Increase of 24% (6.1 million) since 1980
    2. Sex ratio—149 women for every 100 men
        a. Increases with age
        b. Ratio of 123/100 for 65 to 69 age group
        c. Ratio of 259/100 for 85 and older
    3. Older population itself is getting older
        a. In 1992 the 65 to 74 age group (18.5 million) was 8 times larger than in 1900
        b. 75 to 84 group (10.6 million) was 14 times larger
        c. Over 85 age group (3.3 million) was 26 times larger
    4. In 1991, persons reaching age 65 had an average life expectancy of an additional 17.4 years
    5. Factors affecting decreased mortality—improved nutrition, improved sanitation, social improvements, disease prevention, health promotion/ wellness movement
- Marital status and living arrangements
    1. Older men are twice as likely to be married as compared to older women (76% of men; 41% of women)
    2. Half of all older women are widows (48%); 5 times as many widows (8.6 million) as widowers (1.9 million)
    3. Majority (67%) of noninstitutionalized persons live in a family setting
    4. In 1990, 5% (1.6 million) of the 65+ population lived in nursing homes
- Income and Poverty
    1. Median income (1992)—persons over 65 years of age, $14,548 for men and $8,189 for women
    2. Median income (1991)—households headed by persons over 65 years of age, $25,315

3. In 1992, 47% of persons living alone, or with nonrelatives, had an income of $10,000 or less; 8% had incomes under $5,000. Median income was $10,624

4. Major sources of income (1990)

    a. Social Security (37%)

    b. Asset income (25%)

    c. Earnings (18%)

    d. Public & private pensions (18%)

    e. All other sources (3%)

5. Twenty percent of the older population was poor or near-poor in 1992

■ Health and Health Care

1. Number of days in which usual activities are restricted due to illness or injury increases with age; the average is 34 days per year.

2. Six million (23%) older people living in the community have health-related difficulty with one or more personal care activities (bathing, dressing, eating, etc.)

3. 7.6 million (28%) have difficulty with one or more home management activities (shopping, managing money, doing housework, etc.)

4. Most older people have at least one chronic condition and many have multiple conditions; the most frequently occurring conditions

    a. Arthritis (48%)

    b. Hypertension (37%)

    c. Hearing impairments (32%)

    d. Heart disease (30%)

    e. Orthopedic impairments (18%)

    f. Cataracts (17%)

    g. Diabetes (10%)

    h. Sinusitis (14%)

5. In 1987 the over 65 group represented approximately 12% of the population but accounted for 36% of total personal health care expenditures; expenditures totaled $162 billion and averaged $5,360 per year per older person. Approximately 25% came from direct

"out-of-pocket" payments by older persons

6. Hospital expenses are the largest portion of health expenditures (42%); followed by physicians (21%) and nursing home care (20%)

Theories of Aging

- Biological: Attempts to explain three in-vivo biocomponents—cells that undergo miosis throughout life, (e.g., white blood cells [WBCs], epithelial cells); cells incapable of division and renewal, (e.g., neurons); and noncellular material with little turnover and under integrated physiologic control, (e.g., collagen). A unifying theory does not exist that explains the underlying mechanics and causes of aging.

    1. Genetic theories

        a. Gene—one or more harmful genes in the organism become active in later life, causing failure of the organism to survive.

        b. Error—decreased bond over time in protein synthesis; weakening of organic synthesis produces defective cells, leading to successive generations of faulty cells

        c. Somatic mutation—when cells are exposed to x-ray radiation or chemicals, a cell-by-cell alteration of DNA occurs, thereby increasing the incidence of of chromosomal abnormalities

        d. Programmed (biologic clock)—internal, genetic control determines aging process; a set time to live, winds down over time

    2. Nongenetic theories

        a. Immunologic—changes in lymphoid tissue leads to imbalance in T cells and subsequent cellular immune function decrease; results in autoantibody production and immune deficiencies

        b. Free radical—unstable free radicals from environmental pollutants alter biological system, causing changes in chromosomes, pigment, and collagen

        c. Cross-link—collagen molecules and chemicals alter tissue functioning, leading to stiffness and rigidity in tissues

    3. Physiologic theories

        a. Stress adaptation—accumulated damage results from stress response activation

        b. Wear-and-tear—after repeated injury/use, body structures and functions deteriorate from stress

- Social: Behavioristic; examines how one most successfully experiences late life

    1. Disengagement—"aging is an inevitable, mutual, withdrawal or disengagement, resulting in decreased interaction between the aging person and others in the social system he belongs to" (Cummings & Henry, 1961, p. 2)

        a. Progressive social disengagement occurs with age

        b. Mutual, acceptable to individual and society

        c. Studies done since this theory was proposed have found

            (1) Theory does not hold true for the majority

            (2) Degree of disengagement varies with personality and life activity pattern

            (3) Social involvement is a lifelong pattern that remains constant

            (4) Health, energy, income, and roles affect disengagement and activity pattern

    2. Activity theory purports that the maintenance of regular activity, roles (formal and informal), and social supports is positively correlated to life satisfaction and positive self concept

        a. Theory does not take into account diversity of outlook and lifestyle

        b. Studies done since this theory was proposed have found that the quality and meaningfulness of activity are more important than the number of social activities

    3. Continuity—focuses on the relationship between life satisfaction and activity as an expression of enduring personality traits

        a. Assumes stability of patterns over time

        b. Recognizes that the "self" remains the same despite life changes

        c. Focuses on personality and individual behavior over time

- Developmental

    1. Psychosocial

        a. Adult development is based on successful resolution of basic psychosocial conflicts

        b. The crisis facing the mature adult is that of generativity versus stagnation, or self-absorption

    c. Final crisis is integrity versus despair

  2. Developmental tasks—(Erik Erickson, 1963) adult development encompasses a number of developmental tasks

    a. Tasks of later maturity (60-death)

      (1) Adjusting to decreasing physical strength and health

      (2) Adjusting to retirement and reduced income

      (3) Adjusting to death of spouse or partner

      (4) Establishing an explicit affiliation with one's age group

      (5) Adopting and adapting social roles in a flexible way

      (6) Establishing satisfactory physical living arrangements

  3. Adaptation theory—views development as age-appropriate adaptation to social expectations and norms; healthy adaptation is determined within the context of three dimensions of time: historical time, life time (chronological age), and social time, all of which are interwoven (Neugarten, 1968)

  4. Life transitions—the life transitions that occur in adulthood provide a useful framework for explaining adult development; transformation is the central concept of adult development; believes people have an innate drive to grow and change (Gould, 1978); general themes for 50 to 60 year olds

    a. Mellowing and decreased negativeness

    b. Realization of mortality and concern for health

    c. Less responsibility and concern for children (Havinghurst, 1972)

Health Assessment

■ Special considerations to insure an age-specific approach

  1. Normal age-related findings must be differentiated from indicators of disease or disability

  2. There must be an appreciation for the overall decline in homeostatic mechanisms that occur with aging

  3. Norms for health and illness have not been established for this age group

  4. There is often an altered presentation of/or blunted response to specific disease; therefore, the usual signs and symptoms may not be present

- Interviewing and Health History

  1. Establishes the nurse-client relationship

  2. Identifies the chief complaint

  3. Provides a subjective account of current and past health status

  4. Provides medication history including knowledge of drugs, barriers to safe drug taking, system for drug taking, and timing of drug ingestion in relationship to activities of daily living for

     a. Current prescription drugs

     b. Over-the-counter remedies

     c. Home remedies

  5. Provides the personal history & family history

  6. Encompasses review of systems

  7. Identifies topics for health teaching

  8. Provides means for life review

  9. Interviewer concerns

     a. Awareness of age biases and stereotypes

     b. Client centered pace

     c. Positioning to compensate for sensory loss

     d. Adjusting interview in light of fatigue and sensory overload; several interview sessions may be needed to obtain complete information

     e. Tendency for client to reminisce

  10. Client concerns

     a. Visual changes

     b. Hearing changes

     c. Anxiety

     d. Reduced energy level

     e. Pain

     f. Multiplicity and interrelatedness of health problems

- Functional Assessment

  1. Identifies individual needs and care deficits

2. Provides the basis for developing a care plan that enhances abilities in the presence of coexisting disease and chronic illness

3. Provides feedback regarding treatment and rehabilitation

4. Types of functional assessment

   a. Assessment of "Activities of Daily Living"—assesses ability to perform personal care, e.g., bathing, dressing

   b. Assessment of "Instrumental Activities of Daily Living"—assesses the ability to perform more complex personal-care activities, such as cooking, cleaning

5. Functional assessment tools

   a. Katz "Index of Activities of Daily Living" (Katz, Ford, & Moskowitz, 1963)—assesses the functional independence or dependence of clients in bathing, dressing, toileting, transferring, continence, and eating

   b. Barthel Index (Mahoney & Barthel, 1981)—assesses the amount of physical assistance required when a person can no longer carry out activities of daily living

   c. OARS (Older Adult Resource Services): Multidimensional Functional Assessment (1975)—evaluates ability, disability, and the capability level at which a person can function

■ General Survey and Mental Status: The general survey provides an overall impression of the client's general state of health as gleaned from body development, posture, gait, grooming and hygiene, facial expressions and speech. The mental status assessment determines if there are thoughts and mental processes that interfere with optimal level of functioning; an essential component of this assessment is identification of the onset and historical progression of symptoms and behavior. Mental status assessment

1. Is integrated into the interview and physical examination

2. Evaluates client's awareness, orientation, cognitive abilities, mood and affect

3. Mental status tools

   a. Short Portable Mental Status Questionnaire (SPMSQ) (Pfeiffer, 1975)

   b. Mini-Mental State Exam (MMSE) (Folstein, Folstein & McHugh, 1975)

4. If depression is suspected, there are several tools that can be used

    a. Center for Epidemiologic Studies Depression Scale (CES-D) (Radloff, 1977)

    b. Beck Depression Inventory (BDI) (Beck, Ward & Mendelson, 1961)

    c. Hamilton Rating Scale for Depression (Hamilton, 1960)

- Physical Assessment

  1. General Guidelines

    a. Elderly are often cold and at risk for hypothermia; therefore, limit exposure of body parts with careful draping

    b. Pace the examination to accommodate the client

    c. Allow additional time for processing information, if needed, when giving instructions

    d. Determine the appropriateness of some assessment techniques, e.g., deep knee bends and range of motion in clients with total hip replacement or prothesis; range of motion measurements may be required

    e. Allow for client fatigue

      (1) Minimize change of position

      (2) Organize the body into units for head to toe examination

      (3) Integrate information sought by body systems

  2. Integument

    a. Age-related changes

      (1) Wrinkles, folding, sagging, furrowing

      (2) Decreased turgor, loss of fat in face and limbs

      (3) Transparent-like, easy bruising

      (4) Spotty pigmentation in areas exposed to sun (senile lentigines)

      (5) Dryness

      (6) Pallor

      (7) Less sweating, inability to maintain body temperature

      (8) Quality, quantity, and distribution of hair change—thins on

scalp, axilla, pubic area, upper and lower extremities; decreased facial hair in men; women may develop chin and upper lip hair

    (9)   Color of hair may change to dull gray or white

    (10) Nails become dull, brittle, hard, thick, sometimes with splitting of nail surface; nail growth slows

b. Commonly occurring normal skin lesions

    (1)   Seborrheic keratosis—pigmented (light tan to black) macular papular lesion seen on neck, chest, back, and at hair line; can be warty, scaly, or greasy in appearance

    (2)   Senile ectasias (cherry angioma)—bright, ruby-red or purplish papular lesions, 1 to 5 mm, found on trunk, upper chest, and extremities

    (3)   Acrochordons (cutaneous skin tags)—soft, pinkish tan to light brown pedunculated lesions on neck, upper chest, and axillary folds

    (4)   Sebaceous hyperplasia—yellowish, flattened, papular lesion with central depressions, found on forehead, nose, and cheeks

c. Commonly occurring deviations of diagnostic significance

    (1)   Yellowing, cyanosis, or erythema

    (2)   Excoriation over flaking

    (3)   Scaling

    (4)   Excessive thickening, hardening

    (5)   Excessive cold or warm (generalized or localized)

    (6)   Excessive sagging of skin folds and protruding bony prominences (marked weight loss)

    (7)   Crusted skin, foul body odor

    (8)   Skin tears, excessive bruises; note pattern of bruises

    (9)   Hyperemia (pressure area); reddened area persists when pressure is relieved

    (10) Sudden hair loss; patchy balding

    (11) Spoon shaped nails (hypochromic anemias, chronic infections, malnutrition, Raynaud's disease); clubbing

      (12) Excessive thickness of nails (psoriasis, fungal infections, poor vascular supply)

  d. Commonly occurring abnormal skin lesions

      (1)   Actinic or senile keratosis

      (2)   Squamous cell carcinoma

      (3)   Basal cell carcinoma

      (4)   Herpes zoster

      (5)   Seborrheic dermatitis

      (6)   Malignant melanoma

3.   Head, face and neck

  a. Age-related changes

      (1)   Drooping of eyelids (ptosis) and suborbital puffiness

      (2)   Jowls, double chin

      (3)   "Dowager's hump"

      (4)   Thyroid gland may move to a lower position in relation to the clavicles

  b. Commonly occurring deviations of diagnostic significance

      (1)   Marked facial asymmetry

      (2)   Facial expression—dull, sleepy, mask-like, tense, tics, tremors, twitches

      (3)   Unequal muscle contractions; fasciculations

      (4)   Asymmetrical movement during talking or smiling

      (5)   Marked limitation of neck movement

      (6)   Unilateral or bilateral thyroid lobe enlargement or nodules

      (7)   Palpable, hard, firm, large, nodular, irregular lymph nodes

4.   Eyes

  a. Age-related changes

      (1)   Reduced eye movement, deviation of the eyes, jerking eye movement

      (2)   Exophthalmus

      (3)   Increased sensitivity to glare

  (4) Adaptation to darkness—occurs more slowly

  (5) Altered depth perception

  (6) Changes in color vision

  (7) Arcus senilis

  (8) Tendency for grayish or light blue eyes

  (9) Enophthalmos

  (10) Chronic eye dryness

  (11) Decreased visual acuity

  (12) Diminished peripheral vision

  (13) Conjunctiva thins; sclera yellows and may have small, fatty, yellow nodules adjacent to the limbus

  (14) Decreased pupil size; slowed constriction in response to light and accommodation

  (15) Lens yellows and gradually becomes more opaque, resulting in cataract formation

  (16) Retinal changes—blood vessels narrower and straighter, arteries more opaque and somewhat gray in color; drusen (small, round, gray or yellow spots) near the macula

 b. Commonly occurring deviations of diagnostic significance

  (1) Sustained nystagmus

  (2) Asymmetrical light reflections in each eye

  (3) Lid drooping interfering with vision

  (4) Rapid blinking

  (5) Blepharospasm

  (6) Staring

  (7) Marked exophthalmos

  (8) Excessively yellow or dark blue sclera; increased number and size of visible vessels

  (9) Failure of blink reflex

  (10) Pupils of unequal size, irregular shape, absent or unequal convergence or constriction response

  (11) Decrease in or absence of red reflex

(12) Retinal changes—arterioles have enhanced narrowness, A-V nicking, hemorrhages of dark or red stains near vessels

(13) Floaters—usually considered a normal process; can also be associated with retinal detachment

6. Ears, Nose, and Throat

  a. Age-related changes

    Ear

(1) Auricle appears larger, lobule is elongated

(2) Cilia become coarser and stiffer; cerumen production decreases, remaining cerumen much drier

(3) Tympanic membrane is dull, somewhat retracted and white or gray in appearance

(4) Presbycusis—bilateral, progressive, sensorineural hearing loss which affects high frequency sound first

(5) Reduced speech perception

(6) Tinnitus

    Nose

(1) Protrudes more sharply

(2) Diminished sense of smell

    Mouth and Oropharynx

(1) Tooth enamel is abraded, underlying dentin thickens resulting in yellowing of the teeth

(2) Tooth surfaces wear down from long use

(3) Gums recede exposing roots

(4) Balding of tongue

(5) Altered taste perception, sweet and salty taste often blunted; sour and bitter remain intact

(6) Salivary secretion reduced

(7) Saliva more mucoid and thicker

(8) Periodontal structures atrophy and degenerate

  b. Commonly occurring deviations of diagnostic significance

    Ear

(1) Nodules, tophi, lesions

(2) Impacted cerumen, lesions, discharge

(3) Amber, blue, pink to red in color and/or bulging or retracted tympanic membrane

(4) Decreased hearing

Nose

(1) Bulbous appearance

(2) Redness

(3) Increased vascularization

(4) Discharge, crusting

(5) Inablity to identify strong odors

(6) Bright red or pale gray, masses, polyps, lesions

Mouth and Oropharynx

(1) Fissures at corner of mouth; cracked, pale, reddened, or cyanotic lips and/ or oral mucosa

(2) Plaques (*Candida albicans*)

(3) Vesicles, ulcerations, nodules

(4) Malocclusion, missing, darkened, stained, loose or broken teeth

(5) Deteriorated dental work

(6) Tongue or uvula deviates to one side on protrusion

(7) Unclear articulation of sound (phonation)

(8) Absence of gag reflex

(9) Unable to identify common tastes

7. Breasts

    a. Age-related changes

Female

(1) Slightly smaller, less dense, less nodular

(2) Pendulous, elongated, flattened

(3) Nipples become lighter in color, smaller, and flattened

b. Commonly occurring deviations of diagnostic significance

Female

(1) Grossly unequal, recent change in color, or size

(2) Masses, lesions

Male

(1) Gynecomastia, after age 50; usually unilateral (may be associated with testicular or pituitary tumors, cirrhosis, or drug therapy)

8. Thorax and Lungs

a. Age-related changes

(1) Anteroposterior diameter increases; hyperresonance

(2) Respiratory muscles weaken, rib cage becomes calcified, chest wall is stiffer

(3) Epithelial atrophy of cilia

(4) Decreased ability for effective cough

(5) Drier mucous membranes

b. Commonly occurring deviations of diagnostic significance

(1) Costal angle greater than 90 degrees

(2) Barrel chest

(3) Pallor, cyanosis, spider nevi

(4) Chest asymmetry

(5) Tactile fremitus

(a) Increased vibration (pneumonia, compressed lung, tumor)

(b) Decreased/absent vibration (pleural effusion, pneumothorax, emphysema)

(6) Diaphragmatic excursion

(a) Asymmetrical response

(b) Extremely limited excursion overall

(c) Bronchovesicular or bronchial breath sounds over peripheral lung fields

9. Heart and Vascular System

    a. Age-related changes ✗

        (1) Heart (without hypertension) remains the same size or becomes slightly smaller

        (2) Heart rate slows, stroke volume decreases, cardiac output is decreased by 30% to 40%

        (3) Sclerosis and thickening of valve leaflets (mitral and aortic valves); systolic ejection murmur common

        (4) Decreased efficiency of the conduction system leading to arrhythmias

        (5) Decrease in exercise tolerance

        (6) Systolic blood pressure increase (due to increase in response to the loss of elasticity in peripheral vessels and subsequent increase in peripheral resistance)

        (7) Lability of vasopressor action increases, thus raising both systolic and diastolic pressure

        (8) Baroreceptors are less sensitive (orthostatic hypotension)

        (9) EKG—slight prolongation of all intervals

    b. Commonly occurring deviations of diagnostic significance

        (1) Heart rate < 60 or > 90 beats per minute; irregular, bounding, diminished or asymmetrical pulses

        (2) BP of 140/90 to 160/95 mm Hg, coupled with evidence of end-organ damage, left ventricular hypertrophy, diabetes mellitus, smoking history, or family history of hypertension

        (3) BP < 90 mm Hg systolic or 60 mm Hg diastolic; excessively wide or narrow pulse pressure

        (4) BP drop > 15 to 20 mm Hg systolic, 5 mm Hg diastolic, and/or symptoms of dizziness upon standing

        (5) Arterial insufficiency

            (a) Marked pallor in one or both feet

            (b) Delayed color return

            (c) Hair loss on lower legs

            (d) Coolness to touch of extremities

    (e) Marked dusky redness or cyanosis of dependent feet

  (6) Venous insufficiency

    (a) Pain (Homan's sign), redness, thickening and tenderness along superficial vein

    (b) Unilateral or bilateral pitting edema, skin thickening, ulceration, and/or pigmentation

    (c) Distended veins

  (7) Jugular venous pressure over 3 cm—unilateral or bilateral

  (8) Apical pulse displaced laterally and inferiorly, diffuse lifting impulse at left sternal border, thrill

  (9) Auscultation

    (a) S_1 sound—accentuated, decreased, or varying intensity (heard best at apex)

    (b) S_2 sound—accentuated or decreased intensity; wide, fixed, or paradoxical splitting (heard best at 2nd and 3rd interspaces)

    (c) S_3 sound—accentuated intensity, particularly in left lateral position (heard best at apex with bell)

    (d) S_4 sound—normally absent; when heard is a low-pitched sound heard in late diastole or early systole (heard best at apex with bell)

    (e) Systole—early ejection sounds; clicks

    (f) Diastole—pathologic S_3 or S_4

    (g) Murmurs—loud aortic murmurs, systolic murmur at apex

    (h) Pericardial friction rub

10. Abdomen

 a. Age-related changes

  (1) Reduced motility and peristalsis of the esophagus

  (2) Poor relaxation of esophageal sphincter

  (3) Decrease in acid secretions and motor activity of stomach, with mucosal thickening

  (4) Missed defecation signal leading to constipation

      (5)   Diverticulosis

      (6)   Decrease in size of liver

      (7)   Decrease in glomerular filtration rate

      (8)   Increased adipose tissue

  b. Commonly occurring deviations of diagnostic significance

      (1)   Absence of bowel sounds after 5 full minutes of listening

      (2)   High pitched loud sounds, gurgling

      (3)   Bruits (renal, iliac, aortic, and femoral)

11. Musculoskeletal System

  a. Age-related changes

      (1)   Some bony prominences more prominent

      (2)   Decrease of muscle mass, tone, and strength

      (3)   Diminished ease of movement and range of motion

      (4)   Delayed response of deep tendon reflexes

  b. Commonly occurring deviations of diagnostic significance

      (1)   Gross asymmetry or deformities

      (2)   Lordosis, scoliosis

      (3)   Gross hypertrophy, atrophy

      (4)   Gross prominences, swelling, tenderness

      (5)   Crepitation

      (6)   Fasciculation

      (7)   Loss of muscle strength with impaired functional ability

      (8)   Decrease in range of motion with changes in functional ability

      (9)   Changes in gait

      (10) Pain upon movement

12. Neurological System

  a. Age-related changes

      (1)   Decreased sense of touch

      (2)   Increased tolerance to pain

  (3) Overall delayed reaction time

  (4) Slightly decreased deep tendon and superficial reflexes

  (5) Some decrease in short term memory

 b. Commonly occurring deviations of diagnostic significance

  (1) Inability to maintain balance

  (2) Wide-based, shuffling, scissors-like, staggering, reeling, or parkinsonian gait

  (3) Clumsiness of movement

  (4) Inability to perceive superficial touch; asymmetrical response

  (5) Inability to perceive pain; asymmetrical response

  (6) Inaccurate or unequal perception of vibration

  (7) Hyperactive or diminished reflexes; asymmetrical response

  (8) Loss of short term memory affecting functional ability

Drug Therapy and the Elderly (adapted from M. E. Morse, 1993)

■ Drug use

 1. Incidence

  a. 12.7% of population are over 65 years of age

  b. Elderly utilize 40 to 50% of acute hospital stays

  c. Elderly consume over 30% of prescription drugs and 40% of over the counter preparations (OTCs)

  d. 7.5 to 17.9 prescriptions per year are received by people over 65

  e. Elderly spend more than $3 billion per year on medications

  f. Adverse drug reactions are responsible for 27% of hospital admissions of patients 65 or over

 2. Factors responsible for inappropriate drug use in the elderly

  a. Multiple pathologies

  b. Inaccurate diagnosis

  c. Non-specific presentation of illness

  d. Atypical presentation of illness

  e. Multiple providers

  f. Use of OTCs (40% of people > 65 use daily)

 3. Adverse drug reactions (ADRs)

  a. Incidence

   (1) Twenty percent (20%) of readmissions to hospital of elderly patients are related to ADRs

   (2) Occur in 25% of hospital patients > 80 years old

   (3) Contribute significantly to mortality, morbidity, and institutionalization

  b. Most common drugs causing ADRs

   (1) Psychotropics

   (2) Cardiovascular

   (3) Noncompliance—intentional or non-intentional of the above drugs leads to increased incidence of ADRs

    (a) Narrow therapeutic to toxic range of these drugs

    (b) Altered renal excretion

    (c) May nessitate yet another drug to relieve symptoms contributing to polypharmacy

  c. Identifying potential ADRs

   (1) Never assume a change in behavior is the result of aging

   (2) In the elderly, toxic reactions can occur even at low doses

   (3) The likelihood of an adverse reaction increases the longer a person is on the drug

   (4) Consider OTC preparations when evaluating for ADR

   (5) Adverse drug reaction symptoms can occur singly or in symptom clusters (confusion, unsteady gait)

   (6) Be watchful for any signs of involuntary movements; drug-induced Parkinsonism is common

   (7) Assess for signs of tardive dyskinesia (abnormal movement of the lips, tongue, and jaw) and akathisia (restlessness, continuous agitation)

   (8) Evaluate every complaint of dizziness to rule out orthostasis secondary to drug side effect. Drugs are a major cause of

dizziness in persons over age 60

(9) Inappropriate timing of diuretic administration is a common and easily reversible cause of urinary incontinence

(10) Fatigue and weakness can be caused by many drugs commonly prescribed for the elderly (beta blockers, diuretics, tricyclic antidepressants, benzodiazepines, and some antihypertensives)

(11) Ataxia or unsteady gait can be a side effect of drugs such as anticonvulsants, hypnotic sedatives, tranquilizers, and anti-Parkinsonian drugs

■ Other factors influencing drug therapy

1. Pharmacokinetics (what the body does to drugs)

   a. Physiological changes of aging

      (1) Decrease in normal renal function

      (2) Decrease in lean body mass and total body water

      (3) Increase in total body fat per unit of body weight

      (4) Decrease in hepatic blood flow

      (5) Other changes are common but variable, i.e., cardiac function, cognitive function, sensory changes

   b. Absorption

      (1) Mildly decreased gastrointestinal function

      (2) Decreased gastric emptying time

      (3) May be affected by nutritional deficiencies of Vitamin B_{12} or intrinsic factor

      (4) Drug interactions—laxatives, antacids

      (5) Most drugs absorbed in small intestine; notable exceptions are aspirin and alcohol

      (6) Increased gastric pH

      (7) Alterations in absorption common in patients with congestive heart failure, bowel restrictions

   c. Distribution

      (1) Decreased serum albumin production (a major drug binding protein)

(a) Common protein-bound drugs are warfarin, diazepam, phenytoin, tolbutamide, meperidine

(b) Clinical effect—large amount of free unbound drug available for action

(2) Normal aging changes in body composition

(a) Decrease in total body water and lean body mass results on lower volume distribution and higher concentration of drug

(b) Increase in body fat results in increase of volume distribution of fat-distributed or fat-stored drugs

d. Metabolism

(1) Effects of normal aging on metabolism include decreased liver mass, and liver blood flow which may affect metabolism of some drugs such as propranolol

(2) Common diseases of the elderly that affect liver function are hepatitis and congestive heart failure

e. Excretion

(1) Renal function declines by 50% between age 20 to 90; wide variations in individuals

(2) Decreased renal function affects pharmacokinetics if drug is more than 60% excreted by kidney

(3) Drugs that are eliminated by the kidney

(a) Clear body more slowly

(b) Half-lives (and duration of action) are prolonged

(c) Tend to accumulate to higher drug concentrations

(d) Some common drugs that are renally excreted— digoxin, atenolol, lithium, diuretics, NSAIDs, captopril

(4) Serum creatinine does not reflect renal function in elderly as accurately as in younger persons

(a) Decreased muscle mass equals decrease in endogenous creatinine production

(b) Decline in production may give "false normal" serum creatinine

(c) Creatinine clearance is most accurate measure of renal functions in the elderly. Formula for estimating creatinine clearance:

$$\frac{(140 - \text{age}) \times \text{body wt (kg)}}{72 \times \text{serum creatinine (mg/dL)}} = \text{(mL/min)}$$

(for women, multiply result by 0.85)

    (5) Other factors affecting renal clearance

        (a) State of hydration

        (b) Cardiac output

        (c) Intrinsic renal disease

        (d) Number of drugs patient is taking that are renally excreted

        (e) Chronic diseases such as hypertension, diabetes, congestive heart failure

f. Baroreceptor activity

    (1) Decreased sensitivity and responsiveness result in postural hypotension

    (2) Exacerbates orthostatic side effects with short acting nitrates, phenothiazines, diuretics, antihypertensives

g. Fluid and electrolyte balance affected by

    (1) Diuretic use

    (2) Obstructive uropathy

    (3) Diminished fluid intake secondary to functional or cognitive impairments, urinary incontinence, altered "thirst" response

h. Patient evaluation should include

    (1) State of hydration

    (2) State of nutrition

        (a) Of institutionalized elderly 40% are clinically malnourished

        (b) Obtain/monitor serum protein and serum albumin levels routinely

    (3) State of cardiac output

        (a) Decrease in ventricular function without overt heart

    disease

    (b) Diuretic therapy leads to decreased blood volume which can lead to decreased organ perfusion

2. Pharmacodynamics—(what drug does to your body)

    a. Variable in the elderly

    b. Greater tissue sensitivity to central nervous system (CNS)-active drugs

    c. Lesser sensitivity to beta blockers

    d. State of nutrition affects drug effectiveness

■ General principles of prescribing

1. Factors that complicate prescribing for the elderly

    a. Multiple interacting factors which influence age related changes (genetic and environmental)

    b. Each individual must be considered and evaluated each time a drug is considered for use

    c. Limited research available at this time on drug effects on the elderly

2. General recommendations for prescribing for the elderly

    a. Evaluate elderly persons thoroughly in order to identify all conditions that could benefit from drug treatment, be adversely affected by drug treatment, or influence the efficacy of drug treatment

    b. Manage medical conditions without drugs as often as possible

    c. Know the pharmacology of drugs being prescribed. A few drugs should be used well rather than many poorly

    d. START LOW, GO SLOW

    e. When evaluating patient compliance pay special attention to impaired cognition, diminished hearing and vision, and functional deficits

    f. Evaluate entire drug regimen any time a medication is added or discontinued

3. Questions to consider when prescribing an additional drug

    a. Is the drug necessary? Can a non-pharmacological method be tried first?

b. What is the therapeutic purpose of the drug and are we achieving it?

c. Is the dosage correct? Is the dosage form correct?

d. What drug interactions may occur?

e. Is the drug correctly labeled and packaged for this patient's level of function?

f. Who is responsible for drug administration for this patient?

g. Can any medication be discontinued?

Common Selected Problems of the Older Adult

For review of other common health problems that affect the elderly see "Gerontological Nursing Certification Review Guide," published by Health Leadership Associates

Dementia

- Definition

    1. An organic mental syndrome, characterized by impairment in short- and long-term memory with impairment in at least one other aspect of intellectual function, e.g., abstract thinking, judgement, aphasia, or personality

    2. Chronic, insidious, progressive course

- Etiology/Incidence

    1. Can be produced by numerous pathological states that affect the brain.

    2. Affects about 4% of population over 65

    3. Two-thirds of the elderly with dementia have Alzheimer's disease

    4. Some of the states are irreversible, e.g., Alzheimer's disease; others are reversible, e.g., prolonged overdosage of medication or malnutrition

        a. Irreversible causes of dementia

            (1) Alzheimer's disease (most common)

            (2) Multi-infarct dementia

            (3) Jakob-Creutzfelt

            (4) Pick's disease

        (5)   Parkinson's disease

        (6)   Huntington's disease

        (7)   Cerebellar degenerations

        (8)   Amyotrophic lateral sclerosis

        (9)   AIDS

        (10) Down's syndrome

        (11) Korsakoff's syndrome

    b. Reversible causes of dementia

        (1)   Intoxications (drugs, lead)

        (2)   Infections

        (3)   Metabolic disorders (dehydration)

        (4)   Nutritional disorders

        (5)   Vascular problems

        (6)   Space-occupying lesions

        (7)   Normal-pressure hydrocephalus

        (8)   Depression

■ Signs and Symptoms

    1.   Memory impairment, first and most prominent symptom; begins with recent events and then progresses to long-term memory and eventually the person may not even recognize family members

    2.   Impaired abstract thinking

    3.   Impaired judgement

    4.   Impairment of other cortical functions

        a. Aphasia

        b. Apraxia

        c. Agnosia

        d. Constructional difficulty

    5.   Personality change

■ Differential Diagnosis: Diagnosis is not based on a solo evaluation; repeated assessments are done over time to establish a pattern and treat complicating or superimposed conditions

1. Delirium, either alone or occurring with dementia

2. Depression

- Physical Findings: For dementia, there may be no specific physical findings. A comprehensive history and physical examination, which includes a neuropsychological evaluation, extensive laboratory testing, EEG, CT scan, and MRI are required to rule out other diagnoses

- Diagnostic Tests/Findings

1. The diagnosis of dementia is based on the history and evolution of clinical, functional, and laboratory data

2. A progressive decline in memory, other areas of judgement and daily functioning in both instrumental activities of daily living and activities of daily living

3. Although memory loss is prominent, the first sign may actually be visual-spatial abnormalities, such as problems managing a checkbook or following a recipe

4. See Diagnostic Tests and their significance in Neurological Disorders chapter

- Management/Treatment

1. Treatment of underlying disease/disorder

2. Manage behavioral problems with psychosocial and behavioral interventions

3. Discontinue nonessential medications

4. Limit use of restraining devices

5. Anticipate legal and ethical decisions. Assist client and family to make decisions, before need arises, e.g., guardianship, living wills

- General Considerations

1. Maximize client's functional abilities

2. Modify client's environment to compensate for deficits and ensure safety

3. Promote optimal orientation and communication

4. Maintain in home setting as long as possible

5. Promote participation in activities of daily and instrumental activities

of daily living for as long as possible

6. Promote exercise

7. Provide strategies to deal with alterations in sleep-wake pattern

8. Reduce caregiver burden

   a. Family assessment—identify strengths, make appropriate referrals

   b. Patient/family education—effects and progression of disease, strategies for dealing with client's personality and behavioral changes

   c. Provide supportive relationship with family

   d. Respite services

   e. Counseling services

Delirium (acute confusion)

- Definition

  1. Transient state characterized by global disturbance of attention and cognition, reduced level of consciousness, abnormally increased or reduced psychomotor activity, and a disturbed sleep-wake cycle

  2. Rapid onset, brief duration, often occuring at night

- Etiology/Incidence

  1. Results from a widespread reduction in cerebral metabolism and an upset in the neurotransmission process which may be brought on by a wide variety of medical conditions

  2. Most common cause is intoxication due to medications

  3. Several factors, often concurrently, are responsible for delirium in the elderly

     a. Aging process in brain

     b. Reduced resistance to stress and acute illness

     c. Visual and hearing impairments

     d. High prevalence of chronic disease

     e. Sleep loss

     f. Sensory overload

     g. Relocation to unfamiliar environment

4. An estimated 40% (Limpowski, 1989) to 80% (Foreman, 1992) of hospitalized elderly are admitted with delirium or develop it shortly after admission

5. Associated with increased morbidity, increased intensity of nursing care, longer hospitalization, increased rates of nursing home admissions, and increased mortality

6. Can be followed by dementia especially if cause not identified and treated

- Signs and Symptoms

    1. Prominent feature is a disorder of attention manifested by impaired ability to sustain attention to environmental stimuli, carry on a conversation, engage in goal-directed thinking or behavior

    2. Level of consciousness can vary from drowsiness or stupor to excessive alertness and severe insomnia

    3. Perceptual disorders can occur including vivid dreams and nightmares, misinterpretations and illusions, and hallucinations (commonly visual, can be auditory)

    4. Acute paranoid delusions accompanied by fear, anxiety, attempts to escape, or destructive rage episodes

    5. Cognitive impairment often fluctuates with lucid intervals occuring more frequently in the daytime

    6. Disturbance of sleep-wake cycle with insomnia or daytime sleepiness

- Differential Diagnosis

    1. Dementia

    2. Functional psychosis

- Physical Findings

    1. Temperature may be elevated

    2. Focal neurological findings may be present

    3. Restlessness, aggressiveness, dazed expression

    4. Anxiety and lack of cooperation; unpredictable behavior fluctuation

    5. Tachycardia, sweating, dilated pupils, elevated BP

- Diagnostic Tests/Findings

    1. Routine laboratory tests (see chapter on Neurological Disorders)

2. Special tests as needed

   a. EEG to rule out seizure disorder

   b. CT scanning for tumor, hemorrhage, CVA

   c. MRI—multi-infarct dementia

3. Toxicology screen—medication overload

■ Management/Treatment

1. Diagnosis of underlying cause(s)

2. Discontinue or reduce dosage of all medication

3. Treatment should be related to both the cause and the symptoms of the delirium

   a. Remove underlying cause whenever possible or treat

   b. Ensure adequate fluids, nutrition and vitamin supply intake

   c. Provide reassuring, supportive nursing care that assists in reestablishing orientation

   d. Environmental controls to avoid overstimulation or understimulation

   e. Reassure family members that delirium is a transitory disorder

   f. Sedation for agitation and restlessness

      (1) Use short-acting antianxiety agent with no active metabolities (Serax 10-50 mg/day; Ativan 0.5-2 mg/day; Xanax 0.5-4 mg/day)

      (2) Antipsychotics (Haldol 0.25 mg up to three times a day)

4. Preventive measures

   a. Avoid polypharmacy

   b. Monitor drug intake and patient's responses closely

   c. Early recognition of onset of delirium

   d. Anticipate who is likely to suffer delirium

      (1) Persons over age 80 years

      (2) Men are more vulnerable than women

      (3) People living alone, without social supports

      (4) People who have suddenly been relocated

(5)   Sensory deprived persons

(6)   People with disrupted sleep cycle

(7)   People on multiple medications

(8)   People in restraints

(9)   People with pain or discomfort from unmet physical needs

5.   Provide orientation measures

6.   Help maintain sense of body integrity

7.   Provide sense of personal continuity and identity

8.   Provide a safe environment

9.   Assist in dealing with illusions/hallucinations

10. Recognize that confusion often becomes worse in evening and at night; provide supportive environment that enhances sensory input needed for orientation

Depression

- Definition: A syndrome consisting of a constellation of physical, affective and cognitive symptoms that range in severity from mild to severe

- Etiology/Incidence

1.   Multifactorial in nature, involving a combination of psychosocial, biological and genetic factors

    a. Genetic

        (1)   More common in women than men (2:1)

        (2)   Family history

    b. Biochemical

        (1)   Levels of norepinephrine and serotonin decrease with age

        (2)   The enzyme monamine oxidase and the metabolite 5-hydroxyindoleacetic acid increase with age

    c. Dysregulation of the hypothalamic-pituitary-adrenal (HPA) axis

    d. Dysregulation of thyroid axis and growth hormone release

    e. Desynchronization of circadian rhythms

        (1)   Depressive illnesses are cyclic and cause insomnia and diurnal variation of mood

          (2)   Sleep cycle disrupted in old age

    f. Learned helplessness hypothesis

    g. Sociodemograpahic risk factors

          (1)   Female

          (2)   Unmarried, particularly widowed

          (3)   Lack of supportive social network

          (4)   Co-occurrence of physical conditions

          (5)   Lack of exercise

    h. Reactivation of unresolved early losses

2. Fifteen percent of community dwelling elders have depressive illness; major depression affects 3%

3. Seventy percent of clients treated for depression recover; of these 40% have recurrence

4. Fifteen to 25 percent of nursing home residents are estimated to be depressed

5. Undertreated; only 10% of elderly who are in need of psychiatric treatment ever receive it

- Signs and Symptoms
  1. Physical symptoms
     a. Decrease or increase in appetite/weight
     b. Insomnia or hypersomnia
     c. Psychomotor agitation or retardation
     d. Fatigue or lack of energy
     e. Multiple complaints or frequent minor problems
  2. Emotional symptoms
     a. Depressed or dysphoric mood
     b. Anhedonia
     c. Low self-esteem, worthlessness
     d. Feelings of hopelessness, helplessness, or guilt
  3. Cognitive symptoms
     a. Difficulty thinking, concentrating or making decisions

    b. Thoughts of death or suicide

    c. Cognitive deficits ("pseudodementia")

    d. Delusions, often of persecution or incurable illness

- Differential Diagnosis

    1. Medical diagnoses—many medical conditions and medications have depressive symptoms as part of their clinical syndrome; others mask depressive symptoms or lead to a secondary depression

    2. Dementia—depression can be superimposed upon dementia; cognitive deficits can be symptoms of depression and not dementia

    3. Adjustment disorder with depressed mood

- Physical Findings

    1. Resemble depressed person of any age

    2. See chapter on Psychosocial Disorders

- Diagnostic Tests/Findings

    1. Geriatric Depression Scale (Yesavage, Brink, Rose, 1983)

    2. Beck Depression Inventory (Beck, Word & Mendelson, 1961)

    3. Zung Self-Rating Depression Scale (Zung, 1965)

    4. The Hamilton Rating Scale for Depression (Hamilton, 1967)

- Management/Treatment

    1. Goals of treatment

        a. Partial or complete remission of symptoms

        b. Reduce risk of relapse and recurrence

        c. Improvement of pain and suffering associated with physical illness

    2. Antidepressant medications (see Tables 1 and 2 in chapter on Psychosocial Disorders)

        a. Indicated for major depressive episode or recurrent depressive illness; 60% of clients clinically improve with medication

        b. Avoid drugs with anticholinergic, cardiovascular, sedative, and hypotensive side effects

        c. Significant antidepressant responses may take 6 to 12 weeks; some improvement may be noted after 2 weeks

        d. Blood levels of tricyclic antidepressants should be closely monitored

    e. Dosage of antidepressants is generally less than for younger adults

  3. Electroconvulsive therapy (ECT)

    a. Considered when antidepressant medication has been ineffective or medical condition contraindicates its use

    b. More effective than antidepressants in all age groups, although high relapse rate

    c. May cause transient post ECT confusion, especially in very old

    d. All medications should be discontinued prior to receiving ECT

    e. Treatments—3 times/week for 6 to 12 weeks

  4. Psychotherapy

    a. Individual

      (1) Cognitive/behavioral

      (2) Interpersonal

      (3) Psychodynamic

      (4) Life Review

    b. Group

    c. Family

■ General Considerations

  1. Monitor response to antidepressants

  2. Assess suicide risk

  3. Promote adequate nutrition, hydration and elimination

  4. Promote adequate balance of rest, sleep and activity

  5. Assist client to recognize, accept, and verbalize feelings, especially anger

  6. Promote client's feelings of self-worth

  7. Build trust relationship

  8. Collaborate with those involved in client's care (family, other professional providers)

  9. Promote development of social support network

Pneumonia

- Definition: A bacterial or viral lung infection for which the elderly, particularly the frail ill elderly, are at high risk

- Etiology/Incidence
    1. *S. pneumoniae* most comon pathogen; *S. aureus, K. pneumoniae, E. coli* as well as mixed flora account for many cases
    2. Elderly are particularly vulnerable to pneumonia and certain conditions increase the risk, e.g., chronic obstructive pulmonary disease (COPD), congestive heart failure, influenza, alcoholism, pulmonary neoplasm, and smoking
    3. Upper respiratory infections increase the risk of pneumonia; about 60 to 75% of those who acquire pneumococcal pneumonia have had a preceding lower respiratory infection
    4. Aspiration of pharyngeal flora into lower respiratory tract can initiate infectious process
    5. Lower respiratory tract infections are found in 25 to 60 percent of elderly at autopsy
    6. Annual rate of hospitalization for pneumonia (per 10,000 persons)—30 to 60 cases during 3 year period for persons over 65 years compared to 5 to 15 cases for all other age categories
    7. Long term care facilities have an incidence of 100 cases per 1000 patient years

- Signs and Symptoms
    1. Not unusual for the elderly to exhibit rather subtle clinical findings—low grade fevers (or perhaps no fever), no pleuritic pain, non-productive and/or weak cough, and a change in sensorium
    2. Elderly can exhibit a classic bacterial pneumonia syndrome which includes sudden onset, shaking chills, fever, pleuritic chest pain, and productive cough (may be purulent and/or blood tinged)

- Differential Diagnosis
    1. Tuberculosis
    2. Bronchial asthma

3. Foreign body obstruction

4. Atelectasis

5. Pulmonary embolism with infarction

6. Congestive heart failure

■ Physical Findings: May or may not have

1. Cyanosis

2. Intercostal, sub/suprasternal retractions

3. Tachypnea

4. Tachycardia

5. Evidence of dehydration

6. Bacterial pneumonia presents with

   a. Diffuse crackles and wheezes

   b. Bronchial breath sounds

   c. Pleural friction rub

   d. Whispered pectoriloquy

7. Viral pneumonia presents with fine crackles

8. Increase in tactile fremitus over areas of consolidation

9. Dull note over areas of consolidation

■ Diagnostic Tests/Findings

1. Sputum collected before starting antibiotics; Gram stain, culture and sensitivity identify organism and appropriate antibiotic

2. Chest radiograph—PA and lateral chest radiograph are mandatory; bacterial pneumonia is associated with consolidation, effusions, and/or abscess formation; true interstitial infiltrate supports viral etiology

3. WBC count with differential

   a. Normal WBC may be present

   b. May be elevated in bacterial pneumonia

   c. Polymorphonuclear leukocytosis is found in bacterial pneumonia

4. Blood gases—may be abnormal

5. PPD—to rule out tuberculosis

■ Management/Treatment: Strategies directed at early diagnosis and prompt treatment since it is a leading cause of death in older persons

1. Identify and treat causative organism with antibiotics

2. Provide adequate ventilation/oxygenation

   a. Bronchodilators (systemic and inhaled)

   b. Administer oxygen as indicated by arterial blood gases (ABGs)

   c. Reduce metabolic demands (bed rest, long rest periods, light diet, reduce fever)

3. Improve airway clearance

   a. Hydration (oral, intravenous, mist)

   b. Postural drainage

   c. Percussion

   d. Suction

   e. COUGH SUPPRESSANTS ARE CONTRAINDICATED

4. Relieve pain and discomfort

5. Prevention—immunization with pneumococcal vaccine (Pneumovax) to adults age 65 or older as well as for those of any age who have a chronic illness; one vaccination is usually required (Centers for Disease Control and Prevention, 1994)

Congestive Heart Failure (CHF)

■ Definition: Inability of the heart to supply the body and the heart muscles itself with adequate circulatory volume and pressure (Parker-Cohen, Richardson & Haak, 1990, p. 963). Any condition that compromises cardiac function can result in CHF

1. Acute CHF—comes on suddenly and may follow an acute myocardial infarction or cardiac arrest

2. Chronic CHF—the end result of continued strain on a damaged chamber of the heart which has enlarged over time and is no longer able to compensate. Although eventually both sides of the heart fail, there are differences between

   a. Left-sided CHF—initially causes congestion in the lungs, and

   b. Right-sided CHF—causes congestion in the systemic circulation; most evident in the liver and lower extremities

- Etiology/Incidence
    1. May result from conditions that increase fluid volume and lead to circulatory overload, e.g., increased sodium intake, rapid infusion of I.V. fluids, or conditions that increase resistance to movement of blood from the heart, e.g., arteriosclerotic heart disease, hypertensive heart disease, and pulmonary hypertension
    2. Prevalence of this disorder increases progressively with age
    3. One of the most common cardiac conditions in the older adult
- Signs and Symptoms
    1. Left sided CHF
        a. Anxiety, restlessness
        b. Shortness of breath, dyspnea
        c. Orthopnea, paroxysmal nocturnal dyspnea
        d. Cough, hemoptysis
        e. Tachycardia, palpitations
        f. Basilar rales, bronchial wheezes
        g. Fatigue
        h. Weight gain
        i. Cyanosis or pallor
    2. Right sided CHF
        a. Anorexia, nausea
        b. Weight gain
        c. Nocturia, oliguria
        d. Dependent peripheral edema
        e. Weakness
    3. Atypical, nonspecific signs, that can be combined with some of the common symptoms, seen in the elderly
        a. Somnolence
        b. Confusion
        c. Disorientation
        d. Dizziness

e. Syncope

- Differential Diagnosis

    1. Chronic obstructive pulmonary disease

    2. Asthma

    3. Pulmonary embolus

    4. Renal or liver dysfunction with edema

- Physical Findings

    1. Cardiovascular

        a. Abnormal heart sounds—murmurs, S_3, S_4 gallop; may not be heard if cardiomegaly present or may be reduced by one or two grades in intensity due to low output state

        b. Jugular venous distention especially at 90 degree position

    2. Integumentary

        a. Cyanotic lips, pallor

        b. Cold clammy skin

        c. Edema (sacral, peripheral, dependent)

    3. Respiratory

        a. Productive cough, hemoptysis

        b. Wheezes, rales (crackles)

        c. Shortness of breath

    4. Neurological

        a. Anxiety, restlessness

        b. Confusion, memory lapse

    5. Other

        a. Periorbital edema

        b. Vasodilation of vessels and minimal fundal hemorrhages

        c. Abdominal pain

        d. Positive hepatojugular reflux

        e. Obvious fatigue on slight exertion

- Diagnostic Tests/Findings: Tests not specific to CHF itself but provide information on etiology and severity

1. Hematocrit and hemoglobin—anemia

2. Serum electrolytes—hyponatremia, hypokalemia, hyperkalemia

3. BUN and creatinine—decreased renal function

4. Liver function tests—elevated liver enzymes

5. Urinalysis—proteinuria and elevated specific gravity

6. Chest radiograph—may reveal distended pulmonary veins, which reflect redistribution of pulmonary blood flow, with interstitial and alveolar edema

7. EKG—rhythm disturbances

8. Echocardiogram—pericardial effusion, pericardial thickening, hypertrophy, and valvular abnormalities

- Management/Treatment: Overall goals are to decrease workload of the heart, to improve cardiac function, and to prevent complications

1. Physician referral, may or may not require hospitalization depending on severity

2. Non-pharmacological management

   a. Balance rest and activity to promote relief of overworked heart

   b. Bedrest for acute pulmonary edema and failure

   c. Dietary restriction of sodium and fluids

   d. ECG monitoring for arrhythmia

   e. Hemodynamic monitoring

   f. Monitoring of laboratory values

   g. Oxygen for relief of dyspnea

3. Pharmacological management—depends on whether the dysfunction is diastolic or systolic; care needs to be individualized

   a. Diastolic dysfunction when systolic function is preserved

      (1) Calcium antagonists

      (2) Beta-adrenergic blockers

   b. Systolic dysfunction

      (1) Digitalis (digoxin) carefully monitored, check digoxin levels at regular intervals

      (2)   Vasodilators

      (3)   Diuretics

  4. Surgical treatment: Not common in the elderly, but could include

    a. Coronary artery bypass graft, angioplasty

    b. Valve replacement/repair

    c. Left ventricular assistive device

■ General Considerations

  1. Provide assistance with ADLs as needed

  2. Client/family education

    a. CHF, what it is, how it develops

    b. Signs and symptoms to report, e.g., shortness of breath, weakness, sudden unexplained weight gain, confusion

    c. Medications, purpose, dosage and schedule, side effects

    d. Individual activity plan

    e. Dietary instruction

    f. Need for regular medical care

    g. Assessment for home care

Questions

Select the best answer.

1. The older population can be described as being

   a. Predominately female
   b. Becoming a smaller percentage of the total population
   c. Comprised of a decreased number of "old-old"
   d. Enjoying a shorter life expectancy than previous generations

2. Most older adults

   a. Live alone
   b. Reside in a nursing home
   c. Reside in a group home
   d. Live in a family setting

3. Which statement best describes widowhood in the United States?

   a. It is a fact of life for most older men
   b. It is a fact of life for most older women
   c. Widowers outnumber widows in old age
   d. Few women over age 75 are widowed

4. The major source of income for most older persons is

   a. Savings
   b. Earnings
   c. Social security
   d. Pensions

5. Which statement is most accurate?

   a. Older people account for 50% of all hospital stays
   b. The largest portion of health care expenditures for the aged is nursing home care
   c. Approximately 50% of older people living in the community have health-related difficulty with one or more personal care activities
   d. The over 65 age group accounted for 36% of total health care expenditures in 1987

6. Which of the following is not part of a functional assessment?

   a. Assessment of capacity to perform personal care
   b. Identification of care deficits
   c. Assessment of cardiac status
   d. Assessment of capacity to perform instrumental activities of daily living

7. When doing a health assessment with an older client it is imperative that

   a. The nurse do the exam quickly to avoid fatigue
   b. Keep instructions for procedures to a minimum; most older people don't follow instructions well
   c. Use the same techniques that are used with younger adults
   d. Pace the examination to accommodate the client

8. Which of the following is not a normal age-related change of the integument?

   a. Senile lentigines
   b. Yellowing
   c. Dryness
   d. Pallor

9. Commonly occurring skin deviations of diagnostic significance include

   a. Wrinkles, folding, sagging
   b. Yellowing, cyanosis, erythema
   c. Pallor
   d. Dryness

10. Normal age-related changes of the eye include all of the following except

    a. Exophthalmus
    b. Increased sensitivity to glare
    c. Sustained nystagmus
    d. Arcus senilis

11. Commonly occurring head and neck deviations of diagnostic significance include

    a. Facial asymmetry, asymmetrical movement, fasciculations
    b. Jowls, double chin
    c. "Dowager's hump," ptosis
    d. Thyroid gland lower in relation to clavicles

12. Normal age-related changes of the ear include all of the following except

    a. Presbycusis
    b. Nodules, tophi
    c. Dull tympanic membrane
    d. Cilia coarser and stiffer

13. Commonly occurring breast deviation(s) of diagnostic significance in females include

    a. Nipples lighter in color
    b. Smaller, less dense, less nodular tissue
    c. Pendulous, elongated breasts

    d. Palpable masses

14. Which of the following is a normal age-related change of the cardiovascular system?

    a. Heart rate < 60, BP > than 160/95
    b. Marked pallor in one or both feet, hair loss on lower leg
    c. Decreased exercise tolerance, slightly smaller heart
    d. Pain, redness, or thickening along a superficial vein

15. Which of the following has no diagnostic significance in the elderly?

    a. Displacement of the apical pulse
    b. S_4 sound
    c. Slight prolongation of all intervals on the EKG
    d. Pericardial friction rub

16. Which of the following is not a normal age-related change?

    a. Barrel chest, costal angle greater than 90 degrees
    b. Decreased ability for effective cough
    c. Drier mucous membrane
    d. Hyperresonance

17. Commonly occurring deviations of the abdomen that have diagnostic significance include:

    a. Missed defecation signal leading to constipation
    b. Decrease in liver size
    c. Bruits
    d. Increase in adipose tissue

18. Which of the following is not a normal age-related change?

    a. Decrease in muscle mass, tone, and strength
    b. Lordosis, scoliosis
    c. Bony prominences more prominent
    d. Decreased agility

19. Which of the following has no diagnostic significance in the elderly?
    a. A positive Romberg
    b. A Parkinsonian gait
    c. An inability to perceive pain
    d. An overall delayed reaction time

20. Which of the following has no negative effect on drug use in the elderly?
    a. Inaccurate diagnosis
    b. Multiple providers
    c. Method of administration

d. Multiple pathologies

21. Which of these, in a usually healthy individual, could be attributed to an adverse drug reaction?
    a. Dry mouth
    b. Loose stools
    c. Constipation
    d. Confusion

22. Which is not a reversible cause of dementia?
    a. Dehydration
    b. Malnutrition
    c. Infections
    d. Multi-infarct dementia

23. The signs and symptoms of dementia include all of the following except
    a. Loss of memory late in the course of the disease
    b. Apraxia, agnosia, aphasia
    c. Impaired abstract thinking
    d. Personality change

24. Depression in the elderly
    a. Affects men more than women
    b. Can present with an increase or decrease in weight
    c. Presents with somatic complaints related to excessive energy expenditure
    d. Is seldom related to biochemical imbalance

25. The elderly are particularly vulnerable to depressive illness because
    a. Of increased longevity with more years spent in retirement
    b. Of the increases in serotonin and norepiniphrine that occur with aging
    c. Decrease in monamine oxidase causes disequilibrium
    d. Of the physical changes that occur with aging

26. Which of the following is not a characteristic of delerium?
    a. Worse in daytime
    b. Transient state
    c. Rapid onset, brief duration
    d. Disturbed sleep-wake cycle

27. Which of the following puts the elderly at greatest risk for pneumonia?
    a. Decreased activity level
    b. COPD, history of upper respiratory infections
    c. Poor nutritional status
    d. Compromised immune status

28. Congestive heart failure in the elderly will often manifest with atypical, nonspecific

signs that include all of the following except
a. Syncope, dizziness
b. Chest pain
c. Confusion
d. Somnolence

29. Symptoms of CHF vary depending on whether the failure is left or right sided; symptoms of left sided failure include
a. Anorexia, nausea
b. Dependent peripheral edema
c. Orthopnea, paroxysmal nocturnal dyspnea
d. Nocturia, oliguria

Answers

1. a
2. d
3. b
4. c
5. d
6. c
7. d
8. b
9. b
10. c
11. a
12. b
13. d
14. c
15. c
16. a
17. c
18. b
19. d
20. c
21. d
22. d
23. a
24. b
25. d
26. a
27. b
28. b
29. c

Bibliography

A Profile of Older Americans (1993). Washington, D.C.: Program Resources Department, American Association of Retired Persons in cooperation with the Administration on Aging.

Beck, A. T., Ward, C. H., & Mendelson, M. (1961). An inventory for depression. *Archives of General Psychiatry, 4*, 53-63.

Blessed, G., Tomlinson, B. E., & Roth, M. (1968). The association between quantitative measures of dementia and of senile change in the grey matter of elderly subjects. *British Journal of Psychiatry, 114*, 797-811.

Busse, E. W., & Blazer, D. (Ed.) (1989). *Geriatric psychiatry*. Washington, DC: American Psychiatric Press.

Butler, R. N., Lewis, M., & Sunderland, T. (1991). *Aging and mental health*. New York: Merrill, an imprint of Macmillan.

Carnevali, D. L., & Patrick, M. (1993). *Nursing management for the elderly* (3rd ed.). Philadelphia: Lippincott.

Cummings, E., & Henry, W. (1961). *Growing old*. New York: Basic Books.

Ebersole, P., & Hess, P. (1990). *Toward healthy aging: Human needs and nursing response* (4th ed.). St. Louis: Mosby.

Eliopoulos, C. (1991). *Gerontological nursing review: A self-instructional text* (2nd ed.). Baltimore: National Health Publishing.

Erickson, E. (1963). *Childhood and society* (2nd ed.). New York: W. W. Norton.

Folstein, M. F., Folstein, S. E., & McHugh, P. R. (1975). Mini-mental state: A practical method of grading the cognitive state of patients for the clinician. *Journal of Psychiatric Residency, 12*, 189-198.

Gould, R. (1978). *Transformations*. New York: Simon & Schuster.

Hamilton, M. (1960). A rating scale for depression. *Journal of Neurology and Neurosurgical Psychiatry, 23*, 56-62.

Hamilton, M. (1967). Development of a rating scale for primary depressive illness. *British Journal of Social and Clinical Psychology*, 278-296.

Havinghurst, R. (1972). *Developmental tasks and education*. New York: David McKay.

Hazzard, W., Andres, R., Bierman, E., Blass, J. (1990). *Principles of geriatric medicine and gerontology* (2nd ed.). New York: McGraw-Hill

Katz, S., Ford, A., & Moskowitz, R. (1963). Studies of illness in the aged: The index of ADL, a standardized measure of biological and psychosocial function. *Journal of the American Medical Association, 185*, 914-917.

Kopac, C. (1993). Demographics, theories, and nursing process. In C. Kopac and V. Millonig (Eds.), *Gerontological nursing certification review guide for the generalist, clinical specialist, and nurse practitioner*, (pp. 23-39). Potomac, MD: Health Leadership Associates.

Lueckenotte, A. G. (1990). *Pocket guide to gerontological assessment*. St. Louis: Mosby.

Mahoney, F. I., & Barthel, D. W. (1965). Functional evaluation: The Barthel index. *Maryland State Medical Journal, 14*, 61-65.

Morse, M. E. (1993). Drug therapy. In C. Kopac and V. Millonig (Eds.), *Gerontological nursing certification review guide for the generalist, clinical specialist, and nurse practitioner* (pp. 425-478.) Potomac, MD: Health Leadership Associates.

Neugarten, B. (1968). Adult personality: Toward a psychology of the lifecycle. In B. Neugarten (Ed.), *Middle age and aging*. Chicago: University of Chicago Press.

Older Americans Resources and Services (1978). *Multidimensional functional assessment: The OARS methodology—a manual* (2nd ed.). Durham, NC: Duke University Center for the Study of Aging and Human Development.

Parker-Cohen, P., Richardson, S., & Haak, S. (1990). In K. McCance and S. Huether (Eds.), *Pathophysiology: The biologic basis for disease in adults and children* (pp. 916-991). St. Louis: C. V. Mosby.

Pfeiffer, E. (1975). A short portable mental status questionnaire for the assessment of organic brain deficit in elderly patients. *Journal of the American Geriatric Society, 23*, 433-441.

Radloff, L. S. (1977). The CES-D scale: A self-report depression scale for research in the general population. *Applied Psychological Measurements, 1*, 385-401.

U.S. Department of Health and Human Services. (1994). *Immunization of Adults: A call to action*. National Immunization Program, Centers for Disease Control and Prevention, National Center for Prevention Services, Division of Immunization, Atlanta, GA.

Yesavage, J. A., Brink, T. L., & Rose, T. L. (1983). Development and validation of a geriatric depression screening scale: A preliminary report. *Journal of Psychiatric Research, 17*, 37-49.

Zung, W. W. K. (1965). A self-rating depression scale. *Archives of General Psychiatry, 12*, 63-70.

Trends, Professional Issues, Health Policy

Marilyn W. Edmunds
Debra Hardy Havens

Health Policy

Improvement in health is a major policy emphasis in both national goal statements (Healthy People 2000 Objectives) and international policy statements (WHO "Health for All")

■ Purpose

1. Overall objective—all persons to obtain a level of health by the year 2000 that will permit them to lead socially and economically productive lives

2. Specific objectives focus on equal access, acceptability, availability, continuity, cost and quality of care

   a. To achieve equal access to all, focus on

      (1) Establishment of community-based primary health care systems

      (2) Redistribution of health and specialty services to overcome regional inequalities

      (3) Emphasis on self-reliance and participation by the individual and community members in health matters

      (4) Increased emphasis on provision of services to specific target groups

      (5) Increased involvement of existing health organizations and groups

      (6) Expanded education of health professionals

      (7) Expansion of traditional roles

      (8) New focus by government on health rather than cure and on the roles that transportation, housing, and industry can play in bringing about a healthy society (Healthy People 2000, 1990)

   b. Acceptability

      (1) Individuals receive care that they want

      (2) Individuals receive care that is appropriate

   c. Availability

      (1) Individuals have access to health care services and facilities

      (2) Individuals have access to choice of providers

    d. Continuity

      (1)   Individuals have access to primary care providers

      (2)   Individuals have access to follow-up care

    e. Cost

      (1)   Individuals are not denied health care because of lack of money

      (2)   Cost is reasonable for services provided

      (3)   Investment of money in health care leads to improved health

    f. Quality of care

      (1)   Care leads to symptoms reduction or sense of well-being

      (2)   Patients are satisfied with care received

      (3)   Mortality-morbidity indicators show improvement

- Primary health care delivery

  1. First contact with the health care system; implies continuity and coordination of care

  2. Currently in the U.S., health care is fragmented, costly, unavailable to many, with an emphasis on specialty care not primary care.

  3. Nursing has submitted an "Agenda for Health Care Reform" which contains three major parts

    a. A restructured health care system that will focus on the consumers and their health, with services to be delivered in familiar, convenient sites

    b. Basic core of essential health care services to be available to everyone

    c. A shift from the predominant focus on illness and cure to an orientation toward wellness and care (National Leadership Coalition for Health Care Reform, 1991)

- Resource utilization

  1. Attempts to reduce duplication

  2. Attempts to reduce under-utilization/over-utilization

- Policy research utilization/application

  1. Major research trend is in outcome studies. Agency for Health Care

Policy and Research, NIH are funding research with clinical applications

2. National Institute for Nursing Research funds major nursing research

- International health care trends

1. WHO "Healthy People" objectives unite the world

2. Major shift to emphasis on primary care

3. Trend toward earlier preventive efforts

4. Stress on improvements in sanitation, housing, nutrition, and immunization

5. Attention focused on promotion of individual measures to promote health and prevent disease

Nurse Practitioner Role Development

- History of the Role

1. In the early 1960s the Millis Report indicated that because of a physician shortage, many children were receiving inadequate medical care

2. A survey of the American Academy of Pediatrics (AAP) found that most physicians were willing to delegate certain patient care tasks

3. As a result of this response a plan to expand the role of the nurse was developed

   a. In 1964, Dr. Loretta C. Ford and Dr. Henry K. Silver started the first pediatric nurse practitioner program at the University of Colorado Health Sciences Center in Denver, Colorado

      (1) Length of initial program was 4 months of study and 18 months of clinical practice

      (2) Susan Stearly was the first nurse and only student in the Colorado program

   b. Also in 1964 across the country, Priscilla Andrews and Dr. John Connelly began a Pediatric Nurse Practitioner program at Massachusetts General Hospital in Boston, Massachusetts. This class was composed of public health nurses (Murphy, 1990)

4. In 1969 the American Academy of Pediatrics passed a statement saying, ". . . a physician may delegate to a properly trained individual, working under his direct supervision, the responsibility of providing

appropriate portions of health examinations and health care of infants
..." (MacQueen, 1979, p. 31). The American Academy of Pediatrics
also developed training and certificate guidelines for PNPs

5. In 1971 the American Nurses Association and the American Academy
of Pediatrics jointly published "Guidelines on Short-term Continuing
Education Program for PNP/As." This was one of the more formal
attempts at developing standards for the multiple programs that were
developing around the country

6. By 1980 there were almost 300 programs across the country (Bullough,
Sultz, Henry & Fiedler, 1984)

7. Pediatric nurse practitioners, as the first nurse practitioners, served as
the model for the inception of other nurse practitioners, e.g., school
nurse practitioners, family nurse practitioners, adult nurse
practitioners, gerontological nurse practitioners, ob-gyn nurse
practitioners

- Preparation of Nurse Practitioners

  1. Most of the early nurse practitioners were graduated from certificate
  programs offered both within and outside of university settings. By
  1989, 85% of all federally funded nurse practitioner programs were at
  the master's level and only 15% were certificate programs (Mezey,
  1993)

  2. Most evidence now clearly supports master's level preparation for
  nurse practitioners although initially, the appropriate educational
  model was not clear

  3. The evolution from certificate programs to well integrated knowledge
  and skills in master's programs has been fairly consistent across the
  country

- Role of Nurse Practitioner Movement and Professional Organizations

  1. In 1973 a group of pediatric nurse practitioners representing six states
  organized the National Association of Pediatric Nurse Associates and
  Practitioners (NAPNAP)

     a. To set standardized guidelines for PNP practice, NAPNAP and the
     AAP published a "Scope of Pactice Statement" in 1974. This
     statement later resulted in "The Standards of Practice for PNP/As"
     issued jointly by NAPNAP and the Association of Faculties of
     PNP/A Programs (Murphy, 1990)

     b. American Nurses Association was also setting up a PNP Council under the Maternal-Child-Health division the very same year

2. Purpose of Professional Organizations

   a. Benefits

      (1) Provides collective voice for promoting nursing and quality health care

      (2) Monitors and influences laws and regulations

      (3) Communicates information

      (4) Public relations

   b. Relationship to practice

      (1) Study practice issues

      (2) Establish standards for practice

      (3) Act as collective bargaining agent for nurses

      (4) Provides visible presence in the community because of its legitimacy in representing nursing perspectives

■ Changes in the role

1. Originally when the role was in its formative stages it was viewed as

   a. A means to improve the image and stature of nurses within the healthcare and consumer community

   b. A quick solution to the shortage of physician services and access to primary care

2. Originally there was both support and resistance for the nurse practitioner role; research focused on the need to prove the impact of the role

3. Research also originally focused on the need to prove the existence of the role; quality, cost effectiveness, productivity, clinical decision making skills and job satisfaction (McGivern, 1993)

4. Policymakers originally saw nurse practitioners as physician substitutes

5. Nurse practitioners saw the physician maldistribution of the 1960s as an opportunity to increase the availability of primary care services

6. During the 1980s a change took place in the health care environment; the physician shortage of the 60s gave way to a physician glut; nurse practitioners were abandoned in favor of physicians

7. Now, in the 90s, with increased emphasis on primary care and

decreased need for physician specialists and sub-specialists, the nurse practitioner is being looked at as a viable, cost effective member of the health care delivery system

- Types of Roles

  1. Collaborator—establishes communication with other health care professionals to influence care

  2. Researcher

     a. Uses the knowledge of the research process to create knowledge and apply it to practice by sharing it with others

     b. Masters prepared nurse obligated to participate "in activities that contribute to the ongoing development of the profession's body of knowledge" (ANA, 1985, p. 1. Code of Ethics)

  3. Educator—teaches other professionals, family or patients. Requires

     a. Knowledge of the teaching/learning process

     b. Assessment of the learner

     c. Development of teaching plan

     d. Selection of teaching mode

     e. Implementation of plan

     f. Evaluation of teaching and learning effectiveness

     g. See (Teaching and learning in Creasia & Parker, 1991) for a succinct summary

     h. Learning theories

  4. Consultant

     a. Informal—individual draws from personal expertise to advise others, validate current practice, or provide specialized knowledge to help others

     b. Formal—contractual services on a wide variety of health care topics and for a variety of reasons

  5. Clinician—provides direct care or provides clinical information to others

     a. Has expert knowledge

     b. Maintains skills

     c. Evaluates practice

6. Administrator—manages others in the delivery of health care or may case manage the care of a group of patients

    a. Requires knowledge of organizational structures

    b. Requires management styles/strategies

    c. Requires leadership styles/strategies

    d. May require case management skills—administers the care of patients but may not provide the care

7. Independent practice

    a. Legal considerations

        (1) State nurse practice act must be broad and flexible enough to allow for full scope of practice

        (2) Obtain legal assistance in establishing practice

            (a) Small Business Administration Service Corp of Retired Executives (SBA-SCORE) provide free consultation

            (b) Evaluate best legal structure for practice, e.g., corporation, partnership, etc.

        (3) Establish cadre of health professionals to collaborate with

    b. Fiscal

        (1) Consider need for funds to cover 6 to 12 months of operation

        (2) Contact Small Business Administration regarding loan opportunities

        (3) Develop relationshps with your local banker and merchants

        (4) Negotiate directly with major third party payers

            (a) Describe who you are and your credentials

            (b) Describe what you are prepared to do

            (c) Describe the contract you would like to establish

            (d) Discuss fees and terms

    c. Accountability

        (1) Provide for self audit

        (2) Work with local nurse practitioner professional organizations to make certain local standards of practice are met

        (3) Examine quality of clinical documentation

      (4)   Establish open relationship with other nurse practitioners, physicians and health care providers

8.   Other role functions

    a. Advocacy—promotes what is best for the client, ensuring that the clients needs are met, and protects the client's rights (Kozier, Erb, & Blais, 1992)

        (1)   Children/families

        (2)   Nursing profession

        (3)   World health/public health

    b. Ethical actions

        (1)   Ethical decision-making models applied to practice

        (2)   Advocacy, accountability, and loyalty are moral concepts (Fry, 1990)

        (3)   Care/caring, compassion, human dignity also important

        (4)   A discussion of nursing's policy on ethics may be found in Ethics in Nursing: Position Statements and Guidelines (ANA, 1988, Pub. No. G-175)

9.   Marketing the role

    a. Always identify yourself as a nurse practitioner

    b. Use professional cards with your title, credentials

    c. Use brochures, educational materials for descriptions and functions of the role

    d. Take opportunities with radio, television, newspapers to identify yourself as a nurse practitioner and provide information

    e. Volunteer your nurse practitioner service at health fairs, neighborhood center, community functions

    f. List services in the telephone directory under "Nurse Practitioner"

    g. Work with local nurse practitioner organizations to focus media attention upon nurse practitioners

    h. Work with other health care providers on volunteer committees

    i. Donate time to a political campaign

    j. Send announcements of your practice to local medical societies, hospitals, pharmacists, physical therapists, etc. as relevant in your area

    k. Establish referral systems with other nurse practitioners and health professionals

- Legal ramifications

1. The use of malpractice claims for regulating the quality of health care, escalating costs of providing medical care, maldistribution of primary care physicians and growing consumer demand for affordable quality care have created pressure on the health care system to provide low cost alternatives for the delivery of health care services

2. These trends have led to increased use of nonphysician providers (many of whom are nurse practitioners) and new statuatory recognition of these providers (Eccard & Gainor, 1993)

3. Problems arise from the legal perspective when nurses are defined under the nonphysician provider "umbrella" since nurses are separately licensed, contrary to some nonphysician providers, and practice their profession separate from medicine

4. Most states have expanded or amended their nurse practice acts to cover nurse practitioners while others have given physicians more delegative powers

5. Some states have a separate level of licensure for advanced practitioners

6. Individual certification of nurse specialists is the best approach to legal coverage because it makes practitioners accountable for their own practice (Bullough, 1993, p. 274)

7. Legal regulations vary widely from state to state

Knowledge Base

- Scientific content

1. Medicine

2. Physical assessment

3. Statistics and research

4. Physiology

5. Anatomy

6. Microbiology

7. Psychology

8. Sociology

9. Nutrition

10. Pharmacology

■ Elements of theory

1. Development of theory

    a. Relatively specific and concrete set of concepts and propositions that purports to account for or characterize phenomena of interest to the discipline of nursing

2. Application

    a. Theories allow the nurse to assess, plan, implement and evaluate care

3. Evaluation

    a. Use of theories allows the nurse to determine the relevance of the theory to actual practice

    b. Data should be provided to allow the nurse to modify practice

■ Applicable psychosocial theories: The strength of the nurse practitioner is their unique preparation which integrates psychosocial theory into clinical practice

1. Nursing theories

    a. Nightingale's environmental theory

    b. Henderson's complementary-supplementary model

    c. Johnson's behavioral system model

    d. Rogers' science of unitary human beings

    e. King's theory of goal attainment

    f. Neuman's systems model

    g. Orem's theory of self-care

    h. Roy's adaptation model

    i. Leininger's theory of transcultural nursing

    j. Watson's science of caring

    k. Parse's theory of man-living-health

2. For a succinct summary of each of these theories see Creasia & Parker, 1991, pp. 5-18

3. Other theories

   a. Change theory—ability to initiate change or to assist others in making modification in themselves or in the system

      (1) Change theory focuses on how to make change

      (2) Examples of change theorists: Lewis, K.—unfreezing, moving, refreezing; Lippitt, R.—diagnose, assess, select progressive change objectives, terminate; Havelock, R.—build relationships, acquire resources, choose solution, stabilize; Rogers, E.—knowledge, persuasion, decision, decision-implementation, confirmation

      (3) For a concise summary of change theory see Kozier, Erb & Blais, 1992, p. 211

   b. Developmental theory

      (1) Development is patterned, orderly, and predictable with purpose and direction

      (2) Development is continuous throughout life, although the degree of change in many areas decreases after adolescence

      (3) Can occur simultaneously in several areas, e.g., physical and social, but rate of change in each area varies

      (4) Proceeds from simple to complex

      (5) Pace varies among individuals

      (6) Physical and mental stress during periods of critical developmental change, such as puberty, make a person particularly susceptible to outside stressors (Morton, 1989 p. 47)

- Health behavior

  Becker Health Belief Model intends to predict which individuals would or would not use preventive measures based upon perceived susceptibility; perceived seriousness; perceived threat. Health risk appraisal includes a variety of questions about health behavior and attempts to evaluate the patient's risk in a variety of areas. Focus is on decreasing statistical risk by changing behavior through knowledge of risk.

- Stress

  General theory of behavior and response first described by Selye in which the body adapts, as long as possible, to stress. Some degree of stress can be healthy

1. Stress as a stimulus

2. Stress as a response

3. Stress reaction (adaptive response)

4. Stress reaction (sustained response)

5. Stress exhaustion

■ Education

1. Most early programs were certificate programs

2. In the early 1970s, baccalaureate level preparation was considered

3. Seems there is now a general consensus that the nurse practitioner role requires specialized knowledge and skills, which is best acquired in a master's degree program (Mezey, 1993)

4. Continuing education is the obligation of the professional

   a. Participant—many states require continuing education as a condition of continuous licensure

   b. Provider—must meet predetermined criteria to award continuing education credit

■ Credentialing

1. Accreditation—"The process by which a voluntary, non-governmental agency or organization appraises and grants accreditation status to institutions and/or programs or services which meet predetermined structure, process and outcome criteria" (ANA, 1979)

   a. Purpose of accreditation—protects public, by recognizing practitioners who have successfuly completed an approved course of study

   b. Can serve as a mechanism to identify providers who can be reimbursed for services

   c. Accrediting bodies

      (1) National League for Nursing (NLN)—accredits schools of nursing

      (2) Joint Commission on Accreditation of Health Care Organizations (JCAHO)—accredits hospitals and health care organizations and agencies

    d. Establishes standards for the profession

        (1)   Designed initially to improve quality

        (2)   Designed to protect public safety

        (3)   Designed to standardize services and facilities by being explicit about what is expected

2. Licensure: "A process by which an agency of state government grants permission to individuals accountable for the practice of a profession to engage in the practice of that profession and prohibits all others from legally doing so. It permits use of a particular title. Its purpose is to protect the public by ensuring a minimum level of professional competence." (ANA, 1979)

    a. Reciprocity—acknowledgement and acceptance by one state of another state's licensure of a nurse

    b. Registration—individual has met certain criteria and is therefore "registered" within the state and entitled to practice within that state

3. Certification—"A process by which a non-governmental agency or association certifies that an individual licensed to practice as a professional has met certain predetermined standards specified by that profession for specialty practice. Its purpose is to assure the public that an individual has mastered a body of knowledge and acquired skills in a particular specialty." (ANA, 1979)

    a. As of 1991, all but five states recognized National Certification as a means for certifying nurse practitioners and/or nurse midwives. The mechanisms for achieving certification vary by state and include various types of criteria, e.g., treatment protocols, collaborative agreements in addition to national certification requirements

    b. Conditions for certification maintenance or recertification must be met, often involving clinical practice, continuing education, re-examination, periodic self-assessment examinations and peer review

4. Certifying bodies

    a. American Nurses Credentialing Center (ANCC)—specialty examinations in nursing fields, plus adult, pediatric, gerontological, family, and school nurse practitioners

    b. National Certification Board of Pediatric Nurse Practitioners and

Nurses (NCBPNP/N)—specialty examinations for pediatric nurse practitioners and pediatric nurses

c. National Certification Corporation for the Obstetric, Gynecologic and Neonatal Nursing Specialties (NCC)—specialty examinations for Ob/Gyn nurse practitioners, and other maternal, infant and women's health specialties

Professional Issues

- Standards of Practice

1. The development of standards has focused on setting minimum levels of acceptable performance and has attempted to provide the consumer with a means of measuring the quality of nursing care they receive (Eccard & Gainer, 1993)

   a. The ANA defines a standard as an "authoritative statement by which the quality of practice, service or education can be judged"

   b. Standards were developed in 1966 following an organizational revision of the ANA which resulted in the creation of five divisions of practice that corresponded to distinct specialty areas

   c. Both generic standards applicable to all nurses in all areas of practice have been developed in addition to specialty areas

3. Various specialty groups have also developed standards, e.g., National Association of Pediatric Nurse Associates and Practitioners (NAPNAP); Nurses Association of the American College of Obstetricians and Gynecologists (NAACOG) now known as Association of Womens' Health, Obstetric, and Neonatal Nurses (AWHONN); American College of Critical-Care Nurses; American Association of Nurse Anesthetists are but a few of the several specialty nurses organizations with their own Standards of Practice. (Eccard & Gainor, 1993)

4. Legal implications and parameters

   a. Former protocols or standards provide legal protection if nurse practitioner challenged about specific tasks, actions, knowledge

   b. Protocols should be a simple series of steps that will always apply to certain problems or presenting symptoms

   c. Protocols should be the minimum requirements for safe care

   d. Protocols should be updated as scientific knowledge changes

   e. Protocols should be realistic depending on the practice setting in which they will be utilized

f. Protocols must be followed without fail. A deviation from the protocol should be documented in the chart (Moniz, 1992).

g. Informal practice may provide some legal protection if it can be documented that this is the standard of practice within a community or state

- Evaluation of practice

1. Peer review

   a. Provides evaluation which recognizes and rewards nursing contribution

   b. Leads to higher standards of practice within a community and discourages practice beyond the scope of legal authority

2. Quality assurance—a system to evaluate and monitor the quality of patient care and the quality of facility management (JCAHO, 1988)

   a. Provides for accountability and responsibility of individual practitioner in delivering high quality care

   b. Can be used as a means of evaluating and improving patient care

   c. Can serve as a model by which individual nurse practitioners can ensure quality care within their own practice through an organized approach to problem solving

   d. Provides a framework for systematic, continuous evaluation of individual clinical practice

   e. Can reduce exposure to liability

   f. Can identify educational needs of nurse practitioners

   g. Can improve documentation of care provided

   h. Components of quality assurance

      (1) Structure—focuses on organization of client care system

      (2) Process—focuses on activities and performance of care givers in relation to client's needs

         (a) Identifies the person(s) responsible for quality assurance activity

         (b) Delineates the scope of care provided

         (c) Identifies the important aspects of care

        (d)   Evaluates the appropriateness of identified quality indicators

        (e)   Collection and analysis of data

   (3)   Outcome

        (a)   Evaluation of care

        (b)   Client's health care status, welfare and satisfaction

        (c)   Results of care in terms of change in the client

        (d)   Resolution of problem(s)

        (e)   Evaluation of whether general patient care has improved as a result of the evaluation process

        (f)   Communicate process results to appropriate individuals in the institution

   (4)   Effectiveness

        (a)   Are expectations reasonable?

        (b)   Are changes made?

   (1)   Efficiency

        (a)   Are outcomes possible with reasonable effort?

        (b)   Are tasks selected reasonable?

   (6)   Client and provider interactions

        (a)   Is there a mechanism for evaluating patient satisfaction?

        (b)   Is there a mechanism for patient participation in policy development and implementation?

  i. Additional methods

   (1)   Auditing—examining records to see how well they meet established criteria

   (2)   Selected studies—detailed evaluation of information related to a specific disease or process

   (3)   Patient satisfaction—evaluation of subjective response

   (4)   Utilization review—evaluation in which extent of services described or resources used is measured against a standard

   (5)   Peer review—evaluation of care given by similar providers. Focus is on reasonableness of care, what is commonly

expected as care in that setting for that problem

■ Risk management

Includes systems and activities which are designed to recognize and intervene to reduce the risk of injury to patients and consequent claims against health care providers. It is based on the assumption that many injuries to patients are preventable

1. Management liability

    a. Evaluation of sources of legal risk in a practice

        (1) Patients

        (2) Procedures

        (3) Quality of record keeping

    b. Educational or procedural activities in order to reduce risk in identified risk areas

2. Malpractice—any professional misconduct, unreasonable lack of skill, or infidelity in professional or fiduciary duties, or illegal or immoral conduct. Negligence is the failure of an individual to do something that a reasonable person would do, that results in injury to another. Malpractice is the alleged failure on the part of a professional to render services with the degree of care, diligence, and precaution that another member of the same profession in similar circumstances would render to prevent injury to someone else. In order to recover for negligent malpractice, it must be established:

    a. A duty to care by provider to the patient violated the applicable standard of care

    b. Patient suffered a compensable injury that such injury was caused in fact and proximately caused by the substandard conduct (King, 1986)

    c. Safety (client, staff, and volunteers) was compromised

3. Malpractice insurance

    a. Mistakes do happen, despite the best intentions

    b. Malpractice insurance will not protect a nurse practitioner from charges of practicing medicine without a license if they are practicing outside the legal scope of practice within the state

    c. It is universally recommended that all nurse practitioners carry their own insurance

d. The National Practitioner Data Bank collects information on adverse actions against health care practitioners, including nurses. All hospitals must query the data bank every two years regarding health care providers on their medical staffs, those to whom they have granted clinical privileges, or new appointments

4. Personal/professional liability

    a. Many nurse practitioners are covered under a professional liability insurance policy purchased by their employers

    b. This type of insurance covers problems which are of a more general nature; malpractice insurance may be a component of this type of policy

5. General types of liability policies

    a. An insurance contract or agreement between insurer and insured. Two major policy options

        (1) Occurrence coverage—covers events of alleged malpractice which occurred during the policy period, regardless of the date of discovery or when the claim was filed

        (2) Claims made coverage—covers only those claims filed during the policy coverage period, regardless of when they occurred, optional tail coverage contract extends the coverage of a claims made policy into the future to cover all claims filed after the basic claims made coverage period

- Prescriptive Authority

1. Important to ensure adequacy of therapeutic regimens

2. Addressed state by state

3. To date, over 35 boards provide for some degree of prescriptive authority; the degree of authority varies. (Pearson, 1994)

4. Depending on the full scope of the state law a nurse practitioner may obtain a federal DEA registration number

- Testimony as an expert witness in a court of law

1. Standards of care in professional nursing negligence action must be established by expert testimony

2. Nurses are the best people to give testimony on standards of care for nurses

3. Competency of an expert witness is tested by the sufficiency of the

witness's knowledge of the subject matter

4. The degree or depth of the expert's knowledge affects how much weight or credence the jury should give the testimony

5. How to prepare testimony if you are the expert witness or are defending yourself

   a. Prepare thoroughly, with concise, well supported and well documented materials

   b. Know the State Nurse Practice Act and how to apply it to situations

   c. Be aware of existing regulations and how promulgated

   d. Be aware of any Standards of Care written by American Nurses' Association or other professional organizations

   e. Be knowledgeable about reasonable, acceptable, and proper existing practice

   f. Present with confidence, authority and conviction

   g. A professional appearance and demeanor is critical

6. How to deliver and respond to questions

   a. Communicate directly with questioners, directing answers toward the judge and jury

   b. Maintain composure; be relaxed

   c. State opinion and do not change it; do not overtly react to other witnesses that may disagree

   d. Avoid vague imprecise expressions such as "I think" or "I believe;" avoid superlatives such as "always" and "never."

   e. When you know the answer, give it concisely and precisely, but do not answer more than you are asked

   f. When it comes to giving your opinion, it is not always necessary to answer only "yes" or "no." It is often appropriate to say a few more words to explain your opinion.

   g. Take time to allow the question to register and to prepare your answer. This allows the attorney to make appropriate objections before you answer. If an objection is made and overruled, you must answer the question

   h. If you do not understand a question, ask to have it repeated or clarified

i. If you do not remember or know an answer, it is better to acknowledge this than make a mistake. If the answer involves exact time or number and you know the appropriate answer, state your recollection as an approximation (Northrup & Kelly, 1987, p. 531)

■ Interaction with the legal system

1. Evaluate your legal requirements by talking to an attorney or other health care professional

2. Utilize tools available to identify prospective legal counsel

    a. See *Martindale-Hubbell Directory of Attorneys*

    b. Check with friends, colleagues, professional associations

    c. Use Bar Associations and other attorney referral services

3. Interview prospects

    a. Develop rapport between yourself and attorney

    b. Discuss what services the attorney feels may be necessary and services they are willing to perform

    c. Establish the fee structure, payment terms, and estmated total cost. (Northrup & Kelly, 1987)

■ Political activism: Mandatory if nurse practitioners are to remain a viable role. Many policies have the potential to impact on nurse practitioners

1. Analyze health/public/social policy

    a. Determine objective of policy

        (1) What is the problem?

        (2) Problem definition affects policy structure

    b. What are the social dimensions of the policy?

        (1) Who will be affected?

        (2) Examine issues of race, gender, economic class, education, etc.

    c. What are the political dimensions of the policy?

        (1) Is specific legislation required?

        (2) Is it politically feasible to pass legislation?

        (3) How will this policy be implemented?

      d. What are the economic dimensions of the policy?

          (1)   Who will pay for policy implementation?

          (2)   What are the costs involved?

          (3)   What will be accomplished by the money invested?

      e. Who are the opponents and proponents of the policy?

      f. What are other social, political or economic alternatives to the policy?

2.   How to recommend and contribute to development of policy

      a. The process of recommending policy (political process)

          (1)   Provide information or research to legislators who are interested in submitting legislation; they are looking for good ideas

          (2)   Initiate meetings with policy makers to inform them

      b. Formation of community interest groups

          (1)   Numbers of people create visibility for the problem

          (2)   Numbers of people provide more resources in addressing the problem

          (3)   Attract media attention to put issue on the policy agenda

      c. How to form a coalition

          (1)   Define your problem broadly

          (2)   Examine all constituent groups affected by the problem

          (3)   Initiate meetings between members of different constituent groups

          (4)   Determine areas where interests are similar and where interests are different

          (5)   Agree to work together on problems where interests or goals are the same; not work against each other where interests are not the same; work together on interests which are of great importance to some group members but not highly important to others

3.   Advocacy for the establishment and implementation of public policy

      a. Always represent yourself as a nurse practitioner

b. Take the initiative to approach policy makers

c. Coordinate efforts with national associations and other interested parties when appropriate

4. Formal legislative process (usual process)

   a. Federal level

     (1) Issue may be placed on public agenda by interested groups or other means may be used

     (2) Bill introduced into Congress

     (3) Referred to committee for hearings

     (4) Referred to House and Senate for debate and vote

     (5) If both Houses concur, bill goes to President; if they do not, it goes to conference committee

     (6) Conference committee debate and vote

     (7) Legislation either dies or is sent back to both houses

     (8) To President for signature or veto

     (9) If signed by President, bill becomes law. If vetoed, Congress can vote to overturn veto

     (10) After bill becomes law, appropriate agency drafts rules and regulations to implement law

     (11) Draft Regulations published in *Federal Register* for public comment

     (12) After public comment period, final regulations are promulgated and published

     (13) Law is implemented via regulations

   b. State and Local Level

     (1) Basic process is similar although not so complex

     (2) (See Dye, 1992)

   c. Role of Lobbyist

     (1) Professional workers whose job is to get information to policy makers to help influence policy formation

     (2) Assist with developing plan and implementation of achieving goals and objectives

(3)   Expertise is often in knowing who to influence and how to do so

d. Policy often influenced by informal process

(1)   Influence of friends and family

(2)   Associations with church or social clubs

Types of health care delivery systems

- Managed Care

1.   Broad term which describes networks of providers who contractually agree to provide services for particular patient groups

2.   Major dimensions include reviewing and intervening in decisions about health services to be provided—either prospectively or retrospectively; limiting or influencing patient's choice of providers; and negotiating different payment terms or levels with providers

3.   Types of managed care systems

a. Health Maintenance Organization (HMO)—An organized system of health care that provides, directly or through contracts with others, a specified range of comprehensive health services to a voluntarily enrolled population for prepaid per capita payments. They are both insurers and providers of health care

(1)   Emphasizes health promotion and health maintenance

(2)   Patient's choice of health care providers and hospitals, services is limited

b. Preferred Provider Organization (PPO)—A preferred provider organization is an entity through which a partnership is established between a group of "preferred providers"—doctors, hospitals and others—and an insurance company, self-limited employer or its intermediary to provide specified medical and hospital care and sometimes related services at a negotiated price. Providers negotiate lower fees in anticipation of a greater volume of patients and agree to basic managed care principles such as utilization review, accompanying guidelines for hospital admissions, and limited use of facilities and resources

(1)   Marketed to purchasers as opposed to consumers

(2)   Physicians are paid per person or capitated payment depending upon the number of individuals enrolled with

them as primary providers, and patients pay a small co-payment at time of service

- Private practice: Physicians who accept fee for service, third party reimbursement from private insurance plans, Medicare and Medicaid. They are unaffiliated with other physician or organizational groups and charges are based on current market rates

- Home health care: Care provided by a public agency or private organization primarily engaged in providing skilled nursing services and other therapeutic services

  1. Has policies established by a group of professional personnel to govern the services which it provides

  2. Provides for supervision of services

  3. Maintains clinical records on every patient

  4. Has in effect an overall plan and budget

  5. Meets applicable federal, state and local law

- Health centers

  1. Federally funded centers designed to meet specific population needs, e.g., pregnant women, low birth weight babies, the elderly

  2. Provides provision for direct reimbursement to nurse practitioners in rural areas

  3. Examples include Community Health Centers, Federal Qualified Health Centers, Federal Qualified Health Center Look-A-Likes, Rural Health Clinics, Migrant Health Clinics, Indian Health Clinics, National Health Service Corps

- University teaching hospitals

  1. Service and research institutions

  2. Educational training system for health professionals

  3. Quality of care usually high; continuity of care may be decreased

- Hospitals

  1. Clinical service-based facilities of varying size

  2. Often meet special community needs

  3. May develop care specialty for a geographic area

Reimbursement

Types of reimbursement (Provider reimbursement mechanisms). Top agenda item for nurse practitioners. Traditionally, nurse practitioners have not been paid directly for services performed unless authorized by a physician or performed under the supervision of a physician. Nurse practitioners argue that reimbursement should be provided directly to provider and at rate determined for service provided, not by type of provider

- Direct reimbursement
  1. Advantages of direct reimbursement include
     a. Increases the availability and improves accessibility of health care to the consumer
     b. Increases consumer choice of health care providers
     c. Provides for comprehensive or full service health care for the consumer
     d. Provides for cost-effective health care through improved utilization of nurse practitioners
     e. Legitimizes the nurse practitioner role
     f. Decreases restrictions on practice imposed by limited reimbursement mechanisms
  2. Impact of restrictions on direct reimbursement for nurse practitioner services
     a. Reinforces dominance of physicians
     b. Reduces collegial relationships
     c. Limits professional autonomy in nursing
     d. Limits consumer choice
     e. Limits access to services, particularly in underserved areas or with underserved population groups (Labar, 1983)
  3. Government opinion has been that direct payment to nurse practitioners would be inflationary, increasing utilization and fee-inflation. If nurse practitioners provide complimentary rather than substitutive services, both physicians and nurse practitioners could bill for patient services, thus increasing overall health care utilization and costs
- Fee-For-Service
  1. Traditional form of payment made to physicians and health care providers. The provider gets paid a fee for each service that is provided

■ Medicare

1. Provides health insurance protection for over 33 million aged and disabled individuals. The program covers hospital service, physician services, and other medical services for those eligible, regardless of income

2. Medicare is administered by the Health Care Financing Administration (HCFA) in the Department of Health and Human Services. Many of the day-to-day operations, including the reviewing and paying for claims, are performed by organizations such as Blue Cross/Blue Shield plans or private insurers under contract to HCFA. These organizations are referred to as Part A intermediaries and Part B carriers

3. The program has two parts: Hospital insurance (Part A) that covers inpatient hospital and related institutional care; Supplementary Medical Insurance (Part B) covers physician services and other related medical services and supplies

   a. Part A covers inpatient hospital care. In some cases, it also covers short-term skilled nursing facility care after a hospital stay, home health agency visits, and hospice care

      Medicare pays for inpatient hospital services according to a prospective payment system (PPS). Under this system, each Medicare patient is classified according to his or her medical condition into diagnosis-related groups (DRGs). Hospitals are paid a predetermined rate for each patient treated within a given DRG. Hospitals with costs below the payment rates are allowed to keep the surplus, while hospitals with costs above the payment rates must absorb the cost

   b. Part B, the Supplementary Medical Insurance (SMI) program, is a voluntary program; individuals must enroll and pay a premium to receive benefits. All persons are entitled to Part A and all persons over age 65 are eligible to enroll. The program covers the services of physicians, outpatient hospital care, laboratory and x-ray services and other related medical services and supplies. In certain instances, the services of nonphysician providers, like nurse practitioners, are covered

      (1) The program is financed by beneficiary premiums and general revenues. Medicare generally pays 80% of the reasonable charges for covered services, after the beneficiary has met the annual deductible. The beneficiary is liable for

20% of the reasonable charge, an amount that is known as coinsurance

(2) Medicare pays for most Part B services including physician services, on the basis of a reasonable charge. The reasonable charge is the lesser of the actual charge, the physician or supplier's customary charges for the service, and the prevailing charge for the service in the community

(3) By accepting "assignment" on a claim, a provider, (i.e., nurse practitioner, physician, supplier) agrees to accept Medicare's reasonable charge as payment in full. There are incentives for providers to enter into agreements to accept assignment on all Medicare claims. Persons who enter into such agreements are known as "participating" providers

If physician or provider does not accept assignment, the patient is liable for the 20% and difference between what is paid by Medicare and the actual charge

(4) The Omnibus Budget Reconciliation Act of 1989 (OBRA 89), Public Law 101-239, enacted a new payment system for physician's services. Instead of a reasonable charge basis, physician's services will be paid on a fee schedule that uses a resource-based-relative-value-scale (RBRVS). Under RBRVS, physician payments are determined according to the resources and effort (including the physician's time) needed to perform a service. In general terms, the fee schedule will reduce payments for most surgical services, while increasing payments for primary care services such as office visits. Beginning in 1992, the fee schedule is being phased in over a 5-year period

4. Nurse Practitioners: For a Nurse Practitioner's (NP) services to be covered under Medicare, an NP must:

a. Be a registered professional nurse who is currently licensed to practice in the State in which the services are furnished

b. Satisfy the applicable requirements for qualification as NP in the State in which the services are furnished

c. Meet at least one of the following requirements:

(1) Be currently certified as a primary care nurse practitioner by the American Nurses' Credentialing Center or by the National Certification Board of Pediatric Nurse Practitioners

and Nurses

(2) Have satisfactorily completed a formal educational program of at least one academic year that prepares registered nurses to perform an expanded role in the delivery of primary care and that includes at least four months (in the aggregate) of classroom instruction, and awards a degree, diploma, or certificate for successful completion of the program; *or*

(3) Have successfully completed a formal education program (that does not qualify under the immediately preceding requirement) that prepares registered nurses to perform an expanded role in the delivery of primary care and have been performing that expanded role for at least 12 months during the 18-month period immediately preceding February 8, 1988, the effective date for the provision of the services of nurse practitioners as reflected in the conditions for certification for rural health clinics (Medicare handbook 1991)

5. Medicare Covered Services

Coverage is limited to the services an NP is legally authorized to perform in accordance with State Law (or State regulatory mechanism established by State Law). The NP must meet training, education, and experience requirements prescribed by the Secretary of Health and Human Services

The services of an NP may be covered under Part B if all of the following conditions are met:

a. They are the type that are considered physician's services if furnished by a doctor of medicine or osteopathy (MD/DO)

b. They are performed by a person who meets the definition of an NP (See above)

c. The NP is legally authorized to perform the services in the State in which they are performed

d. They are performed in collaboration with an MD/DO. The term "collaboration" means a process whereby an NP works with a physician to deliver health care services within the scope of the NP's professional expertise with medical direction and appropriate supervision as provided for in jointly developed guidelines or other mechanisms defined by Federal regulations and the law of the State in which the services are performed; and

e. They are not otherwise precluded from coverage because of one of the statutory exclusions

6. Medicare Reimbursement for NP Services

Under certain conditions, Medicare will reimburse for services of an NP in the following ways

a. Incident to:

(1) Services of nonphysician personnel, (i.e., nurse practitioners) furnished "incident-to" physician services in private practice is limited to situations in which there is direct physician supervision. Direct personal supervision in the office setting does not mean that the physician must be present in the same room with his or her assistant. However, the physician must be present in the office suite and immediately available to provide assistance and direction throughout the time the assistant is performing services. Such services must be an integral, although incidental, part of the physician's personal professional services, and they must be performed under the physician's direct supervision

(2) Services performed by nurse practitioners "incident-to" a physician's professional services include not only service ordinarily rendered by a physician's office staff person, (e.g., medical services such as taking blood pressures and temperatures, giving injections, and changing dressings), but also services ordinarily performed by the physician himself or herself such as physical examinations, minor surgery, setting casts for simple fractures, interpreting radiographs, and other activities that involve an independent evaluation or treatment of the patient's condition

(3) Services Excluded from coverage:

NP services may not be covered if they are otherwise excluded from coverage even though an NP may be authorized by State law to perform them. For example, the Medicare law excludes from coverage routine foot and dental care, routine physical checkups, examinations prescribing or fitting eyeglasses (except after cataract surgery) or hearing aids, cosmetic surgery and services that are not reasonable and necessary for the diagnosis or treatment of an illness or injury or to improve the functioning of a malformed body member

(4) Billing and payment under "incident-to":

When an NP performs an "incident-to" service in a physician's office/clinic, the service must be submitted to Medicare by the employing physician, under his/her name, provider number, and the most accurate Current Procedural Terminology (CPT) code that describes the treatment being furnished. The payment is made at the full physician rate and paid to the employer

b. Billing and Payment in other circumstances:

Billing and payment for NP services is available only in limited circumstances as follows:

(1) Skilled Nursing Facilities (SNFs): Payment for services furnished in Skilled Nursing Facilities or Nursing Facilities in urban areas, as defined by law. Under the Social Security Act, a SNF must meet certain "conditions of participation" that concern the quality of care provided, proper training for employees, residents' rights, and safety code requirements. Other requirements include that the facility is primarily engaged in providing residents:

(a) Skilled nursing care and related services for residents who require medical or nursing care

(b) Rehabilitation services for the rehabilitation of injured, disabled, or sick persons, and not primarily for the care and treatment of mental diseases.

It is also possible that part of another institution is treated as a SNF

(2) Medicare pays for nurse practitioner and clinical nurse specialist services in SNFs in non-rural areas on a reasonable charge basis. This amount, however, may not exceed the physician fee schedule amount for the service. The payment is made to the NP's employer

c. Rural Health Clinics: Nurse practitioners can own rural health clinics where reimbursement is covered under the Medicare program. In addition, services of NPs and CNSs in rural health clinics are paid to the clinic on a reasonable cost basis. Payment is made to the clinic

    d. Rural Areas:

        (1)   A rural area is defined as any area outside of an urban area for which an urban area is defined as a "Metropolitan Statistical Area" (MSA) or New England County Metropolitan Area (NECMA) as defined by the Executive Office of Management and Budget or otherwise defined by law

        (2)   Rural Inpatient Settings: The payment amount for the services provided by a nurse practitioner is limited to 75% of the physician Fee Schedule amount when they are performed in a hospital setting. In this case, the payment is made only under assignment and made to the hospital

        (3)   Rural Outpatient Settings: For all other services, (outpatient), an 85% limit is applicable. Payment is made only under assignment. Also, payment can be made directly to an NP providing services in a rural area or to his or her employer or contractor

■ Medicaid

1. Program is authorized by Title XIX of the Social Security Act, which is a Federal-State matching program providing medical assistance to approximately 25 million low income persons who are aged, blind, disabled, or members of families with dependent children

2. Federal funds account for 56% of total program expenditures

3. Each state designs and administers its own Medicaid program, setting eligibility and coverage standards within broad federal guidelines. There is substantial variation among the states in terms of eligibility requirements, range of services offered, limitations placed on those services, reimbursement policies

4. Every state except Arizona participates, as well as District of Columbia, American Samoa, Guam, Puerto Rico, the Virgin Islands, and the Northern Mariana Islands

5. At the state level, Medicaid is administered by a designated state agency

6. Federal oversight of the Medicaid program is the responsibility of the Health Care Financing Administration (HCFA)

7. There are proposals to increase provider participation, improve coordination between Medicaid and other programs, and provide

outreach, education, and social services to pregnant women and children

8. Reimbursement regulations

   a. Providers must accept Medicaid payment as payment in full and may not collect from beneficiaries

   b. Medicaid pays only after any other insurance or third party payment sources available to the beneficiary have been exhausted

   c. Payments must be sufficient to enlist enough providers so that covered services will be available to Medicaid beneficiaries to the extent they are available to the general population in a geographic area

   d. Payments are either prospective or retrospective for institutional care; payments are usually the lesser of the provider's actual charge for the service and maximum allowable charges established by the state for physician services. Some states have a flat fee schedule and payments may be unrelated to actual provider charges

9. Medicaid reimbursement to nurse practitioners

   a. Budget Reconciliation Act of 1989 (H.R. 3299) required states to cover the services of certified pediatric and family nurse practitioners beginning July 1, 1990 when practicing within the scope of state law and regardless of whether they are under the supervision of, or associated with a physician or other provider (*Congressional Record*, 1989)

   b. Level of payment determined by state Medicaid Agency. Current reimbursement at 60 to 100% of physicians' rate (Pearson, 1993)

   c. Pediatric and Family nurse practitioners may directly bill Medicaid for their services and may apply for a provider number from their state

   d. States may pass regulations for direct payment for Medicaid to other nurse practitioners not identified in the federal statutes. Currently, 42 states pay nurse practitioners (Pearson, 1993)

■ Prospective Reimbursement to Hospitals

1. Payment mechanism based upon the projected costs of caring for a patient with a particular problem. Under this system, each Medicare patient admitted to a hospital is classified according to his or her medical condition into a diagnosis-related group (DRG). Hospitals are paid a predetermined rate for each patient treated with a given DRG.

Hospitals with costs below the payment rate are allowed to keep a percentage of the surplus, while hospitals with costs above the payment rate must absorb the loss

2. Nurse practitioners not paid directly for services delivered in hospital

■ Third-party payers

1. Two-thirds of total health care revenue comes from third party agencies—private insurance companies or government

    a. Public sources (federal, state, local) pay for 40% costs

    b. Private sources pay for 60%

        (1) Includes direct out-of-pocket expenses

        (2) Includes amount paid for insurance

■ Other third party payers

1. Civilian Health and Medical Program of the United Services (CHAMPUS)

    a. Federal health plan that provides coverage to the military personnel and their families

    b. Program is a means of cost sharing authorized health care services and benefits for dependents of active duty personnel and retirees, dependents and surviving dependents of service members

    c. Program utilizes a variety of health personnel and reimburses them for their services

    d. Nurse practitioners are reimbursed for services

2. Federal Employees Health Benefit Programs

    a. FEHBP is the largest employer-sponsored group health insurance program in the world, serving 10 million participants and offering over 250 insurance plans

    b. Offers wide variety of plans

    c. Nurse practitioners are recognized as designated health care providers under the system

Questions

Select the best answer

1. Healthy People 2000 is

   a. A report on the health status of 2000 people in the U.S.A.
   b. An international health policy paper
   c. A statement of national health policy goals to help all people live socially and economically productive lives
   d. A research analysis of what makes people healthy

2. WHO "Health for All" is

   a. A report on who is healthy in the world
   b. A general policy statement on improving the world's health care
   c. A research study on the components of health in all countries
   d. A discussion of who is healthy

3. Nursing has submitted an "Agenda for Health Care Reform" which includes

   a. A restructured health care system that will focus on the consumers and their health, with services to be delivered in familiar, convenient sites
   b. A predominant focus on illness and acute care
   c. The insistence on more specialty training for physicians
   d. A two-tiered system of health care for the wealthy and the poor

4. The major trend in health policy research is now

   a. Outcome studies
   b. Process studies
   c. Structure studies
   d. Primary care studies

5. Which of the following is not considered in the overall cost reduction strategy in the delivery of health care services

   a. Individuals are not denied health care because of lack of money
   b. All individuals may have free care
   c. Cost is reasonable for services provided
   d. Investment of money in health care leads to improved health

6. The process of quality assurance focuses on

   a. Activities and performance of care given in relation to client's needs
   b. Accessibility of care
   c. Organization of client care

d. Outcome of care

7. Which of the following methods is not appropriate in evaluating care?

    a. Examining records to see how well they meet established criteria
    b. Detailed evaluation of information related to a specific disease or process
    c. Evaluation of patient satisfaction
    d. Evaluation of care given by other institutions for the same disease process

8. The predominant component of malpractice is

    a. Negligence in providing professional care
    b. Overcharging fees
    c. Provider uses acceptable standards of care
    d. Patient suffers no injury

9. In preparing to give testimony as an expert witness you should

    a. Be aware of existing regulations and how promulgated and implemented within the state
    b. Be aware of all other relevant legal cases
    c. Give as much information as possible each time a question is asked
    d. Make certain the judge understands what you are saying, even if you have to repeat it

10. The trend for nurse practitioner prescriptive authority is

    a. The majority of states allow nurse practitioners to write prescriptions for controlled substances
    b. There is a large degree of variability among states regarding the prescribing authority of nurse practitioners
    c. The majority of states have not drafted legislation or regulations which deal with NP prescribing
    d. To use presigned prescription pads

11. The most important major components which should be considered in examining health/public/social policy include

    a. Political, social, economic and professional components of the policy
    b. How powerful are the opponents of the policy
    c. How to sell the policy to the media
    d. What kind of supporters exist for the policy

12. In working to form a coalition

    a. Keep policy focus very narrow
    b. Include all groups remotely involved in the problem
    c. Do not work with groups who do not totally agree on every issue of the problem

d. Agree to not work against each other where interests are not the same

13. The federal legislative process includes

    a. The President refers the Bill to committees for hearings
    b. Bill becomes law when passed by Congress
    c. President may sign or veto Bill submitted to him
    d. Draft regulations are published in *Congressional Record* for public comment

14. The legislative process

    a. Does not follow a formal legislative path
    b. Is often influenced by informal processes
    c. Makes it illegal for paid, professional workers to give information to policy makers to help influence policy formation
    d. Is ended if President vetoes the Bill

15. Managed care is a broad term which describes

    a. The manager in a health maintenance organization
    b. The type of care provided in a Preferred Provider Organization
    c. Networks of providers who contractually agree to provide services for particular patient groups
    d. Networks of hospitals who provide patient care for acutely ill patients

16. A Health Maintenance Organization is an organized system of

    a. Health care facilities
    b. Health care that provides through contracts, a specified range of comprehensive health services to a voluntarily enrolled population for prepaid per capita payments
    c. Health care which must provide health care to all clients in a geographic area
    d. Health care providers who provide specialty services on an out-patient basis

17. A Preferred Provider Organization is an entity through which

    a. Providers negotiate lower fees with insurance companies in anticipation of a greater volume of patients
    b. Providers all work in the same clinic and admit to the same hospital
    c. The providers work on a "fee-for-service" basis
    d. Services are marketed to consumers

18. Characteristics of University Teaching Hospitals include

    a. Focus on hospital is clinical services
    b. Cost of care is lower because provider services are given by individuals in educational training curricula
    c. Quality of care is often low because of inexperienced clinicians

    d. Continuity of care may be a problem because of staff rotation and turnover

19. The term accreditation means

    a. The process by which a voluntary, non-governmental agency or organization appraises and grants accreditation status to institutions and/or programs or services which meet predetermined structure, process and outcome criteria

    b. The process by which a governmental agency appraises and grants accreditation status to institutions and/or programs or services which meet predetermined structure, process and outcome criteria

    c. Professional regulations which oversee the conduct and function of a profession's affairs

    d. A process by which an agency of state government grants permission to individuals accountable for the practice of a profession to engage in the practice of that profession and prohibits all others from legally doing so

20. The term licensure means

    a. The process by which a voluntary, non-governmental agency or organization appraises and grants accreditation status to institutions and/or programs or services which meet predetermined structure, process and outcome criteria

    b. The process by which a governmental agency appraises and grants accreditation status to institutions and/or programs or services which meet predetermined structure, process and outcome criteria

    c. Professional regulations which oversee the conduct and function of a profession's affairs

    d. A process by which an agency of state government grants permission to individuals accountable for the practice of a profession to engage in the practice of that profession and prohibits all others from legally doing so

21. The purpose of licensure is to

    a. Standardize programs or facilities

    b. Protect the public by ensuring a minimum level of professional competence

    c. List programs or facilities which meet certain standards

    d. Designate professional standards of practice

22. Certification is

    a. Process by which a non-governmental agency or association certifies that an individual licensed to practice as a professional has met certain predetermined standards specified by that profession for specialty practice

    b. Process by which an agency of state government grants permission to individuals accountable for the practice of a profession to engage in the practice of that profession and prohibits all others from doing so

    c. The process by which a voluntary, non-governmental agency or organization appraises and grants accreditation status to institutions and/or programs or services which meet predetermined structure, process and outcome criteria

d. The process by which a governmental agency appraises and grants accreditation status to institutions and/or programs or services which meet predetermined structure, process and outcome criteria

23. The purpose of certification is to

a. Assure the public that an individual has mastered a body of knowledge and acquired skills in a particular study
b. Improve quality of programs
c. Have a list of qualified candidates
d. Recognize outstanding performance

24. Standards of practice are

a. The prevailing set of professional knowledge and skills established by an informal evaluation of practice within a community
b. Authoritative statements by which the quality of practice, service or education can be judged
c. Composed of informal discussions among health care providers within a community
d. A scientifically documented "gold standard" against which all practice is measured

25. Quality assurance programs can

a. Provide for accountability and responsibility of individual practitioners in delivering high quality care
b. Be tied to revenue generation
c. Increase exposure of practitioner to liability
d. Only evaluate the quality of records kept

26. Malpractice insurance

a. Will not protect a nurse practitioner from charges of practicing medicine without a license if they are practicing outside the state legal scope of practice
b. Will protect against entries into the National Practitioner Data Bank
c. Will protect a nurse practitioner from making a clinical mistake
d. Will pay for legal defense in the alleged failure on the part of a professional to render services with the degree of care, diligence, and precaution that another member of the same profession in similar circumstances would render

27. Personal/professional liability insurance covers

a. Liability issues of a more general nature
b. Items such as homes, automobiles in addition to malpractice insurance

    c. Areas not covered by employer insurance

    d. Malpractice incidents exclusively

28. You are an Ob/Gyn nurse practitioner and you care for a baby whose parents sue you 10 years later because they claim your care damaged their child. You would want to have

    a. Malpractice insurance

    b. Occurrence coverage

    c. Claims made coverage

    d. Personal liability insurance

29. Advantages of direct reimbursement to nurse practitioners include

    a. Reinforces dominance of physicians

    b. Limits professional autonomy in nursing

    c. Limits consumer choice

    d. Provides for cost-effective health care through improved utilization of nurse practitioners

30. Medicare is

    a. Legislation from Social Security Act, Title 19

    b. Provides health insurance to low income persons

    c. Administered by Health Care Financing Administration

    d. Administered by a designated state agency

31. Medicare Part A provides for

    a. Inpatient hospital care, short-term skilled nursing facility care

    b. Outpatient physician services

    c. Laboratory and radiography services

    d. 80% of reasonable charges for covered services

32. Medicare Part B provides for

    a. Inpatient hospital care according to a prospective payment system

    b. Short-term skilled nursing facility care following hospitalization

    c. Home health agency visits and hospice care

    d. Services of physicians, outpatient hospital care, laboratory and radiography services

33. Which of the following services of nurse practitioners are covered by Medicare, part B

    a. All services delivered to Medicare patients

    b. Only those provided with a physician physically present at all times

    c. Only routine physical examinations performed for prevention of illness and wellness promotion

d. "Incident to" physician services in private practice with physician supervision and with physician consultation immediately available

34. Medicaid is

a. Authorized through Social Security Act, Title 18
b. A Federal-State matching program providing medical assistance to low income persons
c. A program designed primarily to assist patients who are elderly
d. Administered by insurance company or organization

35. Medicaid reimbursement to nurse practitioners

a. Covers the services of gerontological and adult nurse practitioners
b. Level of coverage determined by state Medicaid Agency with considerable variation among states
c. Payment is always directly to agency and not to provider
d. Payment is based on usual and customary charge

36. Nationally nurse practitioners are reimbursed through which of the following programs?

a. DRGs
b. Private insurance companies
c. CHAMPUS and FEHBP
d. Blue Cross-Blue Shield

37. The nurse practitioner role originally began

a. In Colorado in 1975
b. As an experimental program in an Internal Medicine Clinic
c. With the pediatric nurse practitioner movement in an effort to expand traditional nursing functions to overlap those traditionally performed by physicians
d. As a Ph.D. program in human development

38. The nurse practitioner role has focused on

a. Provision of care to ambulatory patients with an emphasis on primary health care
b. Diagnosis and management of unstable acutely ill patients
c. Diagnosis and treatment of major acute illnesses
d. Specialty role development

39. Legal authority for nurse practitioner is granted by

a. State law and regulations (usually Nurse Practice Act)
b. Federal law

c. Health Care Financing Agency
d. Medical and Pharmacy Practice Acts

40. Knowledge base of nurse practitioners is composed of

a. Scientific content
b. Applicable theory
c. Scientific content and Theory
d. Nursing Theory and Psychosocial Theory

41. Developmental theory is an example of a theory which

a. Proceeds from the simple to the complex
b. Theory which is in the early phase of developing
c. Nursing theory which has developed to guide the practice of nurses
d. Scientific content which is taught in all nursing schools

Answers

1.	c	22.	a
2.	b	23.	a
3.	a	24.	b
4.	a	25.	a
5.	b	26.	a
6.	a	27.	a
7.	d	28.	b
8.	a	29.	d
9.	a	30.	c
10.	b	31.	a
11.	a	32.	d
12.	d	33.	d
13.	c	34.	b
14.	b	35.	b
15.	c	36.	c
16.	b	37.	c
17.	a	38.	a
18.	d	39.	a
19.	a	40.	c
20.	d	41.	a
21.	b		

Bibliography

1992 Medicare Explained. Commerce Clearing House: Chicago, IL.

American Nurses Association. (1979). *The study of credentialing in nursing: A new approach*, Staff working papers, (pp. 2, 28). Kansas City: ANA.

American Nurses Association. (1985). *Code of ethics*. Kansas City: ANA.

American Nurses Association. (1988). *Ethics in nursing: Position statements and guidelines*. Pub. No. G-175. Kansas City: ANA.

Bullough, B. (1993). State nurse practice acts. In M. D. Mezey & D. O. McGivern (Eds). *Nurses, nurse practitioners: Evolution to advanced practice* (pp 267-280). NY: Springer Publishing.

Bullough, B., Sultz, H., Henry O. M., & Fiedler, R. (1984). Trends in pediatric nurse practitioner education and employment. *Pediatric Nursing, 10*, 193-196.

Congressional Record. (1989).

Creasia, J. L., & Parker, B. (1991). *Conceptual foundations of professional nursing practice*. St. Louis: Mosby Yearbook.

Dye, T. R. (1992). *Understanding public policy* (7th ed.). Englewood Cliffs, NJ: Prentice Hall.

Eccard, W. T., & Gainor, E. E. (1993). Legal ramifications for advanced practice. In M. D. Mezey & D. O. McGivern (Eds.), *Nurses, nurse practitioners: Evolution to advanced practice* (pp. 281-321). NY: Springer Publishing.

Edmunds, M. W. (1991). NPs who replace physicians: Role expansion or exploitation? *Nurse Practitioner, 16*(9), 46, 49.

Fry, S. T. (1990). Measurement of moral answerability in nursing practice. In C. F. Waltz and O. I. Strickland (Eds.). *Measurement of clinical and educational nursing outcomes*. Vol IV. New York: Springer Publishing.

Health Law. (1990). Committee on Energy and Commerce. U.S. Government Printing Office. Washington, D.C. Committee Print 101-104. 101st Congress 2nd Session.

Joint Commission on Accreditation of Healthcare Organizations. (1988). *Overview of quality assurance and monitoring and evaluation*. Chicago: JCAHCO

King, J. H. (1986). *The law of medical malpractice* (2nd ed.). St. Paul: West Publishing Co.

Kozier, B., Erb, G., & Blais, K. (1992). *Advocacy and change in concepts and issues in nursing practice* (2nd ed.). Redwood City CA: Addison-Wesley.

Labar, D. (1983). *Third party reimbursement for services of nurses*. Kansas City, MO: American Nurses Association.

MacQueen, J. C. (1979). The challenges of the PNP/A movement. *Pediatric Nursing, 5*, 31-35.

McGivern, D. O. (1993). The evolution of advanced nursing practice. In M. D. Mezey and D. O. McGivern (Eds.). *Nurses, nurse practitioners: Evolution to advanced practice* (pp. 3-30). NY: Springer Publishing.

Medicare Carriers Manual Part 3—*Claims Process* issued by Department of Health and Human Services, Health Care Financing Administration, Transmittal No. 1463, HCFA Pub. 14-3.

Mezey, M. (1993). Preparation for advanced practice. In M. D. Mezey & D. O. McGivern (Eds.), *Nurses, nurse practitioners: Evolution to advanced practice* (pp. 31-58). NY: Springer Publishing

Mittelstadt, P. M. (1993). Federal reimbursement of advanced practice nurses' services empowers the profession. *Nurse Practitioner, 18*(1), 43-49.

Moniz, D. (1992). The legal danger of written protocols and standards of practice. *Nurse Practitioner*, 17(9), 58-60.

Morton, P. G. (1989) *Health assessment in nursing*. Springhouse, PA: Springhouse Corporation.

Murphy, M. A. (1990). A brief history of pediatric nurse practitioners and NAPNAP 1964-1990. *Journal of Pediatric Health Care, 4*, 332-337.

National Leadership Coalition for Health Care Reform. (1991). *A comprehensive reform plan for the health care system.*

Northrup, C., & Kelly, M. (1987). *Legal issues in nursing,* St. Louis: Mosby Year Book.

Pearson, L. (1994). 1993-1994 Update: How each state stands on legislative issues affecting advanced nursing practice. *Nurse Practitioner, 19*(1), 16-25.

Pearson, L. (1993). 1992-1993 Update: How each state stands on legislative issues affecting advanced nursing practice. *Nurse Practitioner, 18*(1), pp. 23-28

Public Health Service. (1990). *Healthy People 2000.* (DHHS Publication No. PHS 91-50212). Washington, DC: U.S. Government Printing Office.

The Medicare 1991 Handbook, U. S. Department of Health and Human Services, Health Care Financing Administration. Publication No. HCFA 10050, SSA ICN-461250.

Wilkinson, M. G. (1991). Teaching and learning. In J. L. Creasia and B. Parker, (Eds). *Conceptual foundations of professional nursing practice.* (pp. 263-266). St. Louis: Mosby Yearbook.

INDEX

For information on Certification Review Courses, Home Study Programs and Review Books contact:

Health Leadership Associates, Inc.
Post Office Box 59153
Potomac, Maryland 20859

1-800-435-4775

REVIEW BOOK/AUDIO CASSETTE ORDER FORM
HEALTH LEADERSHIP ASSOCIATES, INC.

PLEASE PRINT OR TYPE

NAME: _____

ADDRESS: Street _____ Apt. # _____ City _____ State _____ Zip Code_____

TELEPHONE: _____ (HOME) _____ (WORK)

Section 1: AUDIO CASSETTES

Professional "live" audio recordings of Review Courses are approximately 15 hours in length unless otherwise noted and include detailed course handouts. Continuing Education contact hours are available for these audio cassette Home Study Programs.

QTY	REVIEW COURSE TITLE	PRICE	
____	Adult Nurse Practitioner	$150.00	_____
____	Ambulatory Women's Health Care Nursing	$150.00	_____
____	Clinical Specialist in Adult Psychiatric and Mental Health Nursing	$150.00	_____
____	Family Nurse Practitioner	$330.00	_____
	(Consists of ANP, PNP & Childbearing Management courses)		
____ *	Generalist Gerontological Nurse	$ 75.00	_____
____	Generalist Medical-Surgical Nurse	$150.00	_____
____ *	Generalist Pediatric Nurse	$ 75.00	_____
____ *	Generalist Psychiatric and Mental Health Nurse	$ 75.00	_____
____	Gerontological Nurse Practitioner	$150.00	_____
____	Home Health Nurse	$150.00	_____
____	Inpatient Obstetric/Maternal Newborn/Low Risk Neonatal/Perinatal Nurse	$150.00	_____
____ **	Obstetrics/Childbearing Management	$ 45.00	_____
____	Pediatric Nurse Practitioner	$150.00	_____
____ **	Test Taking Strategies and Techniques	$ 30.00	_____
____	Women's Health Care Nurse Practitioner	$150.00	_____
	(Formerly Ob/Gyn Nurse Practitioner)		

* 8 Hour Course, ** 2-4 Hour Course

SUB TOTAL:		_____
Maryland Residents add 5% sales tax:		_____
CEU FEE ($10/course):		_____
Shipping: 2-4 Hour Course	$ 4.00	_____
All other Courses	$10.00	_____
TOTAL:		_____

PAYMENT DUE METHOD OF PAYMENT

☐ Check or money order (US funds, payable to Health Leadership Associates, Inc.) A $25 fee will be charged on returned checks.

☐ Purchase Order is attached. P.O. # _____

☐ Please charge my ☐ MasterCard ☐ Visa

Credit Card# _____ Exp. date _____

Signature _____

Print Name _____

REVIEW GUIDES & AUDIO CASSETTES

1) Section 1 Total $ _____

2) Section 2 Total $ _____

3) Section 3 Total $ _____

TOTAL PAYMENT DUE $ _____

Section 2: REVIEW BOOKS

QTY	BOOK TITLE	PRICE	
____	Adult Nurse Practitioner Certification Review Guide (second edition)	$ 47.75	
____	Family Nurse Practitioner Certification Review Guide Set (Includes ANP, PNP, and Women's Health Care NP Guides)	$123.25	_____
____	Generalist Pediatric Nurse Certification Review Guide (second edition)	$ 47.75	
____	Gerontological Nursing Certification Review Guide for the Generalist, Clinical Specialist, and Nurse Practitioner (revised edition)	$ 47.75	
____	Pediatric Nurse Practitioner Certification Review Guide (second edition)	$ 47.75	
____	Psychiatric Certification Review Guide for the Generalist and Clinical Specialist in Adult, Child, and Adolescent Psychiatric and Mental Health Nursing	$ 47.75	
____	Women's Health Care Nurse Practitioner Certification Review Guide (Formerly Ob/Gyn Nurse Practitioner)	$ 47.75	

SPECIAL OFFERING

____	TODAY and TOMORROW'S WOMAN - MENOPAUSE: BEFORE AND AFTER (Girls of 16 to Women of 99) (Author: Virginia Layng Millonig)	$ 19.95	

SUB TOTAL:		_____
Maryland Residents add 5% sales tax:		_____
CEU FEE ($10.00)		_____
Shipping $5.00 for one book:		_____
$2.00 for each additional book: (Except $1.00 for each add'l. *Today and Tomorrow's Woman*)		_____
TOTAL:		_____

For orders of 10 or greater call 1-800-435-4775.
(All prices subject to change without notice)

Section 3: REVIEW BOOK/AUDIO CASSETTE DISCOUNT PACKAGES

A discounted rate is available when purchasing Review Book(s) and Audio Cassettes together. When purchasing packages, indicate Book/Audio Cassette selections in sections 1 and 2. Calculate amount due in this section.

QTY	PACKAGE SELECTION	PRICE	
____	8 Hour Course / 1 Review Guide	$120.00	_____
____	15 Hour Course / 1 Review Guide	$190.00	_____
____	FNP Package	$415.00	_____

FNP Package consists of Adult NP, Pediatric NP, Women's Health Care NP Guides & Audio Cassettes of the ANP, PNP, and Childbearing Management Courses.

SUB TOTAL:		_____
Maryland Residents add 5% sales tax:		_____
CEU Fee ($10)		_____
TOTAL:		_____
(Shipping charge included in package rate)		

RETURN POLICY
Due to the nature of the material contained in the review books and audio cassettes, returns on books ONLY will be accepted one week post delivery. No returns on audio cassettes except for defective audio cassettes which will be replaced.

MAIL TO:	Health Leadership Associates, Inc. P.O. Box 59153 Potomac, MD 20859
OR PHONE:	(800) 435-4775; (301) 983-2405
OR FAX:	(301) 983-2693

Health Leadership Associates,

*the nation's foremost provider, publisher
and producer of Nursing Certification Review
Courses, Books, and Home Study Programs,
announces the launching of their*

WOMEN'S HEALTH DIVISION

with

Today and Tomorrow's Woman, Menopause: Before and After
(Girls of 16 to Women of 99)

At Last! You Can Face the Future Informed and Prepared.

This is the book that women of all ages, the men who care about them, and the health professionals who advise them have needed for years. *Today and Tomorrow's Woman* shatters the myths about menopause and describes the reality . . . clearly, honestly, and accurately.

Separates Fact From Fiction So You Can Make Better Choices. *Today and Tomorrow's Woman* presents page after page of easy-to-understand information on every aspect of menopause.

Dr. Millonig has filled this book with concrete information and advice . . . supported with real programs you can follow for a healthier lifestyle.

Most important, *Today and Tomorrow's Woman* is a book about health, not politics. There is no hidden agenda, no guilt trips, and no unusual philosophy. Dr. Millonig wrote this book to give the reader the information needed to make the right choice.

Order Today!
Call Toll-Free 1-800-435-4775